Errors and Interaction

Pragmatics & Beyond New Series (P&BNS)

ISSN 0922-842X

Pragmatics & Beyond New Series is a continuation of Pragmatics & Beyond and its Companion Series. The New Series offers a selection of high quality work covering the full richness of Pragmatics as an interdisciplinary field, within language sciences.

For an overview of all books published in this series, please see *benjamins.com/catalog/pbns*

Volume 309

Errors and Interaction. A cognitive ethnography of emergency medicine
by Sarah Bro Trasmundi

Errors and Interaction

A cognitive ethnography of emergency medicine

Sarah Bro Trasmundi
University of Southern Denmark

John Benjamins Publishing Company
Amsterdam / Philadelphia

The paper used in this publication meets the minimum requirements of the American National Standard for Information Sciences – Permanence of Paper for Printed Library Materials, ANSI Z39.48-1984.

DOI 10.1075/pbns.309

Cataloging-in-Publication Data available from Library of Congress:
LCCN 2020013599 (PRINT) / 2020013600 (E-BOOK)

ISBN 978 90 272 0704 3 (HB)
ISBN 978 90 272 6103 8 (E-BOOK)

John Benjamins Publishing Company · https://benjamins.com

To my two sons, Victor and Luca, with pride and love

Table of contents

Preface

Doing cognitive ethnography in emergency medicine involves dealing with a complex and wrinkled authentic world, and any given particular situation offers endless details the analyst can attend to. In my case, many people have helped iron out the wrinkles and made this work both possible and intriguing. First, I would like to express my deepest thanks to my friend and colleague, Sune Vork Steffensen, who always encourages me to do better, and who has been – and continues to be – my biggest inspiration in my academic career. Working with him is difficult: He is a perfectionist, he is the cleverest person I know, and he is extremely ambitious, which is why I also enjoy working with him. Many thanks to the employees of the emergency ward at Køge Hospital, who trusted me and carried out their job when the cameras were recording. Special thanks to Anne Grethe Mølbak, Marlene Schneekloth, Henning Jans and Poul Mossin. You all have my deepest respect both professionally and personally. Much of this work has been discussed with outstanding colleagues around the world, whom I have been able to visit, many of them for a longer period of time. In particular I worked with Michael L. Anderson at *Center for Advanced Study in the Behavioral Sciences* at Stanford University, David Kirsh at University of California San Diego, Claire Kramsch at Berkeley University, Mark Bishop at Goldsmith, University of London, and finally Per Linell at Gothenburg University. I cannot emphasise enough how much Per Linell has inspired me, how much he has taught me and how grateful I am for the many discussions we have had about our works both in Copenhagen and in Gothenburg. I truly cherish and value those moments and he has become a close friend and an amazing work buddy. Some of my nearest colleagues have been supportive even when they did not know, and even when they were not present. Special thanks go out to my original, teasing *and* thoughtful friend and colleague, Christian Benne, and to Charles Goodwin, Stephen Cowley and Per Linell, who all strongly encouraged me to write this book. Their recommendation to do so is what made it a reality. The fact that I am no longer able to engage with Chuck Goodwin is a huge loss, and I hope with this edited volume, it is clear how big an inspiration he has been and how his works still inspire me. Thanks to members of the *Centre for Human Interactivity* and the *Advanced Cognitive Ethnography Lab*. Also, a heartfelt thank you to my friend, Tanja Isabel Aebischer, an indescribable support in my life, and a strong, ambitious woman, who keeps inspiring me.

Above all, there are my family. They have been my private emergency room in so many caring ways, for instance by showing no mercy in ensuring I got this book written. I will not spell out in great detail what they already know but let me finally say to the men in my life – Martin, Victor and Luca Bro Trasmundi – *Grazie*. It is the best word that comes to mind.

Introduction

Healthcare practitioners instantly know when an error has occurred, but the conditions and the path that lead to such damaging outcomes are often blurred to them or at worst impossible to recall. For instance, I observed a doctor interacting with a patient about medication issues. After the doctor left, the patient mentioned to his wife that he did not understand what the doctor had tried to tell him, in fact he was unsure whether he should continue with his medication or not. While the doctor later characterised the rapport between him and his patient as troublesome, distrustful and filled with misunderstandings, he was unable to point to why this pattern emerged, and what enabled those interpersonal challenges.

In this case, as in many other similar situations, I also observed that the practitioners preferred to describe such situations metaphorically: The interaction crashed, it went downhill, it was heated, broken etc. But what actually happened (what was said and done) was difficult for all parties to grasp and hence act successfully upon. This example is more than just an example; it is an exempl*ar* of how healthcare practitioners in the ward act and perceive their work performances and it leads to the crucial question: How do healthcare practitioners manage cognitive events in patient treatment and diagnosing in a way that yields cognitive results? This question is the main subject within the framework of cognitive ethnography that I investigate in this volume. The question entails multiple nested questions such as: How do healthcare practitioners anticipate and counter errors? That is, how does an emergency medical team function to prevent errors in complex diagnostic situations? How do errors emerge and escalate in a (dys)functional social system? Further, how does medical culture affect real-time interaction and how is the culture itself shaped by the exact same dynamics?

Professional action underlines various forms of cognitive and social life that involves language, tools, organisational procedures, shared expertise, cultural values and social rules. In that view, action is enabled by more than what is visible for us in the here-and-now situation. Everyone knows that it is impossible to understand current events in a specific organisation without understanding the history of that organisation and how it is managed. Doing the right thing is an ability of enacting local and historical resources and building new actions that enable practitioners to deal with the unexpected. Yet, what this enactment *looks like* is still underexplored in a naturalistic setting of emergency medicine. This book is therefore a contribution to the fields that study human errors related to communication in emergency medicine. The book provides the reader with a new take on this heavily investigated topic, both theoretically and methodologically. First, let me introduce you to this field, why it is important and what I intend to do throughout the book.

Within the literature and in public debates, interest falls on the extent of human errors, the types of errors made and their consequences (Amalberti 2013), but the dynamics involved in error anticipation or error prevention are often underestimated or even overlooked in the existing literature (Reason 2008; Amalberti 2013). The extent of human errors related to miscoordination is immense; in the Western world, approximately 70% of all human error in healthcare is related to lack of coordination and communication (Amalberti 2013; Kohn et al. 2000). Intriguingly, most of these errors have proved to be avoidable but at the same time difficult to grasp (Leape et al. 1993), and often such errors have been linked with cultural challenges in the ward, for instance those of role hierarchies. Thus, the most common recommendation based on those studies encourages healthcare institutions to start with a cultural change in the social practice of medicine. But what does it mean to change a culture or a medical practice? The book explores how cultural accounts are grounded in real-life situations, just as it describes how they can be investigated through concrete video observation of local interaction.

The overarching focus of the book is how human cognition in medical interactivity relates to human errors and successes. The main challenge is to account for how multiple timescales affect local action, both at a theoretical and an empirical level. This interest manifests itself through a cognitive ethnographic study, which investigates that while practitioners immediately feel the consequences of their actions, they often lack an understanding of what leads to specific outcomes. There is, quite simply, a missing link between what the literature and healthcare practitioners think happen and what actually happens in the specific context in which healthcare practitioners are embedded. Only when we learn about why and how errors emerge and develop, does it become possible to intervene effectively and successfully. Thus, this subject needs to be investigated further if the aim is to reduce the number of human errors and to contribute to dialogical and caring healthcare practices. I argue that cognitive ethnography is a useful framework for investigating the emergence and management of human error in emergency medicine. Further, by doing so, this book provides a perspicuous site for demonstrating the relevance of such an approach far more generally.

At an empirical level, the book unfolds real-life video recorded processes that lead to human error in a medical emergency ward. It does so by using an ecological, interactivity-based approach, which treats interaction and cognition as distributed activities that emerge in coordination within a system of people, artefacts and socio-cultural patterns. With this approach new empirical results enrich the reader's understanding of what happens in the medical ward and the results can be used in the design of education programmes in the field of emergency medicine. In fact, this is already the case in the emergency ward that provides the data for this particular study. The book is divided into three parts. Here is a brief overview of what will follow.

Part I, *Investigating errors in healthcare interaction*, consists of two chapters. Chapter 1 presents the emergency ward, an important setting and an exemplar case for demonstrating the value of cognitive ethnography and cognitive event analysis. It opens with a discussion of public expectation to healthcare and general debates, which has shaped the literature on human errors in emergency medicine. It elaborates the argument that there is a missing link between what happens in real-life settings and the findings provided by research thus far. Chapter 2 presents Cognitive Ethnography and Cognitive Event Analysis. It presents cognitive ethnography in relation to distributed cognition by tracing the discipline back to Hutchins' earliest work on cognition "in the wild". It links Hutchins' notion of distributed cognition to Steffensen's account of human interactivity to account for human coordination in its ecological entirety. An ecological perspective of human coordination involves a multi-scalar view on how cognitive results are achieved in a cognitive system. Methodologically, the project uses a non-experimental design to investigate the core features in medical interactivity. Empirical work is based on the use of video ethnography at the department of emergency medicine at a Danish Hospital. As a cognitive ethnographic fieldwork, the study combines methods ranging from research that links video observation with qualitative interviews and participant observation on how material culture influences action. Given this constellation of methods, the research design allows for a focus that spans both micro and macro scales of medical interactivity. The chapter finally presents a new and promising analytical method, the Cognitive Event Analysis, which is suitable for analysing pico-events in cognitive task performances.

Part II, *Behind the scenes: Welcome to the emergency ward*, constitutes the analytical corpus of the book. It consists of seven Chapters (3–9). The initial chapter in Part II, Chapter 3, introduces the reader to the empirical setting. It presents the empirical work that has been conducted "in the wild" at an emergency medicine ward as well as the methodological, practical and ethical concerns that have been raised prior to and during the study. Based on an initial coding process, six themes were defined and further investigated as organising principles of the interactions in the following analysis, which includes six Chapters (4–9). Overall, the analytical chapters provide a fine-grained investigation of interactivity in the emergency ward. The main findings are based on analyses of how a medical team links agents, artefacts and expertise. This analysis balances between (potential) medical error cycles and, more generally, how practitioners undertake treatment as a team-based, problem-solving and decision-making activity. Each chapter investigates an analytical topic. The topics are (a) medical visual systems, (b) interruptions, (c) diagnostic procedures (e.g. anamnesis and patient examination), (d) medical cultural dynamics, (e) sense-making teams and (f) writing the electronic medical record. The analysis of each topic demonstrates how team members enact expertise-in-action, and also how lack of coordination and communication can lead to human errors. In particular, it describes that non-routine events are crucial to what goes on in the emergency ward: Anomalous events function as affordances and trigger feedback mechanisms, which prompt team members to anticipate possible changes of plans. To provide an example it will be demonstrated that interruptions are handled differently depending on the practitioners' level of expertise, team constellation and situational and material circumstances.

Part III, *The Aftermath: The scientific enterprise*, synthesises the results, and the final Chapter 10 is a point of reference for future research on human interactivity – not only within the domain of healthcare, but also more broadly in organisational contexts. The empirical investigations provide a thorough understanding of what actually happens as healthcare teams diagnose and solve problems – or fail to do so. This insight has a direct impact on the design of training programmes in the ward, and such interventions may lead to a safer and more caring practice for all parties involved. The chapter also discusses how the book, as an empirically grounded methodological and theoretical contribution to the field concerned with human interactivity in emergency medicine, opens up for new projects and investigations.

Lastly, the prospective impact of the book is mentioned. By showing the results of using cognitive ethnography to the study of human errors, the chapter illustrates the benefits of treating language and cognition as distributed and intertwined in interactivity. In so doing, it challenges traditional approaches in linguistics and cognitive science to adapt their methods in accord with these foundational assumptions.

PART I

Investigating errors in healthcare interaction

But as strange as it may sound, there is beauty in our imperfections. How boring would our lives be if each of us were a purely rational, perfect specimen? Our flaws are what make us who we are. - Nathan H. Lents (2018: xiii)

CHAPTER 1

The ecology of human errors in emergency medicine

1. Background: Errare humanum est?

In the Western world, approximately 70% of all human error in healthcare is related to lack of coordination and communication (Amalberti 2013; Kohn et al. 2000). Intriguingly, most of these errors have proved to be avoidable but at the same time difficult to grasp (Leape et al. 1993).

> Even more disturbing, communication failures are the leading root cause of the sentinel events reported to the Joint Commission [...] specifically, the Joint Commission cites communication failures as the leading root cause for medication errors, delays in treatment, and wrong-site surgeries, as well as the second most frequently cited root cause for operative and postoperative events and fatal falls. (O'Daniel and Rosenstein 2008: 271)

According to Eisenberg et al. (2007), the most difficult task for hospitals is to improve communication processes (Eisenberg et al. 2007: 391). Eisenberg et al. (2007) report that medical errors are ubiquitous, and many of the errors are linked to communication failure. Furthermore, it is argued that there is a "need for research about communication and information sharing among healthcare providers" (Nemeth et al. 2004: 726).

The level of human error is alarming, and healthcare is under massive pressure from many sides. First, technological and sociological development increases both workload and complexity, which, in turn, raises the risk of human error. Second, public expectations of healthcare are increasing while tolerance of errors is diminishing (Reason 1995; Horsky et al. 2005). As a consequence of this pressure, multiple initiatives have been implemented in order to streamline and control decision-making in healthcare. Many of such initiatives are based on quantitative studies that presuppose that errors are grounded in error prone individuals who need fixed operational procedures to scaffold cognitive processing:

> We have seen an expansion of intervention studies to design, implement, and evaluate either an interprofessional checklist or clinical guidelines or protocols [...] linked to a specific clinical issue [...] A key limitation of these outcome-based

> often retrospective, quantitative studies is that we know little about the processes whereby interventions work or fail, and little about the way culture or context shapes practices, constraining or facilitating interprofessional collaboration. (Paradis et al. 2014: 235)

Given the need for qualitative research, a reduction of negative outcome is not achieved by adding even more procedures into the work practice. According to Leape: "The most fundamental change that will be needed if hospitals are to make meaningful progress in error reduction is a cultural one" (Leape 1994: 1857). Leape (1994) argues that an error intolerant culture has emerged in healthcare institutions. He describes the consequences of socialising doctors in a medical educational system that has an immense focus on perfection: Society, media and healthcare institutions expect that a good doctor is a doctor who makes no mistakes (Leape 1994). The individual has been viewed as a peril and a distinct system component whose erroneous choices lead to disastrous breakdowns, primarily due to a lack of attention, unsafe acts or ignorance (Reason 2008: 3). Leape furthermore holds that such an error free ideology affects sense-making processes and attitudes in real-life treatment situations as the fear of making mistakes essentially leads to an error prone practice. Expectations of an omnipotent healthcare practitioner naturally affect how healthcare practitioners perceive themselves. Thus, according to Leape (1994), the organising principle should be turned around so that practitioners are acknowledged as caring individuals working in complex and dynamical systems. Based on this view, healthcare professionals are not insensitive, rule-following creatures that operate in a vacuum (Madsen 2014). According to Leape, among others, it is only when healthcare institutions, the media and society acknowledge that doctors are not just rational but also moral beings, emotionally attached to what they do together with team members and patients, that errors can be investigated, understood and reduced in a fruitful way (Leape 1994; Reason 2000; Kohn et al. 2000; Pedersen 2010, 2012). In other words, a positive and tolerant approach to making mistakes in medicine is crucial. Recent evidence from neuroscientific studies supports this line of argumentation (Moser et al. 2011). Specifically, it reveals how individuals with a positive, flexible approach towards learning and intelligence are less prone to repeating mistakes than those with a negative, fixed view on learning and intelligence (Moser et al. 2011). If intelligence is treated as malleable and is developed through engagement, then mistakes and errors are seen as opportunities to learn and improve rather than as shortcomings (cf. Moser et al. 2011; Mangels et al. 2006). When practitioners' attitudes towards performance are a decisive factor in how well they bounce back from errors, this will, in turn, give an indication of how errors will be dealt with in future incidents. The attitude of a practitioner is not solely a phenomenon inherent in the individual; culture and norms affect how professionals deal with error.

Leape encourages healthcare institutions to acknowledge this and to nourish the education of practitioners in a way which deals with errors in a realistic manner rather than denying their existence.

Such insights are valuable and provide an understanding of practitioners' working conditions at a general level. However, they do not fully explain what happens in the local encounter when culture is re-enacted and shaped. For healthcare institutions to be able to enhance practice they need better explanations and more specific advice than general statements such as Leape's broad recommendation to start with cultural change. Again, what does it mean to change a culture? How does one systematically generate cultural changes in a socio-technical system? To characterise the mechanisms of cultural changes, one needs to explore the enabling conditions of medical sense-making in great detail. This means that explanations of why healthcare professionals act the way they do are a prerequisite for efficient and capable intervention. What do practitioners see, feel, think, do and say? How do they manage decision-making? How do they avoid getting overwhelmed? What exactly prompts them to break or follow a rule? How are sociocultural norms enacted through bodies in action?

A widespread problem exists in the field of healthcare concerning how we conceptualise human errors in interaction. The field of human error is titanic. In the following sections I briefly define the classical view on human error within cognitive psychology, leading to the argument that a broader perspective on human error is needed and that such redefinition changes the object of study remarkably.

1.1 Two models of human error

When one seeks to understand human error, ontological, epistemological and methodological questions come to the fore. Explanations vary depending on the perspective one has on human error. Thus, a definition of human error is needed. The following definition is based on recent literature about human error and particularly on James Reason's book *The Human Contribution* (Reason 2008), which builds on his previous books *Human Error* (1990) and *Managing the Risks of Organizational Accidents* (1997). Reason, a psychologist, is one of the most quoted authors within the field of human error in medical settings. In the introductory part of his 2008-book, he admits that defining error is a challenging task: "Although there is no one universally agreed definition of error, most people accept that it involves some kind of deviation" (Reason 2008: 29). In a similar vein Sandars and Esmail (2003), in an attempt to understand the diversity of definitions across studies, report in a review on the frequency and nature of medical error in primary care that "there are a wide variety of definitions and methods used to identify the frequency and nature of medical error" (Sandars and Esmail

2003: 231). Reason links his preliminary categorical challenge to how taxonomies are shaped to fulfil specific purposes:

> Just as there are several possible definitions, so there are also many ways in which errors may be classified. Different taxonomies serve different purposes. These depend upon which of the four basic elements of an error – the intention, the action, the outcome and the context – is of greatest interest or has most practical utility. (Reason 2008: 29)

The division of errors into four elements serves as a functional heuristic that allows investigations of one error domain at a given time. As such, it gives rise to detailed descriptions of the multiple aspects involved in the emergence of an error from its starting point in an error cycle to its negative outcome.

Notwithstanding the many different definitions of error and error taxonomies, the literature has been divided into two main positions that ascribe causality of human errors to very different sources. The two positions are denoted as the *person model* and the *system model* respectively (Reason 2000, 2008). It is argued below that each position conveys a specific model of causality and an underlying understanding of the nature of human error that provides very different explanations and philosophies of error management (Reason 2000, 2008). Challenges concerning the localisation of error in space-time remain, and these will be discussed further in the Sections 1.3 and 1.4 after the presentation of the two models.

1.1.1 *The person model*

According to Reason, 'the person model'[1] of human error originates from the occupational health and safety approach to industrial accidents, "but it is also deeply rooted in folk psychology" (Reason 2008: 71). This approach focuses on specific occurrences and, when errors occur, blames individuals for either moral weakness or lack of attention as a result of aberrant mental processes. On its own, Reason suggests, a person approach can only deal with symptoms: "Instead of dwelling upon the last accident and trying to find local fixes for what was probably a unique occurrence, the attention of safety managers is now directed towards eliminating the worst of the current latent problems" (Reason 2005: 60). In this view, individuals have been viewed as free agents who independently choose what to do and what not to do, or simply choose between safe and unsafe modes of behaviour. Unsafe acts are traced back to individual forgetfulness, inadequate knowledge, lack of skills, inattention, etc. (Reason 2008: 72). As a consequence, when errors

1. Reason's use of the term *person* in his "person model" is hardly compatible with a humanistic understanding of the concept of person, who is normally thought of as a human being with a cultural belonging. In Reason's view, the "person model" seems to refer to what, in a humanistic perspective, would be called an "individualistic model".

are traced back to how individuals make decisions, blame is placed on independent individuals without considering how organisational and cultural aspects of an operation affect decision-making. As a self-perpetuating force, a blame culture is maintained by its own inherent logic of linear causality. This logic is also fed by public expectations of infallibility, which emerge in parallel to doctors' abilities to extend the boundaries of what is possibly as medical technology advances. When seeking to minimise error prone practices through the person model, individual cognitive scaffolding is targeted. Consequently, reward and punishment mechanisms are used to prompt individuals to perform flawlessly. While the approach reflects the expectations coming from society, politicians, etc., it explains errors as linear sequences of incidents related to a single timescale and location. It overlooks how errors emerge as people orient to past events and anticipate what comes next "on the basis of individual and collective intentions, aspirations and expectations" (Steffensen and Pedersen 2014: 86). As Leape emphasises, the medical culture is mired in an error free ideology that affects how decisions are made in local situations. This culture stems from the consumer relation between healthcare services and the public, because medical experts are viewed as omnipotent and according to Reason and others, it entails an urge to place blame on individuals when errors occur (Reason 1997, 2000, 2005, 2008; Merry and Smith 2001).

However, since errors have multiple causes, it is misguided to blame individuals or groups in the medical sector, as is often done in public media. In short, "the problem is not bad people in health care – it is that good people are working in bad systems that need to be made safer" (Kohn et al. 2000: 49). The literature acknowledges that doctors are neither failure prone nor arrogant, but rather educated in a tradition and operating in a system that predisposes them to behave and use skills that may not fit current requirements. So why do we blame them? Reason proposes several reasons for blaming individuals for specific human errors. He points out that a person or team at "the sharp end" or "in the loop" is closest to the error in time and space. Psychologically, we often react by ascribing causal efficacy to the entity closest in time and space to the effect; when the doctor is closest to the error (as damaging outcome), he or she is seen as the "last" and most visible defence layer (Reason 2000). To track the error to its organisational roots is difficult (Reason 2008) and "blaming individuals is emotionally more satisfying than targeting institutions" (Reason 2000: 768).

Reason has successfully argued that to embrace the complexity of human errors, one must address the issue of how and when blame is to be placed on specific individuals (Reason 2005; Merry and Smith 2001). He argues that the person model, as it looks at single individuals in a vacuum, is only able to contain information about error as output and not about its complex root system running beyond individual action. Finally, the person approach might not just be incomplete, but simply flawed, as its reductionist outlook breaks down a failure into smaller and smaller parts until the elements of error are simple and localised. But, according to Reason, this operation motivated the comparison of the Canadian invented CANDU reactor with the Chernobyl RBMK reactor, where the defence features were reduced to small elements that were "compared on a one-to-one basis" (Reason 2008: 84). Chapman (2004) addresses the crucial point that this comparative endeavour misses:

> What if essential features of the entity are embedded not in the components but in their interconnectedness? What if its complexity arises from the ways in which its components actually relate to and interact with one another? The very act of simplifying by sub-division loses the interconnections and therefore cannot tackle this aspect of complexity. (Chapman 2004: 35)

Reason thus argues for a systemic perspective that incorporates the complexity that the person model misses.

1.1.2 *The system model*

To get beyond the error frontline, Reason proposes a new error model that enables the identification of what he defines as *error traps* to explain how errors draw on latent conditions (Reason 2000). The Swiss cheese model visualises how an error emerges when holes in multiple defence layers align with particular latent conditions and active failures. (Reason 2008: 101)

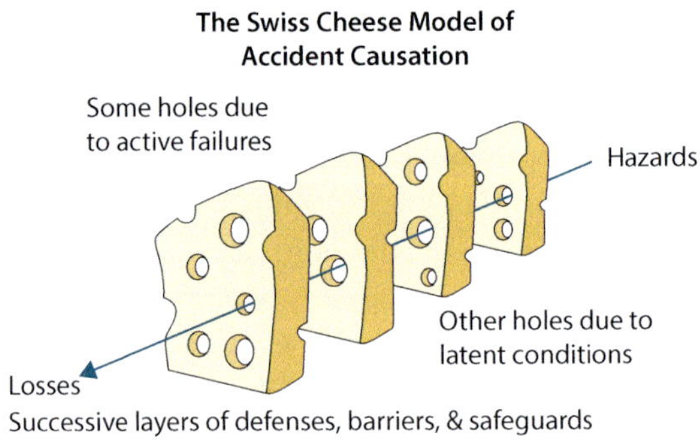

Figure 1.1 The swiss cheese model of how defences, barriers and safeguards may be penetrated by an accident trajectory (Reason 2008)

While the person model recognises errors as failure output, the system model emphasises how failure emerges in a process of momentary alignment. Failure happens as a hazard passes through the trajectory of accident opportunity (Reason 2008). Reason's model, thus, traces errors to multiple causes that are connected on several levels. From this perspective, errors should be investigated at the levels of person, team, task, workplace and institution. He emphasises that modern healthcare exploits high technology systems and procedures whose defensive layers are designed to protect patients from human errors. While some of the layers are engineered (alarms, automatic shutdowns, patient surveillance technology, etc.), others depend on procedures (regularly performed checks, administrative controls, etc.), and yet others rely on people in their formal roles (surgeons, control room operators, etc.). Unlike an actual Emmental, the cheese layers in the model are continually working, breaking down and shifting location, so the holes are constantly moving from place to place (Reason 2008). One ineffective defence layer rarely causes human errors; errors are rather conditioned by several ineffective defence layers that bring off negative outcomes (Reason 2005, 2008). The model, however, is rather deterministic in that it places practitioners within a system without allowing them to either affect how it works or act against the system's logic. If this were to occur, there would have to be bidirectional relations. However, Reason has recently added a slice of cheddar at the left of the model to symbolise coping resources, which may recover the critical event even after many defence layers have been penetrated. Thus, recovery abilities are symbolised by a cheddar slice without holes that serves as a negative feedback mechanism[2] blocking the critical event trajectory (Reason 2008).

The model builds on a "new view" of human error (Dekker 2002), which (a) treats error as a symptom of deep and complex conditions within the system, (b) believes that safety is not an inherent system condition but something practitioners must create within the system and (c) links errors with how tools are used, how tasks are achieved and what the environment affords. Progress on safety systems only emerges as the understanding of multi-causality and interconnectedness of system mechanisms increase (Dekker 2002; Shappell and Wiegmann 2001). This new view contrasts with the old view, which considers that the system is safe and that only people are unreliable, and that automatisation, training and discipline are the means for protecting the system (Dekker 2002). The system approach on the other hand treats human errors as inevitable yet also manageable, and individuals are viewed as resources rather than as latent, dysfunctional components.

Instead of placing people within a flow of one-way procedures, it can be recognised that there are various means of engaging and disengaging with people, procedures and equipment (Hutchins 1995a; Hazlehurst et al. 2008). Much has been gained from focusing on the patient as "the little person" against "the big

2. I use the term negative and positive feedback mechanisms for describing a cognitive system's activities that either reduce or increase complexity and eventually leads to errors, breakdowns or new solutions. For instance, when frustration emerges and leads to desperate actions that continue to worsen the cognitive process, this can be explained as positive feedback within the system (Bertalanffy 1968; Flach 1999).

system"; however, there has also been a tendency to forget the well-being of the practitioner(s). Sometimes practitioners are blamed for acting as well as they can because, judged in terms of optima, this is not "good enough". One benefit of a system perspective is that it makes it possible to consider *both* the patient *and* the practitioner. The focus falls on whether, in a given environment, medical teams *can* act satisfactorily. This leads to an important insight. It is meaningless to present an analysis of a single situation without relating that analysis to a pattern on a level that illuminates cultural and organisational affordances for specific ways of acting. The problem is complex and multifaceted, and this complexity needs to be incorporated into research.

However, in the literature and in public debates, interest falls on the extent of human errors, the types of errors made and their consequences (Amalberti 2013). As the dynamics involved in error anticipation or error prevention are often underestimated or even overlooked within the existing literature (Reason 2008; Amalberti 2013), Reason (2008) provides an alternative perspective: to study the human as a hero that adapts and compensates for what is lacking in a way that leads to a heroic outcome. Reason's interest falls on *the human contribution*, rather than errors (or successes) in isolation (Reason 2008: 3). Not only is the focus on errors caused by a prejudiced motivation, it is also problematic because it focuses on the one side of the story (what goes wrong). By merely looking into error processes, we only learn part of what errors are about because anticipatory actions that prevent errors from happening are easily overlooked. The argument presented here is: if one wants to learn about human errors, one needs to study the variety of human contributions, and not just negative outcomes. This idea is pursued in this study. In a similar vein, Lundberg et al. (2009) argue that the consequence of linear person approaches is related to the WYLFIWYF principle (What You Look For Is What You Find) (Lundberg et al. 2009). In line with Reason's system model, Hollnagel presents the Functional Resonance Analysis Method (FRAM), which is a tool for modelling complex socio-technical systems in healthcare (Hollnagel 2012). It builds on the principle of functional resonance, paying attention to the functions involved in medical events and investigating outcomes as results of resonance that emerge from variability of work routines (Hollnagel 2004). Further, Hollnagel argues that to understand human error and risk performance, one must investigate common functions and processes as the basis for both failures and successes. FRAM generally focuses on how functions are carried out and not just on how they fail, as established approaches tend to do (Hollnagel 2012). Finally, it is worth mentioning one of the reasons to why the system model gained ground in research. In 1989, the psychologist, Gary Klein, presented the Naturalistic Decision Making (NDM) framework at a conference in Dayton, Ohio (Klein 2008). The NDM framework was developed as a reaction to the existing approaches to the study of human decision-making, which mostly carried out their research in experimental settings as, for instance, simulation-based settings. The traditional framework gained valuable insights into how people did *not* make decisions, but not what they *did* (Klein 2008).

> Researchers were not likely to find out how people actually made decisions by conducting experiments to test hypotheses derived from statistical and mathematical models of ideal choice strategies. Even the decision researchers who performed studies in field settings, using experienced participants, primarily assessed performance according to formal standards. (Klein 2008: 1)

The NDM framework works on different grounds. It requires field research of how people make decisions in naturalistic settings. Researchers within the NDM framework developed different models of human decision-making:

> People were not generating and comparing option sets. People were using prior experience to rapidly categorize situations. People were relying on some kind of synthesis of their experience – call it a schema or a prototype or a category – to make these judgments. The categories suggested appropriate courses of action. The static notion of decisions as gambles, which portrays people as passively awaiting the outcomes of their bets, did not fit leaders who were actively trying to shape events (Klein 2008: 2)

With Reason, Klein and Hollnagel as front figures, the scope of human error is expanded from dealing with individual outcome to error traps and, more recently, to human contributions in general. In line with the system perspective, the current study is not fixated on outcomes (e.g. final diagnosis); rather, it turns its attention to the positive and negative feedback mechanisms in diagnostic and treatment events in emergency medicine. According to Flach (1999), it is vital to investigate how a system adapts and coordinates as the unanticipated occurs in a way that challenges conventional actions and standard procedures. He encourages an investigation of how decisions are made when practitioners navigate across the frontier of the automatic and unknown, where conventionalised procedures become constraints for proper action. Flach (1999) suggests that under these circumstances, the agent becomes more of a problem solver than a rule follower. This flexibility allows the agent (a) to observe and coordinate the flow of actions and (b) to think creatively, allowing for boundary reconstruction of the system and (c) to respond appropriately to the unexpected even if it means sacrificing local stability and performing on "the edge of chaos" (Flach 1999: 125). Altogether, this new view on human errors provides a systemic perspective that involves a bidirectional focus on human errors and successes. The new focus is, in short, on how feedback mechanisms operate in a complex environment, for good and for ill.

2. Critique: Research incommensurability

While recognising the importance of agency beyond the agent, Klein, Reason – and other proponents of the system approach – remain focused on information processing in the individual, computational brain. Reason, amongst others, locates and reduces the human mind to internal cognitive schemas: "The human mind has an extraordinary ability to store the recurrences of the world in long-term memory as schemas (knowledge packages), and then to bring their products into play whenever they correspond to the current contextual calling conditions" (Reason 2008: 18). Such a concurrent processing view is limited to descriptions of how separate though interacting subsystems operate in isolation with individual intentions: "All operators make errors, but the best of them have the ability to compensate for adverse effects. This ability depends on their skill and experience, as well as the extent to which they have mentally rehearsed the detection and recovery of their errors" (Reason 2001: 30). As cognition is located within single individuals, the approach leaves aside how the overall system is enabled to act as a cognitive system. Both the person approach and the system approach are inadequate for investigating what happens beyond the level of individual belief or social behaviour. At best, the person approach deals with cognitive aspects of individual human error, while the system approach investigates the social behaviour of a large, complex system.

As the investigation of communicative issues in healthcare has generally been preoccupied with the role of individuals (and individuals within systems), it is either concerned with individuals' internal cognitive skills and their functions, or individuals' communicative skills as they are used in external information exchange processes. According to this segregational view, individuals use their communicative skills to gain information that enables them to make decisions which can be right or wrong, and these two sequential processes are studied separately. In cognitive science, the classic view of cognition (cf. Boden 2006) as confined to individual brains has focused on internal information processing as practitioners interact with information systems and carry out predefined tasks (Kushniruk et al. 1997). For instance, extensive descriptions of situation awareness and decision-making emphasise the competences of the individual without relating them to sociocultural organisations (Fioratou et al. 2010).

Regarding the conversational features in interaction, fields such as ethnography, sociology, and ethnomethodology have studied the social and interactional order in conversations (e.g. individuals' use of sequential patterns in verbal interaction), treating this as the sole explanatory framework for human interaction (e.g. Goffman 1974, 1983; Heritage and Clayman 2010). Thus, the theories of cognition and interaction that are embedded in the aforementioned approaches do not correspond with recent understandings of cognition and language as distributed and ecological (see Chapter 2). Basically, this means that errors as they emerge and are experienced in practice do not correlate with empirical findings based on conventional approaches to human errors. This incommensurability entails a scientific gap. This book hypothesises that this gap is due to a misconceived view on the nature of cognition and language, and thus also of human errors related to interaction.

Finally, both the person approach and system approach fall short of explanations that deal with errors in a multi-scalar view, both in space and time. However, recent studies underline how enabling conditions of human interaction are also tied to timescales beyond the conversational level – such as, for instance, the ones tied to the bio-mechanics of living bodies (Thibault 2011; Steffensen 2012, 2013; Cowley et al. 2013; Linell 2009; Jensen 2014b; Chemero 2009; Di Paolo et al. 2018). These impending, ecological, intellectual semblances challenge traditional approaches to human interaction. By opening up to deal with both faster and slower timescales than those concerned with words, human errors can be dynamically linked with history, culture and knowledge in situated interaction. The transgression of timescales is pivotal in the study of human interaction, because culture emerges and materialises in the relationship between here-and-now and slower timescales. In what follows, an ecological understanding of human errors is presented.

3. An ecological approach to human error: From errors to error cycles

An ecological account of human error deals with *error cycles* consisting of (a) conditions for errors, (b) real-time occurrences and (c) development due to the (lack of negative) feedback mechanisms of the system. When moving from error as a local phenomenon to error cycles as a process, the ecology of errors expands local boundaries in time and space. An error cycle is characterised as dysfunctional dynamics within a cognitive system with a functional agenda. From this perspective, errors are *not* solely defined by their negative outcome, but as the process in which tensions, frustration and fixation biases can emerge. Sometimes, such processes are balanced as the system adapts flexibly when changes are anticipated. Cowley (2007) describes human behaviour as flexible and adaptive, meaning that humans use: "*cognitive dynamics* to control how they coordinate the world. Humans extend this general capacity by cooperating in cultural settings. Using resources that constitute our perceived worlds, biology becomes enmeshed with history" (Cowley 2007: 1). A cognitive system's flexible adaptive behaviour can be described as an ability to change and expand its ecological niche[3] as it recalibrates its boundaries. For instance, the system flexibly adapts when a practitioner innovates, finds a new solution to a well-known problem, or when a novice doctor relies on an experienced nurse, distributing the responsibility between the parties rather than turning to individual problem-solving. As will be explicated in Part II (in particular Chapter 4–9), coaction is a meshwork shaped by what has happened before, what the environment offers, capabilities for action and the expectations related to the joint professional project (Rączaszek-Leonardi 2011). Hence, errors are related to how practitioners interact and manage cognitive events by manipulating their environments and each other. By widening the scope of attention to include abstract information structures (Baber et al. 2006), people, relationships and material environmental structures, a more nuanced description of what actually happens and how errors are tied to multiple timescales is revealed. From this perspective, intention and thinking are not internal local processes; they are distributed (Hutchins 1995a; Hutchins 2014; Hollan et al. 2000) and non-local (Steffensen 2013; Steffensen and Cowley 2010), i.e., linked with experience, culture and norms.

Conditions for errors can be latent systemic properties and real constraints on action. Moreover, an ecological definition of human error necessarily deals with the mesh of multiple timescales (latent conditions, emergences and responses) in a cognitive system. The crucial element in this definition is the coupling between the subsystems. The coupling precludes reductionist analysis of single components in the system. The cognitive powers of the overall system emerge in interaction. Even though results are achieved as a consequence of coordinated interaction, the enabling (latent) conditions for coordination are important for the overall system operations. In a professional organisation these latent conditions relate to (a) individual capabilities as skills, experience, ideologies and beliefs, (b) the socio-culturally shared norms, rules, values, experience and belief, (c) the physical environment and (d) local interaction.

Sociocultural norms and rules afford a range of behaviours that practitioners and patients use to interact in an expected way. Such expectations enable successful outcomes but may also entail fixation biases that prevent practitioners from solving a problem and moving on. Depending on the system's capability for action, specific

3. From an ecosystemic perspective, niche construction describes the process of how an organism modifies its environment through its metabolism and its interactions (Laland et al. 2013). As such, a functional relation between a species and its environment is maintained in niche construction: "What human beings do together arise in a specific ecological niche (cognitive-natural-sociocultural) and feeds back into that very niche: structures and resources arise in ecologically embedded interactivity, just as they integrate into human interactivity, across time and space." (Steffensen and Fill 2014: 19)

feedback mechanisms contribute to or constrain the error process. Thus, how a technological artefact facilitates diagnostic processes or not depends on situated action, sociocultural rules for using the device and whether it is a functional part in a given situation. As such, interaction, as the coupling energy, becomes the guiding element in analysis. This is important since patterns of behaviour can be traced to how a practitioner alters the environment. Such alteration is an interaction between historical and physical characteristics such as the level of skill, the level of knowledge information, the history of experience and local affordances for action (how the setting is organised, what is being said, which cognitive aids are visible to whom etc.), see e.g. Goodwin 1994, 2007, 2018. Specifically, a practitioner modifies the functional relationship between himself and his environment, or rather, he adapts to the changes in the system of which he is a part. A doctor can move around in the system, but there are constraints on actions. The cognitive ecosystem is defined by its bounded and dynamic possibilities for action (Hodges and Baron 1992; Hodges 2007a, 2007b, 2009). As a heuristic the constraints relate to ontogenetic development (including personal history, level of skill, educational level, etc.), physical structures and artefacts available (electronic devices etc.) and sociocultural norms (e.g. what is usually done by whom). An understanding of each element, as considered by the person approach, for instance, is not crucial for grasping how such constraints work. If a doctor lacks communicative expertise, an experienced nurse can compensate for this and, if a problem is solved in a functional way, it might not be relevant to understanding the system. How such an interaction has contributed to situational development is the relevant starting point, directing attention to the system as a whole and beyond the components within the system. Thus, some actions can be traced to cultural patterns, and others are explained as ecosystemic. But importantly, cultural explanations are not based on an outside-in perspective; rather, they are grounded in embodied actions in the situation itself. Thus, part, II takes its starting point in real-time situated particularities and identifies local dynamics that can be traced to patterns beyond the local situation.

Acknowledgements

This volume is an edited version of my 2015 PhD thesis (Pedersen 2015). I am highly indebted to the external reviewers in the PhD committee: Per Linell, Charles Goodwin, and Stephen J. Cowley. I owe them many thanks for their critical and valuable comments in terms of their written evaluation and continuous feedback on my work. Their comments have been integrated into the edited version. This edited version further includes earlier published versions of some of the analyses. I happily thank the original publishers as well as – in a few cases – co-authors for permission to reuse previous published works in this volume. Information about reuse of published work will be found in the relevant chapters and sections where they appear.

CHAPTER 2

A cognitive ethnography of emergency medicine

Many of the foundational problems of cognitive science are consequences of our ignorance of the nature of cognition in the wild [...] The first part of the job is, therefore, a descriptive enterprise. I call this description of the cognitive task world a "cognitive ethnography." One might have assumed that cognitive anthropology would have made this sort of work its centerpiece. It has not. Studying cognition in the wild is difficult, and the outcomes are uncertain. - Edwin Hutchins (1995a: 370ff)

1. How errors, interaction and cognition can be studied *in the wild*

Imagine you are a patient who enters the emergency ward. You expect to be treated as a *person* with a history. Your history is to some extent relevant to your current medical condition and the way you respond to the overall situation. You also expect that the healthcare team is well equipped to identifying and making sense of your symptoms and that they are capable of managing the situation in relation to a certain area of medical expertise and experience. Similarly, the medical team expects you, the patient, to reveal relevant information and to be honest and cooperative. In sum, in the medical encounter multiple assumptions are tacit, and the interaction is to a large extend based on reciprocal trust. While patients expect a professional and dialogical interaction at the emergency ward, time is limited, information can be difficult to discern, and circumstances vary to a high degree within this organisational domain. As mentioned in the previous chapter, the circumstances often lead to an increased risk of human errors, and often the stressful and varied circumstances impair the ability to engage dialogically and reflect systematically about what happens. Expertise develops intuitively as practitioners engage in repeated task performances in the ward. While expertise is based on intuition or skilled embodiment, practitioners struggle to explain exactly how it manifests itself in local interaction: *they just know what to do*, they explain. That is why investigations of what happens in a narrow local timescale are incomplete. Rather, a broader lens is needed which allows the analyst to zoom in and out in the organisational domain of emergency medicine.

Cognitive ethnography provides such a longitudinal lens. By using specific analytical tools, the possibility for exploring real-time dynamics of human behaviour within a macro-framework, allow the analyst to investigate different temporal scales that together impact local interaction and cognition. In theoretical terms, the non-local trajectory impacts local action. Cognitive ethnography thus lives through interactions over time, and the context around interactions (such as past and future) plays a crucial role for professional interaction. Cognitive ethnography continues to refer and relate to manifest data only, but it is liberal and radical as it extends the unit of analysis to include a broad range of data and approaches.

Chapter 1 argued for the need of an ecological investigation of human errors in emergency medicine. The main focus of this chapter is to introduce such an ecological framework that enables investigations of the ecology of human errors in the emergency medical ward. Specifically, it introduces the framework of cognitive ethnography and secondarily the method of Cognitive Event Analysis.

The chapter does not intend to provide a systematic review of cognitive ethnography and its related methods. It does not give an account of all cognitive-ethnographic works that have been carried out within the situated field. Rather, it provides an introduction to where cognitive ethnography comes from and how it can be used as a framework for real-life investigations of human error in a complex organisational setting.

2. Cognitive ethnography and its roots in distributed cognition

This following part of this chapter introduces cognitive ethnography, which serves as the framework for this study, and secondly, it presents the method of Cognitive Event Analysis, an analytical method apt for investigating cognitive events. The presentation of cognitive ethnography involves a presentation of distributed cognition. Despite the value of a distributed cognition perspective, this chapter critically engages in some of the challenges that follow in the wake of the approach. I thus introduce the interactivity perspective as a complementary and needed anti-representationalist take on cognition. However, in order to understand the motivation and theoretical assumptions underpinning cognitive ethnography, it is relevant to elaborate on its origins in distributed cognition. We thus venture 40 years into the past to get a sense of how cognitive ethnography became a distinguished discipline.

In November 1980, Edwin Hutchins conducted cognitive anthropological fieldwork on a U.S. navy ship that was on its way into the open North Pacific. As he stayed on the navigation bridge, he had access to the work procedures of the navigation team. After completing the first study of the navigation team, he realised that situated cognition was not individual but a social, distributed phenomenon. Hutchins thus coined the term, *distributed cognition*,[1] and he articulated its main principles in his seminal 1995 book, *Cognition in the Wild*. He describes first and foremost how the distributed cognition perspective is needed. It is radical as it offers a new way to tie cognition with sociocultural practice. For instance, Hutchins discloses the distributed traits of cognition as they emerge in interactions and through coordination within a cognitive system (Hutchins 1995a). In his study of how a navigation team serves as a cognitive, computational system, interest falls on the interaction within the system rather than on individuals and their internal information processing. His findings are based on observations of naturally occurring events, which, according to Hutchins his colleagues were not interested in. The majority of his colleagues focused exclusively on experimental research detached from naturally occurring situations and it caused frustration:

> I became disillusioned with my field I lost interest in it. The choice of naturally situated cognition as a topic came from my sense that it is what cognitive anthropology really should have been about but largely had not been. Clifford Geertz (1983) called for an "outdoor psychology," but cognitive anthropology was unable or unwilling to be that. The respondents may have been exotic, but the methods of investigation were largely borrowed from the indoor techniques of psychology and linguistics. When cognitive and symbolic anthropology split off from social anthropology, in the mid 1950's, they left society and practice behind.
>
> (Hutchins, 1995a: xii)[2]

Distributed cognition is a contemporary product of intense development in cognitive science. As part of the historical grounding of distributed cognition, the

1. Already in the late 80s Hutchins was using the term "distributed cognition". It appears in the title of the concept paper *Distributed cognition in aviation* for a NASA project (Contract No. NCC 2–591), and Hutchins later revealed that the project led to – in his view – the most important paper on distributed cognition, (the paper is: Distributed cognition in an airline cockpit (1996)) not because it has been cited a lot, but because "it was the first time I really made a consistent application of my ideas to data from my ship study" (personal communication: 13 September 2015). He further emphasises that it took Engestrom and Middleton years to get the edited volume out, which is why it does not appear as an early publication (it was published in 1996); however, it was produced in the late 80s.

2. It is worth mentioning that Gary Klein's (2008) NDM-framework (see Chapter 1) is a result of a similar dissatisfaction with the way cognitive scientists conducted their studies in simulation-based settings. However, Klein is rather conventional in his understanding of cognition as a mental process (see Klein 2008), and his conceptual work on cognition is less radial than Hutchins' conceptual framework. Therefore, I emphasise Hutchins' work here as his conceptual idea of cognition as distributed within cognitive systems impacts on how it can be demarcated and studied.

radical transformations that cognitive science has undergone in the last decades are briefly scrutinised before the perspective is elaborated further.

These transformations concern the nature of cognitive processes, which have a direct impact on methods and theories about cognition. Retrospectively, the transformations have been defined as first, second and third wave developments in cognitive science (Steffensen 2012). In the classic view on cognition (the first wave) held by mainstream cognitive science during the 1960s and until the mid 1970s, computational models of internal manipulations of symbolic representations treat cognition as the link between perceptual input and behavioural output that occurs in a mental realm (cf. Boden 2006). Behind this view resided the idea that cognition is reduced to symbol manipulation processes (information processing) identical to how a computer process information (cf. Newell et al. 1958). With advances in neuroimaging, brain scientists leapt into the domain of the human mind. Anderson et al. (2012) explain how such approaches, when relying on fMRI scans, propose that separate brain regions contain local information about cognitive faculties. For instance, faculties such as memory, reason and conceptualisation are traced to separate brain areas, and cognitive abilities are experimentally investigated in isolation, for instance in relation to attention (cf. Anderson et al. 2012). In this perspective, neural firings in the brain enable the individual to make mental representations of an outer world: This process was defined as cognitive. Such research explains important, useful features of the brain. However, if the aim is to understand how human cognition works in real life, the brain-bound view misguides this scientific endeavour (Anderson et al. 2012). This modular view on cognition was soon replaced with connectionist models of cognition, defined as second wave development (Steffensen 2012; Jensen, 2014b). During the 1970s, 1980s and 1990s, empirical findings pointed to how cognition was embodied in a way that challenged the inner-outer dichotomy radically. Although cognition was no longer treated as purely brain-bound, it remained body-bound, and as the locus of interest for cognitive scientists the individual endured. The second wave cleared the way for phenomenological studies in cognitive science, allowing for new discussions about perception based on Merleau-Ponty's thinking, among others: "We encounter the world neither as data-crunching information processors, nor as ghostly apparitions floating over the surface of things like a fog. Perceptual perspective is *bodily* perspective" (Carman 2008: 11). The brain was understood in relation to a historical body where perception of being in the world is intertwined with cognitive processes.

Incorporating a growing range of parameters outside the brain and body, the tendency to expand the location of cognition seems to continue in this ongoing cognitive development. Thus recently, a branch of cognitive science has again reframed the status of brains, bodies and the world to achieve a more ecological and systemic view of cognition (Norman 1993; Salomon 1993; Hutchins 1995a, 2014;

Kirsh 1997, 2009, 2013; Vallée-Tourangeau 2013; Anderson et al. 2012; Chemero 2009; Di Paolo et al. 2018). This ecological perspective on cognition has been described as a third wave of development in cognitive science. Several researchers have provided the field with various concepts that all share the criterion that cognition is not limited to a neurological substrate. In the third wave development, Andy Clark's The Extended Mind Hypothesis (Clark 2008) and Hutchins' Distributed Cognition (Hutchins 1995a) have particularly crystallised.

Having moved from an internal, localisable and brain-bound view on cognition to an embodied one, and then finally to a broader ecosystemic and distributed view, the object of analysis has been redefined dramatically (Hutchins 1995a). Moreover, such a redefinition changes theory and methods as it opens to interdisciplinary research. Within third wave cognition, distributed cognition has manifested itself as a valid perspective, which is elaborated on in the following.

In the field of distributed cognition, Hutchins (1995a, 2014), Hollan et al. (2000) and Kirsh (1997, 2009, 2013) qualified the perspective and applied it in other areas – specifically in the domain of human-computer interaction. The distributed cognition perspective is distinct in the sense that it seeks to describe environments of interactions (Hollan et al. 2000). For instance it deals with interactions between participants and technologies rather than taking one of them in isolation. As a result, cognition is defined as distributed in and among people and material artefacts, and through time (Hollan et al. 2000). Hollan et al. (2000) argue that when one seeks to grasp cognitive processes from this perspective, three interdependent ways in which processes of cognition can be distributed are identified:

- Cognitive processes may be distributed across members of a social group
- Cognitive processes may involve coordination between internal and external (material or environmental structure)
- Cognitive processes may be distributed through time in such a way that the products of earlier events can transform the nature of later events. (Hollan et al. 2000: 176)

Cognitive events can play out when individuals draw on material artefacts and exploit future events. As they do so, they constitute a distributed cognitive system, which is "a system that produces cognitive outputs, just as an agricultural system yields agricultural products. The operation of a cognitive system is a cognitive process" (Giere 2004: 771). The distributed cognition perspective radically changed the understanding of where cognition flows, but it also forced researchers and designers to rethink design and design settings in general (Hollan et al. 2000). While distributed cognition, as well as other cognitive perspectives and theories, seek to unveil the organising principles in cognitive systems, distributed cognition innovates as it defines cognition beyond the individual:

> Cognitive science has a long history of studying the relationship between individuals' internal organizations and their behaviors in terms of information processing properties of the central nervous system [...] Distributed cognition, by contrast, treats the activity system rather than the individual as the unit of cognitive analysis and considers the properties of this system that determine performance. (Hazlehurst et al. 2007: 540)

In a similar vein, the interaction analyst, Charles Goodwin, expands the cognitive locus to "situated activity systems that make up the lifeworld of a work group. Within such systems, human cognition is embedded not only in biology and linguistic structure, but also in history, culture, and the details of local, situated interaction" (Goodwin 2000b: 33). In all cases, interest falls on the cognitive system rather than the individual. A cognitive flow permeates brain and body in an environment and cannot be localised in a fixed space time. However, in particular cases, the boundaries of a cognitive system are not temporally or spatially predefined. For instance, distributed cognition emphasises that sometimes the individual is the right unit of analysis, sometimes it is too much, sometimes (and often) too little. The definition of the object of analysis is determined by a criterion of systemic function:

> A process is not cognitive simply because it happens in a brain, nor is a process noncognitive simply because it happens in the interaction among many brains. For example, we have found it productive to consider small sociotechnical systems such as the bridge of a ship [Hutchins, 1995a] or an airline cockpit [Hutchins 1995b; Hutchins and Klausen 1996; Hutchins and Palen 1997] as our unit of analysis. In distributed cognition, one expects to find a system that can dynamically configure itself to bring subsystems into coordination to accomplish various functions. A cognitive process is delimited by the functional relationships among the elements that participate in it, rather than by spatial colocation of elements. (Hollan et al. 2000: 175)

Thus, turning to the place where cognition flows is a process guided by a principle of function and not by boundaries of the body or the skull. In grouping them, distributed cognition demonstrated its particular theoretical traits and strengths when analysing human computer interaction. It has a focus on developing design and technological solutions that make possible flexible adaptive behaviour. Thus, with distributed cognition comes cognitive ethnography:

> Cognitive ethnography is a methodology developed specifically to explore distributed cognition (Ball and Ormerod 2000; Hutchins 2003). It allows researchers to explore how cognitive activity is distributed across social and material artifacts (people and objects that aid, enhance or impede cognition) as well as over time. A cognitive ethnography involves integrating data across observations, interviews

> and exploration of social and material artifacts. By conceptualizing material and social artifacts not only as aids to individual cognition, but also as integral elements of distributed cognitive activity, i.e. activity grounded in the interaction between individuals and their environment (Hutchins 1995a), a cognitive ethnography provides a process analysis of cognition as it is enacted in the real world. (Mylopoulos and Farhat 2014: 374)

Cognitive ethnography studies, therefore, focus on how activity systems achieve goals and manage decisions. Many distributed cognition studies have investigated the function of artefacts (Pedersen 2015; Pedersen and Steffensen 2014; Trasmundi 2019). Overall, they show how they serve as important cognitive aids, which over time may function in different ways depending on the situation. The abilities of the individual in a local situation are pivotal to how action is tied to external structures. The studies provide a rich body of information about how artefacts either constrain or facilitate cognition and how distribution of information enables individual cognitive offload as information is shared in an environmental observable structure, which is maintained with a minimum of cognitive effort. Cognitive ethnography is linked with the qualitative cognitive sciences and hence is different from traditional ethnography in a number of important ways. Traditional ethnography can be defined as:

> a particular method or set of methods which in its most characteristic form [...] involves the ethnographer participating overtly or covertly in people's daily lives for an extended period of time, watching what happens, listening to what is said, asking questions – in fact, collecting whatever data are available to throw light on the issues that are the focus of research. (Hammersley and Atkinson 1995: 1)

It is crucial to underline that sociologists and anthropologists define ethnography differently. Some equate it with almost any kind of study relying on participant observation while others argue that its characteristic features are its epistemological stance grounded in a socio-cultural paradigm (Hutchins 1995a). Ormerod and Ball (2017: 581) state:

> that no encompassing definition of ethnography exists that denotes a set of necessary and sufficient attributes. As such, ethnography may best be seen as a 'radial category' that involves a core 'prototype' –encompassing features such as situated and rich observation, openness, reflexivity, personalization, historicity, observational intensity and participant autonomy – as well as variations from this prototype.

Regardless of the different definitions the aim has been akin compared to ethnomethodologists. While traditional ethnographers are interested in how members of a group see society and construct their own perspective and reality through that particular vision, ethnomethodology is more attentive to how members *do* things, especially through language use (Seale 2012: 247). The ethnomethodological approach is concerned with the reality that people construct as well as the reality in which they are embedded. A cognitive ethnography is therefore different from traditional ethnography as it refers to how cognitive psychologists through observational fieldwork reveal how people coordinate their behaviour to achieve results. While this cognitive objective allows for investigations of rapid timescales, it also goes beyond descriptions of the member's perspective.

2.1 Beyond the representationalist view of distributed cognition: The role of interactivity

While distributed cognition has moved away from internal information processing, it maintains the representationalist view of cognition. The process *per se* is not changed; only the location of cognition is negotiable due to the task to be accomplished:

> In particular, we treat the 'propagation of representational state' through activity systems as explanatory of cognitive behaviour and investigate the organizing features of this propagation as explanation of system and human performance. A representational state is a particular configuration of an information-bearing structure, such as a monitor display, a verbal utterance, or a printed label, that plays some functional role in a process within a system.
>
> (Hazlehurst et al. 2007: 540)

However, at a basic level, an ecological paradigm embraces a phenomenon in its wholeness – that means as part of a larger system than that which appears in real time. Moreover, any individual is in direct relation with its environment, which means that the relation is not mediated by representations (Gibson 1979/86). Instead, action is a result of a relational, structural coupling between an individual and its environment (Maturana and Varela 1987; Baggs and Chemero 2018). An explanation of behaviour, therefore, requires an investigation of a system rather than of individual components within the system. From an ecological perspective, due to its emergent properties, a system is open and complex. Recently, Hutchins (2014) has refined his argument of an ecological take on cognition. He introduces the notion of cultural ecosystems to exhibit the non-local and supra-individual aspects of human cognition. He explicitly distinguishes distributed cognition from the extended mind hypothesis. He argues that, instead of the individual, distributed cognition takes a distributed cognitive system as the centre for cognition. In contrast, the extended mind hypothesis deals with a mid-level spatial scale for cognition in which the human being is always the centre of analysis. Moreover, the extended mind hypothesis distinguishes between extended cognitive processes and purely internal, mental cognitive processes. This is important as distributed cognition "is not a kind of cognition; it is a perspective on cognition [...] Distributed cognition begins with the assumptions that all instances of cognition *can be seen* as emerging from distributed processes" (Hutchins 2014: 36). This claim makes distributed cognition a perspective on cognition rather than a hypothesis of how cognition flows to the most economical place, which is Clark's focus (Clark 2008). Hutchins' proposal to treat distributed cognition as a perspective is aligned with Steffensen's concept of human interactivity (Steffensen 2013). Steffensen (2013) argues that at the core of human action, one finds sense-saturated coordination defined as interactivity:

> Defining interactivity as sense-saturated coordination that contributes to human action characterises three aspects of the relevant phenomena. First, coordination refers to a reciprocal flow of minuscule, pico-scale interbodily movements that link and lock human beings in self-organised systems. [...] Second, this coordination is sense-saturated, that is, it is pervaded by our species-specific capability for sense-making (Linell, 2009). We engage in sense-making as our bodies integrate present circumstances with autobiographic memories and sociocultural histories: through sense-making the not-here and the not-now saturate our here-and-now coordination. Third, sense-saturated coordination constrains what we do and how we do it. (Steffensen 2013: 197)

While interactivity has a primordial quality, to *explain* interactivity in all its complexity by single perspectives coming from distinct fields is to no avail. The framework presented in this chapter seeks to provide an ecological account for human interactivity by allowing multiple perspectives to capture different temporal dynamics in interaction. These perspectives are interdependent descriptions that inform each other in the analytical process such that non-local situations are understood in relation to the local and vice versa. Steffensen adds:

> Underlying each perspective, one finds interactivity: it is an ontological substrate that each discipline has turned into an 'object.' While all three perspectives [cognitivist, microsociological and biological] may yield descriptively adequate models within an epistemological domain [...] they cannot, in themselves, provide an explanatory model of interactivity, i.e. of what really happens in the flow of human existence. (Steffensen 2013: 196)

The interactivity-based perspective does not operate with a clear distinction between language and cognition. Rather, it prioritises what individuals actually *do* in real-life situations as they draw on experience and non-local constraints (Loaiza et al. forth; Thibault 2011; Love 2004). Following Cowley (2011), attention must be paid to how individuals orchestrate speech, thinking and gesture by turning to bodily dynamics *and* symbols (Cowley 2011; Rączaszek-Leonardi 2011). By viewing language as ecological, distributed (Cowley 2011; Love 2004; Thibault 2011; Steffensen 2011, 2013) and grounded in coordinating bodies, the synchronic system view on language must be rejected as too shallow (Cowley 2011). Preferably, language must be investigated as a diachronic, whole-bodied skill that enables action, perception and cognition in the here-and-now situation (Steffensen 2011; Cowley 2009; Loaiza et al. forth; Di Paolo et al. 2018). Language is not reducible to biology; nevertheless, it cannot be understood without its biological grounding. Additionally, human language is unique since it has "catapulted and stabilized human cognition in ways that are unequalled in the ecology of any other species. The human ecology is radically *extended*" (Steffensen 2011: 204). Trasmundi (2019) adds:

> An interactivity approach, therefore, requires that we turn to investigations of how people "find their way" (Thompson 2007) in the process of dealing with ideas, tasks, and obstacles in their lives, in this case during patient treatment. In order to understand how people are able to coordinate and align actions to achieve a certain task, Meyer et al. (2017) argue that we need to integrate the fast and microscopic perspective on unfolding events in time with a slower perspective on the sedimentation of habits and culture as well as the emergence of artifacts and methods. (Trasmundi 2019: 632)

While conventional approaches to human interaction and cognition have prioritised and simplified what appears to happen in real time and reduced it to few causal frames often fixated on one local timescale, recent trends pay attention to how lived experience are enacted in the here-and-now. By showing how language and cognition shape sense-saturated coordination over time, culture, norms and intentions can be dynamically linked with real-time perception and action. Embodied, ecological approaches to human coordination are gaining ground, and Meyer et al. (2017) have described the growing attention to the human as a "becoming person" as a paradigm shift in the language sciences. Meyer et al. (2017) describe how an embodied focus on human action demarcates the old view of language as a mental, abstract and synchronic phenomenon represented by Saussure's wired and disembodied 'talking heads' from a recent ecological view, which grounds language in embodied experience and gives room for intercorperal, fleshy, lively and dynamic models of human coordination. They propose to exchange Saussure's 'talking heads' with the more corporeal metaphor 'perceiving bodies', inspired by for instance Ruben's Baroque paintings of "*people's limbs and flesh entangled and pushing and pulling one another*" (Meyer et al. 2017: xviii). Meyer et al. (2017) further argue that intersubjectivity is the natural and immediate form of human existence because the human being, over time, becomes skilled in withdrawing and distancing oneself from others, and we can, in turn, experience ourselves as being decoupled, isolated beings who communicate individual intentions through verbal articulation. Solipsism, thus, biases our understanding of how our bodies are shaped by historical relationships with others. This fact makes an embodied approach to language epistemologically complex as we perceive utterances as words that translate our individual thinking. The remaining question is then: How can we investigate interactivity? How can we provide descriptions of the whole array of human coaction spanning from its enabling conditions to how it is managed and how it causes cognitive results? An investigation of such ranges allows for a multi-scalar view on local interaction and cognition conducive to the notion of timescales and temporal ranges (Uryu et al. 2014, Steffensen and Pedersen 2014; Pedersen and Steffensen 2014), which will be elaborated in detail below. If we choose understanding human interactivity, we cannot escape the notion of timescales:

> There simply is no single time scale of an ecological phenomenon. [...] Acknowledging that such ecological phenomenon as brain activity [...] cognitive performance, human conversations, and social practices all and each unfold on multiple time scales, we need a model that does not reduce time scales to a tiered hierarchy of duration. (Steffensen and Pedersen 2014: 87)

Steffensen and Pedersen (2014) argue that time is a phenomenon, which relies on emergent dynamics of human systems. *Lived time* of ecological, living systems is governed by complex and multiple causal frames (Enfield 2014), which relate to biology, cultural narratives, purposive behaviour and situated awareness (Steffensen and Pedersen 2014). An ecological paradigm emphasises the systemic features of human coaction, which was claimed in Chapter 1. It thus changes the focus from social interaction to human interactivity as a mode of social and ecological cognition that flows as inter-bodily dynamics on multiple timescales (Kirsh 1997). Because ecological systems are governed by multiple causal frames, external criteria (specific research questions within a specific scientific domain such as geological change or human interaction) help define, which *temporal ranges* should be investigated further (Loaiza et al. forth). A temporal range is defined as a "limited range of time scales within which self-similarity appears" (Steffensen and Pedersen 2014: 87). Thus, in the study of human interaction and cognition, it makes sense to focus on the temporal range of a dialogical system encompassing conversational timescales, inter-bodily timescales and event timescales. However, as individuals recruit sociocultural resources, enabling conditions for local sense-making is complex and multi-scalar. Thus, an awful lot more can happen in a situation than a conversational timescale explains. Because human beings are time rangers (Pedersen and Steffensen 2014, 95, (Loaiza et al. forth) they know how to recalibrate dialogical systems and achieve relative stability in the organism-environment system, which they are part of. This view is what is pursued in the investigation of how healthcare professionals manage complex events. With the method of Cognitive Event Analysis (see Chapter 3), focus is on how such recalibrations are managed, that is, how disturbances, fixations and other constraints on action affect functional coordination. It is hypothesised that such moments, when a system experiences boundary constraints, reveal much about how sociocultural timescales and embodied, situated activity co-direct action in the context of what happens.

2.1.1 *Methodological challenges when studying authentic ecologies of emergency medicine*

As Hutchins reveals in the chapter's initial quote, studying cognition "in the wild" is difficult. Observation of multiple gradations are needed to account for interactivity, or in other terms, the distributed processes involving the complex pool of what people say, do, think, feel, accomplish, etc. But few studies have paid attention to the cognitive dynamics of decision-making, problem-solving or sense-making as those processes traditionally have been regarded as private, inner, mental states, which cannot be observed in real-life settings. Automation, for instance, is generally regarded as intrinsic dynamics of expertise and is linked to, let alone described with, the concept of recognition-primed retrieval (Klein 1998; Kahneman and Klein 2009) in situations involving cognitive task performances such as medical decision-making. However, with *state of the art* cognitive science, cognition is – as mentioned above – distributed, observable and grounded in natural actions of behavioural coordination (Hutchins 2014; De Jaegher 2007). Following Hutchins' suggestion, grounding cognitive research in the domain of natural, real-life, cognitive events makes one immediately aware of the methodological challenges that follow such a decision. To exchange the laboratory setting for a natural habitat of a sociocultural practice entails considerable repercussions for how the research design should be framed (Hutchins 1995a). It invites more ecological and ethnographic research forms that favour non-experimental, though resource demanding, research designs (Streeck et al. 2011). While experimental designs are driven by hypotheses, they cause the researcher to suppose *a*) what the problem is, *b*) how it can be identified, *c*) which variables are needed to test specific cognitive abilities and *d*) how experimental results contribute to an understanding of how people solve problems in real-life situations. While experimental research carried out in laboratories has other strengths (strictly-controlled and demarcated tests and measurements), they obviously tell different things about a given phenomenon, *or* they investigate different kinds of cognitive processes that leave out the coordinative dynamics involved in cognition:

> the conventional approach in which perception, decision making, and action are treated as functionally distinct elements within the closed-loop system will not be appropriate to the study of coordination. This conclusion is supported by recent work in naturalistic decision making. This research has indicated that the decision making of experts in natural environments is intimately linked to perception (or recognitional processes) and that laboratory research in which decision making is uncoupled from perception has little value for predicting performance in these natural settings. (Flach 1999: 122)

Laboratory studies using experimental approaches based on quantitative measurements are limited to investigate "cognitive processes that extend over long periods of time (days, weeks or months), as arises in tasks associated with professional design or scientific exploration" (Ormerod and Ball 2017: 575). Unlike the decontextualised approaches, ecological, contextualised and grounded methods – as ethnography – grasp the situated dynamics in a cognitive system (Hutchins 1995a; Hammersley and Atkinson 1983). Traditionally, those methods have been the preserve of anthropologists and sociologists, and this renders them sensitive to the aims of exploring knowledge used in particular social practices. In this view, it can be argued: "that just as ethnographers typically seek to demonstrate a key theme from different "views", so too do cognitive psychologists need to provide accounts of cognitive activity based on both de-contextualized and contextualized methods and the converging evidence they afford" (Ormerod and Ball 2017: 577).

The cognitive ethnographic fieldwork underlying this study, involves a combination of methods ranging from observational research such as video and participant observation as well as observing material culture over time and collecting qualitative interviews (Seale 2012: 163). The design allows for a dual focus on both the micro and macro scale of interactivity in the medical settings as well as a registration of an experienced and observed level of behaviour and sense-making. The overall focus of the study is on the micro-timescale that includes what happens in real time by the use of video observation. Thus, on a micro-scale it investigates how professionals accomplish cognitive results and especially how fluid medical teams integrate skills in interaction, cognition and teamwork. On a macro-scale it investigates how the structural and cultural organisation of these teams influence cognitive output. Both dimensions are designed to use cognitive ethnographic fieldwork (Hutchins and Nomura 2011) in generating a *thick description* (Geertz 1973) or investigation of what happens in the light of the overall cognitive ecology (Hutchins 2014) and the organisational culture of the ward (cf. Chapter 7, Section 3).

While cognitive ethnography reveals how people coordinate their behaviour to get results, it links with an ecological cognitive science that aspires "to understand how organisms make their way in the world" (Reed 1996: 11). Specifically,

Reed (1996: 184) states: "From an ecological approach, psychology must take an animal's encounters with its surroundings as the fundamental phenomenon to be explained". To observe how people make their way in the world requires an intentional interest into how they adapt flexibly to changes in their environment relations. Crucially, cognitive ethnography is especially well-suited for pursuing a *naturalised* view on what happens, providing accounts of coordination that go beyond the ethnomethodologists' focus on the "member's perspective" (Ormerod and Ball 2017). Cognitive ethnography fits the interactivity-perspective as it allows for studies of how human beings make their way in various situations. The framework allows for the generation of multiple data with a focus on cognitive and coordinative behaviour over time.

While there are many views of embodied cognition that are more or less radical in their assumptions (Wilson and Golonka 2013), it is clear that emerging support for the notion necessitates methodologies amenable to studying situated interactions as people engage in high-level cognition in real-world activities (Ormerod and Ball 2017). Investigations of multiple timescales in interaction require methods for treating data that are yet to be qualified in a coherent analytical model. One promising model is, as mentioned above, the Cognitive Event Analysis. This model will be presented below.

2.2 Cognitive Event Analysis (CEA)

CEA emerged from a need to grasp human interactivity and sense-making as ecological and multi-scalar. Its theoretical roots are thus grounded in the ecological and dialogical framework described above (Steffensen 2013). That means that sense-making is investigated as coordination between agent(s) and an environment extended in time and space. CEA thus extends its unit of analysis to the organism environment system (Järvilehto 1998, 2009) and guides attention to the multi-scalarity of interaction (Steffensen 2013; Steffensen et al. 2016; Steffensen and Pedersen 2014; Pedersen and Steffensen 2014; Cowley 2014a; Trasmundi 2016). At its core, CEA is an ecological method, which investigates how distributed cognitive systems (Giere 2004; Hollan et al. 2000) achieve results as they rely on real-time dynamics and non-local conditions for coordination (Steffensen et al. 2016; Steffensen 2013; Cowley 2014a; Trasmundi 2016; Trasmundi and Linell 2017; Trasmundi and Steffensen 2016; Trasmundi and Harvey 2018). In practical terms, a distributed cognitive system includes all components that contribute to cognitive processes and results, including people (self and others), material artefacts, environmental structures, cultural conditions, rules etc. As a result the achievements of human actions, which enable the individuals to manipulate the ecological setting in accordance with a particular goal.

Theoretically, CEA builds on insights from ecological psychology (Gibson 1979/86), distributed language (Cowley 2011; Love 2004) and distributed cognition (Hutchins 1995a; Hollan et al. 2000). The method is grounded in the humanities and builds on an ecological perspective to human interaction and cognition, which favours a microscopic focus on inter-bodily dynamics, for instance, prosody (inspired by work of Cowley (1998)), gesture and movement (inspired by work of Goodwin (1994, 2000a, 2002, 2007, and Gibson (1979/86)). CEA therefore finds its starting point in local coordination of flexible, adaptive behaviour within a distributed cognitive system. When such behaviour is constrained in ways that inhibit progression within the system, it relates to what Anderson (2014) defines as the main cognitive problem of human behaviour, namely, deciding "what to do next" (Anderson 2014: 135). Drawbacks emerge when immediate solutions to what to do next are suspended, requiring recalibration of the cognitive system (Steffensen et al. 2016). In my data, it is relevant to zoom in on events that are characterised by stress and constrained possibilities for action, for instance in situations where the unexpected happens. In that respect, CEA is useful. For instance, in a recent study (Steffensen et al. 2016), it is demonstrated how the method is apt for scrutinising the very specific problem space around an interruption of fluent action perception cycles to explain how individuals overcome the *suspended nexts*. Automatised action perception cycles are based on experience and they work until interruptions, fixations and suspended nexts force the agent to think and act differently. Many cognitive resources are allocated to testing new solutions because the process lacks a known trajectory and useful experience, which can be enacted *in situ*. Already in 1910 the philosopher John Dewey defined such suspended nexts as *forkedroad situations* and as the core conditions for reflective thinking:

> Thinking begins with in what may fairly enough be called a forkedroad situation, a situation which is ambiguous, which presents a dilemma, which proposes alternatives. As long as our activity glides smoothly along from one thing to another, or as long as we permit our imagination to entertain fancies at pleasure, there is no call for reflection. Difficulty or obstruction in the way of reaching a belief brings us, however, to a pause. [...] Demand for the solution of a perplexity is the steadying and guiding factor in the entire process of reflection. Where there is no question of a problem to be solved or a difficulty to be surmounted, the course of suggestions flows on at random [...] Thinking is not a case of spontaneous combustion; it does not occur on "general principles." There is something specific which occasions and evokes it. [...] Reflective thinking, in short, means judgement suspended during further inquiry; and suspense is likely to be somewhat painful. (Dewey 1910: 11ff.)

When automaticity and habits are uncertain in a particular situation, a breakdown or a disturbance appears to individual(s) within the system and makes them think differently because the activity-system experiences (painful) constraints. When a flow is disrupted, an agent will look for a fixed viewpoint from which one can see new solutions and connections (Dewey 1910). Moreover, a *forkedroad situation* affords a separation of processes into meaningful categories. According to Dewey, this is analogous to Heidegger's hammer example, in which it is argued that we only experience a hammer *as* a hammer in the moment the system becomes dysfunctional: when the hammer breaks, hits your finger or something else changes the flow within the system (cf. Dewey 1910).

In a somewhat similar vein, Steffensen (2013) highlights that what agents tend to do in such situations can be described as action perception cycles of solution-probing activities rather than modelling of inner mental representations. At an empirical, analytical level, CEA explores such cognitive trajectories of cognitive systems. A trajectory is a dynamical activity path that emerges as agents move through a problem space towards a cognitive result (Steffensen et al. 2016). The visual outlook of a CEA trajectory is shown below in Figure 2.1 before it is elaborated further.

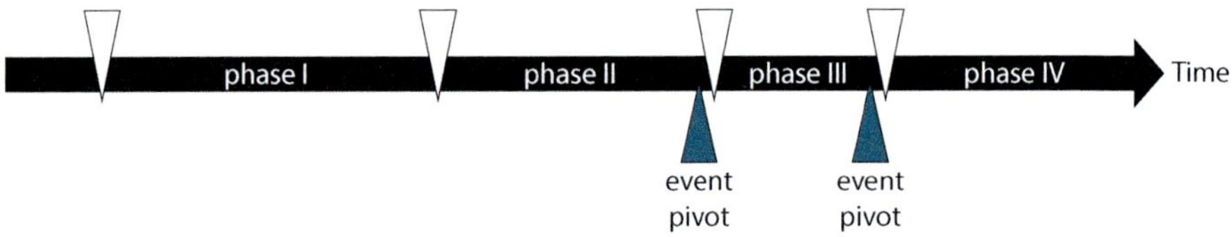

Figure 2.1 CEA – Event trajectory inspired by Steffensen et al. (2016)

Transition points (the white triangles in Figure 2.1) define an interactivity path, which can be characterised as an event. An event covers a change that emerges in the relation between agent and environment. Within the change process, multiple transition points emerge, but often just one or few points are "pivotal for making this event happen. Such transition points are in CEA termed *event pivots* (Steffensen 2013: 201). An event pivot (the blue triangles in Figure 2.1) is thus functionally defined as a transition point, which is a *conditio sine qua non* for identifying a segment of a cognitive trajectory as a specific (kind of) event" (Steffensen et al. 2016: 82). The methodological procedure of CEA consists of five steps based on video recordings (Steffensen 2013; Steffensen et al. 2016). The steps are visualised in Table 2.1 below:

Table 2.1 Five steps of a Cognitive Event Analysis (Steffensen et al. 2016)

Procedure	Description
Cognitive Event Identification	Identification of a cognitive event, typically an organism-initiated change in the layout of affordances in the organism environment system, in a video record of a naturalistic or experimental data set. The event may be defined from an observer's or a participant's point of view
Event Pivot Identification	Identification of the critical transition point (or "phase transition") without which the cognitive event would not be an event
Data Annotation	Segmentation and annotation of (peri-pivotal) video sequence, using multiple (hierarchical or coordinated) tiers, with or without a constrained set of annotation values
Cognitive Trajectory Segmentation	Segmentation of video sequence into *functionally* and/or *behaviourally* defined phases
Cognitive Trajectory Analysis	Analysis of how specific segments of the cognitive trajectory (particularly the event pivot) are enabled by preceding segment and behavioural tendencies

While CEA allows for detailed investigations of local problem-solving, its analytical focus remains on the microscopic dynamics of human interactivity. The bio-cognitive dynamics that are scrutinised emerge as changes in an overall cognitive system. While such changes may not necessarily be experienced as changes for the participants, they are important for the understanding of how errors are encountered and can be managed successfully both in the local situation and in future situations (cf. Chapter 7, Section 3).

By drawing attention to other causal frames in local interaction, the stabilised, conventionalised and socially coordinated behaviours that emerge on slower timescales can support analyses of how and why practitioners manage problems as they do: For instance, how do they avoid getting overwhelmed, how do they cope with the unexpected, and what enables them to see new solutions or what prompts them to get out of a fixation bias? While these questions can be dealt with on various timescales, no single timescale allows for a comprehensive answer. CEA focuses on how disturbances, fixations and other constraints on action affect functional coordination in the here-and-now. CEA-style investigations of the dynamical coordination go beyond the enchronic scale of interaction. It thus allows an integration of such investigations with theoretical perspectives on human cognitive, emotional and linguistic capabilities for action, as well as with the moral obligations that prompt us to engage in certain behaviours rather than in others. However, CEA does not equip us with a comprehensive basis for answering, say, *why* a patient interruption prompts practitioners to either ignore or respond to the comment. CEA cannot explain what constitutes enabling conditions, but it can point to them as conditions for sense-making, which leads to results. Arguably, a method for investigating how human beings animate dialogical systems in order to achieve results is not only valuable for interaction analysts and cognitive psychologists. Sociologists, anthropologists and other social scientists may also benefit from methods that allow them to study the texture of the interface between human agents and their environment (Trasmundi and Steffensen 2016) While CEA enables investigations of human interactivity in organisational settings, it is the main analytical method used in the analysis. This analytical method constitutes the second part of the book.

PART II

Behind the scenes

Welcome to the emergency ward

There is a common misconception among cognitive scientists, especially those who do their work in laboratory settings, that research conducted outside the laboratory is necessarily "applied" work. I will argue in what follows that there are many excellent reasons to look at the "real world" that are not concerned with hoped-for applications of the research findings [...]. Pure research on the nature of real cognitive practices is needed. - Edwin Hutchins (1995a: xiii-xiv)

CHAPTER 3

Presenting the case of the emergency ward

1. Stepping into the emergency ward

An emergency ward is a medical treatment unit which specialises in acute care and treatment of patients who arrive often by the means of an ambulance and without any prior appointment. Due to the unknown patient flow as well as the patients' medical histories, the work environment is often stressful and highly unpredictable. Often, decisions must be reached immediately and on insufficient grounds, which can lead to human errors. While the chaotic, dynamic work environment provides the healthcare practitioners with various work conditions, work performances often reflect such challenges, for instance through stressful communications and hurried procedure-following.

The analyses presented in this second part of the book are based on a dataset from such an emergency ward. Specifically, the dataset derives from a large cognitive, video-ethnographic study conducted by Pedersen (2015) over a three-month period. It was carried out in collaboration with the emergency ward at a Danish hospital (Køge Hospital).[1] The main corpus of data consists of a large set of video-recordings of diagnostic events, fieldnotes, and interviews with healthcare practitioners.[2]

1. This volume is a result of an independent research project established in cooperation with the emergency ward at Køge Hospital. The Department of emergency medicine at Køge Hospital receives 47,000 patients annually, of which 30,000 are treated for minor casualties (small burns, strains etc.) and then discharged. Of the remaining 17,000 patients, 2,000 are high-emergency cases that demand treatment by a multi-disciplinary emergency team, a resuscitation team or a trauma team. For ethical reasons, trauma cases are excluded from the project. Small teams of 1–2 doctors and 1–2 nurses treat the remaining 15,000 patients; these patients are triaged, given an initial treatment, and referred to further treatment, either at home, in a specific specialist ward or in the ward's observation beds.

2. Specifically, 17 diagnostic treatment situations were video-recorded with up to three cameras. One of the cameras was handheld to cover blind angles or zoom in on specific aspects. I video-recorded alternately at two wards: a sub-emergency and an acute emergency ward. A 70 pages long research protocol that covered relevant practical, ethical and legal aspects of the project as well as relevant documents, e.g. documents concerning written consent, and information

1.2 Coding, visualisation and data presentation

A few comments on the data selection are made prior to the analyses. The overall coding process was an iterative process that uses a two-phased inductive approach, only framed by an external criterion of function in relation to work tasks: how cognitive events are managed in relation to the overall task. Based on this initial coding process, six themes were identified and chosen for further investigations (a) medical visual systems, (b) interruptions, (c) diagnostic procedures, (d) medical cultural dynamics, (e) sense-making in teams and (f) writing the electronic medical record.[3] Each chapter in this second part of the book thus focuses on a thematic aspect related to the systemic function of cognition and, at an overall level, the analytical chapters contribute to the overall interest in understanding the emergence and conditions for human errors and contributions. That is, each chapter investigates the diversity of enabling conditions in the interactive social ecology of human errors and contributions in emergency medicine.

The analysis primarily uses video-data to examine the real-time dynamics of medical cognition. The rich corpus of audio-visual data needs to be transformed into meaningful representations on paper. As the analysis deals with events played out on very rapid timescales, transcriptions of verbal utterances require a detailed and well-developed transcription method that accounts for the various dynamics in verbal utterances. This project applies the transcription system developed by Gail Jefferson for the analysis of conversation (Jefferson 1983, 1985, 2005). Some basic elements from the transcription system that are used are shown in Table 3.1 below.

In the transcriptions as well as in the figures, *D* and *P* are abbreviations for *doctor* and *patient*, respectively. Inspired by Streeck (2010) and Goodwin (2014, 2018), amongst others, I apply edited pictures of the participants in the text to visualise embodiments in action. Non-verbal utterances are either visualised by pictures inserted in the text document or they are marked in the transcription followed by an explanation in a footnote. The major challenge is to visualise movements and the dynamical flow of small-scale changes. However, for lack of anything better, a gallery of static representations is used to indicate such rapid changes, and they are often supported by markings, verbal explanations etc.

Different software programs were used to edit, annotate and present the data. All pictures are edited in Photoshop. The editing includes (a) blurring of the practitioners' and patients' faces (due to ethical and legal concerns), (b) the use of arrows to indicate gaze and movements and (c) other visual markers to direct

papers to all involved participants, were worked out. The data made public are anonymised and all patient and practitioner identifiers are removed.

3. See Pedersen (2015) for at detailed description of the exact coding process.

Table 3.1 Transcription system

Transcription system	
CAPITAL LETTERS	Indicate remarkable loudness of verbal utterances
Degree signs around a word, e.g. °hi°	Illustrate verbal utterances articulated in a special low volume (tone of voice)
Left square bracket [	Illustrates the onset of overlapping verbal utterances
Numbers in closed parentheses (1.2)	Specify the length of silence in seconds and tenths of seconds
(.)	Micro pause (<0.2 seconds)
=	Latched talk/rush through
Underlined words or sounds	Indicate if utterances are articulated with a special prosodic emphasis.
Ascending or descending arrows ↑ ↓	Illustrate rising or falling local intonation
Pro:::longation	Indicates prolongation of preceding sound
.	Stopping fall in tone
.hh	Hearable in-breath
hh	Hearable out-breath
(xxx)	Non-audible speech
(laugh)	Non-verbal utterances
[comment]	Transcriber's comment

attention to a specific element in the picture. The annotation tool ELAN is used to annotate multiple and simultaneous dynamics in interactivity.[4] Before a task is investigated in detail, data is imported into the programme that allows for precise annotation of simultaneous actions including verbal and non-verbal actions such as: gaze, gesture, body movement, verbal utterance, activity type and interruptions as the most common tiers. The ELAN annotation tool enhances the analysis process and ensures exact measurements of multiple, overlapping actions in time, for instance a team's gestures and gaze orientation during verbal utterances.

After the annotation process, relevant events from the interactivity trajectory were chosen for further analyses primarily by the use of CEA. As mentioned above, CEA operates with an event trajectory that illuminates relevant event pivots. The layout of CEA is adopted in the analyses (see Steffensen et al. 2016; Steffensen

4. ELAN is a professional annotation tool developed by researchers at the Max Planck Institute for Psycholinguistics, The Language Archive, Nijmegen, The Netherlands. It is developed for the creation of complex annotations on visual data (Sloetjes and Wittenburg 2008).

2013). In one case (see Chapter 8, Section 2), the computer software Praat,[5] which was invented for analysis of speech in phonetics, was used to annotate the exact measurement of vocal pitch attractors. These measurements are visualised in the text with the aid of Praat tools.

5. The software was designed by Paul Boersma and David Weenink, University of Amsterdam. For an introduction to Praat, see: praat.org January 15, 2019.

CHAPTER 4

Medical errors and visual perception

1. The hypothesis of visual perception[1]

Reaching a diagnosis is the overarching shared goal at the emergency ward. How this is done depends on multiple factors such as the practitioners' abilities to relate symptoms to causes, interpret patients' narratives, and connect experience and knowledge to real-time occurrences. How these processes unfold is especially interesting when challenges emerge and creative strategies must replace the usual procedures. In the dataset, there is a striking difference in the way practitioners handle the diagnostic process when faced with challenges. Indeed, their actions do not indicate that their perceptions rely on objective representations. Rather, they tend to imply situated initiatives based on direct perception (Gibson 1979/86; Noë 2004). The chapter is based on the hypothesis that perception does not only depend "on the eyes in the head on a body supported by the ground" (Gibson 1979/86: 1) but just as much on sociocultural constraints, individual experience and local dynamics, which makes perception a result of a sense-saturated visual system. Furthermore, if perception is sense-saturated and depends on local and non-local coordination, different people use different strategies in order to achieve the same output. If this hypothesis is supported, it has educational consequences for how practitioners are trained. The complexity that follows such a view leads to a deeper investigation of a practitioner's level of expertise in relation to environmental affordances for proper action. In the light of this, designing medical materials or focusing on an individual's knowledge level, only deals with part of the cognitive ecology of medical problem-solving.

Working from this hypothesis I investigate three cases from the dataset that all share some core features and also represent different degrees of constraining elements in the process of diagnosing. Common to all three cases is the emergence of local constraints that force the practitioner to perceive and act on changes in the layout of affordances (Gibson 1979/86; Chemero 2000, 2003). The way the

1. Sections 4.1–4.3.3 were originally published as "Temporal Dynamics in Medical Visual Systems" in *Cybernetics & Human Knowing*, 21, 2014. It is republished here with the permission of Cybernetics & Human Knowing: http://chkjournal.com/about and the co-author, Sune Vork Steffensen.

practitioners adapt to the changes is related to feedback mechanisms and error cycles. The cases differ with respect to types of constraints, the medical and clinical situation and the level of expertise amongst the healthcare staff.

Generally, the chapter investigates how medical practitioners make use of a visual system that goes beyond local and individual interaction. It underlines how medical decision-making is determined by local dynamics, sociocultural patterns and individual experience. It argues that explanations of human interactivity cannot be confined to only the social timescale, e.g. Enfield's enchronic timescale (Enfield 2014). I exemplify this by investigating three cases from emergency medicine where problem finding and problem-solving are related specifically to vision. The focal point of the investigations is on how problem finding and problem-solving are constrained by a medical visual system. The function of a visual system is directly related to the conditions of error cycles, which will be demonstrated in the analyses and discussed in the conclusion of this chapter.

The first case emphasises (a) that the novice doctor prioritises a sociocultural timescale, which furnishes her with retrospective information, over the real-time timescale of local interaction, which *ceteris paribus* could have contributed with valuable knowledge, (b) that cultural artefacts in the medical arena, which are themselves material products of past sociocultural events, can both facilitate and obstruct conducive cognitive processes, and (c) that medical novices during their education have acquired a deep, specialised knowledge of medical procedures and categorisation via medical textbooks and classes. However, in real-life medical encounters, such abstract knowledge may be at odds with the experiences and aspirations of the interlocutors at the peril of a dialogical medical practice.

The second case describes how an experienced doctor and his medical team mould the optic array as he draws on interactivity. The sense-saturatedness allows for an immediate and intentional, but at the same time automatic locomotion that serves as a positive feedback mechanism in the interactivity trajectory. The team's anticipatory actions feed back on the latent conditions for errors in a functional way. Finally, the third case demonstrates an element of learning as a doctor seeks to perceive new possibilities by moving, probing and manipulating the problem space within the environment. Before I present the cases, I discuss how the ecological approach to visual perception is related to the hypothesis and the analytical methods used in the analyses.

2. Distributed visual systems: What makes human perception special

When doctors act in a medical environment, they depend on vision, i.e., what and how one sees, feels and perceives in action. With Gibson I reject the hypothesis that we perceive the environment with our eyes: "We are told that vision depends on the eye, which is connected to the brain. I shall suggest that natural vision depends on the eyes in the head on a body supported by the ground, the brain being only the central organ of a complete visual system" (Gibson 1979/86: 1). Seeing is a distributed activity that requires a whole visual system to work (Gibson 1979/86; Noë 2004). Gibson's approach has proven itself useful and it has intrigued many scholars by arguing against mental representation as the key to understanding visual perception. However, Gibson's objective was to show the automaticity of real-time action-perception-cycles of an organism-environment system (Järvilehto 1998, 2009) constituted by both the embodied effectivities of the organism and the functional affordances of the environment (Gibson 1979/86: 36). Gibson did not seek to explain the historicity of perception, nor its symbolic or cultural aspects. Rather, he focused merely on the timescale of real-life perception:

> Human observers cannot perceive the erosion of a mountain, but they can detect the fall of a rock. They can notice the displacement of a chair in a room but not the shift of an electron in an atom. [...] emphasis will be placed on events, cycles and changes at the terrestrial level of the physical world. The changes we shall study are those that occur in the environment. (Gibson 1979/86: 12)

Gibson's approach to perception expanded the perceptual system in space but not in time. Gibson derives his explanatory power from what happens in an animal's physical encounter with the physical environment. Contrary to this local time view on perception, Goodwin (1994, 2002, 2003, 2007) scrutinises the sociological aspect of how the environment affords various perceptions amongst different groups of people. For instance, he links situated cognition of professionals to processes of classification that guide relevant action-perception cycles to achieve a successful outcome in real-time. In the following statement he exemplifies this line of thought by describing how archaeologists use coding schemes to provide equivalent observations in a way that literally transform nature into culture:

> by using such a system a worker views the world from the perspective it establishes. Of all the possible ways that the earth could be looked at, the perceptual work of students using this form is focused on determining the exact color of a minute sample of dirt. They engage in active cognitive work, but the parameters of that work have been established by the system that is organizing their perception. In so far as the coding scheme establishes an orientation toward the world, it constitutes a structure of intentionality whose proper locus is not the isolated, Cartesian mind, but a much larger organizational system. (Goodwin 1994: 609)

When repetitive interaction sculptures categorical patterns and forms over time, they provide the interlocutors with a *professional vision* (Goodwin 1994), an expert view that is often materialised into "objects of knowledge that become the insignia of a profession's craft: the theories, artefacts and bodies of expertise that are its special and distinctive domain of competence" (Goodwin 1994: 606). In the following analysis, it is underlined how human perception stems from cultural knowledge and real-time flexible, adaptive behaviour. Relating Goodwin's term 'professional vision' to Gibson's 'visual system', I account for how perception is embedded in an extended space-time. In other words, a distributed visual system defines the ecological array of enabling conditions for perception. Hence, what a doctor sees, feels and perceives is both socially pre-organised through material-cultural artefacts and the implementation of procedures and narratives, and it is dynamical, anticipative and situated.

3. Case 1: Temporal dynamics and visual perception

3.1 The distributed patient

The interlocutors in the first case are a novice, female doctor and an alcoholic, male patient. The patient's GP has sent him to the hospital primarily because of his yellow eyes, which is an indication of a hepatic disease. He is lying in a bed facing the doctor, who is seated right beside him. In her hands she holds the patient's medical record. See Figure 4.1 for an overview of the layout.

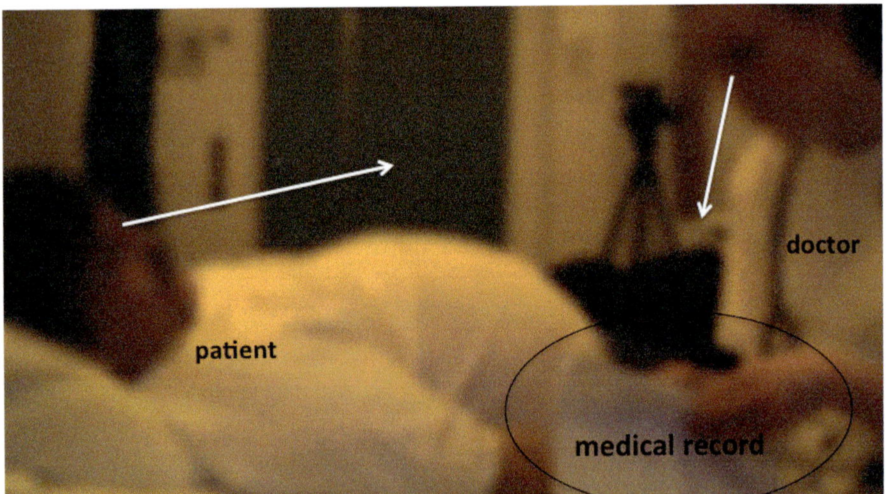

Figure 4.1 Overview of the layout: Visual attention

As we enter the conversation, the doctor has just examined the patient, and next she asks the patient what colour his faeces have been over the last few days. This is important because it gives a further indication of the functionality and condition of the liver. In this case, I scrutinise how they relate to the topic of his faeces.

As stated, the doctor is holding the patient's medical record in her hands. In the record, she has information about the patient's history, partly from the GP, partly from previous encounters at the hospital. As she starts interrogating the patient on his faeces, a problem of clarification emerges, because the patient does not confirm what the medical record says:

Transcript 4.1[2]
Danish original

1. D: dels så har du: fortalt at du har noget hvid afføring (.) o:g (0.1)
2. P: noget hvad
3. D: =NEJ (0.3) nu skal jeg lige se igen (.) noget SORT afføring (0.3)
4. P: nå:rh jamen han spurgte hvad farve det var og så siger jeg det er både den ene og den anden
5. D: jamen for det er både hvidt og sort >indimellem er det BLEG- eller blegt< ↑ ik
6. ps: (1.0)
7. P: °°jo[h altså ø:h°°
8. D: [det er det
9. Ps (1.6)
10. P: jeg har som regel altid tynd mave men altså:
11. D: ↓mm
12. P: el lidt tynd mave ik (0.2) men øh
13. D: har du afføring hver dag
14. P: jah
15. ps: (1.6)
16. D: og de:t okay
17. ps: (0.5)
18. D: men ha- d ka det være °sån b bleg° nogen gange
19. ps: (0.5)
20. P: °nej blegt° altså hvad mener du (0.3)
21. D: jamen det de:t er nemlig os t (.) et tegn på at man kan være noget galt med leveren eller galde(.)bl[æren
22. P: [ja
23. ps: (0.5)
24. P: altså de[t er ik øhh der er ikke øh hvidt eller uden farve eller↓
25. D: [eller er det mig der husker forkert
26. D: ↓mm men det kan være sort nogen gange (0.3)
27. P: ja:eh så er det det mørkere mere eller mindre altså det ka så [normalt er det sådan mørkegult ik (.) eller jeg ved ik hva (0.2) [hva det er normalt at

2. When the text is marked in grey, it indicates that the doctor gazes in the clinical record. Otherwise, she looks at the patient.

være
28. D: [↓mm
[mm
29. D: MØRKEGULT (0.2)
30. P: altså sådan gulligt eller j[a
31. D: [ja okay
32. P: altså
33. ps: (0.6)
34. D: så det vil sige lidt blegere
35. ps: (0.8)
36. P: phh[h
37. D: [eller kitfarvet (.) sådan lerfarvet måske
38. ps: (1.0)
39. P: °°nja°° (.) [hvis det sku-
40. D: [?fedtet
41. ps: (1.0)
42. P: <u>det</u> tror jeg ik (0.2)
43. D: nej okay (.) det er ps de:t er øh lidt (.) underligt din læge har skrevet det her det må jeg ærligt indrømme det (xxx) aldrig hørt [før

English translation

1. D: and then you: have told that you have some white faeces (.) a:nd (0.1)
2. P: some what
3. D: =NO (0.3) let me see again (.) some BLACK faeces (0.3)
4. P: oh yes but that is he asked what colour it was and then I say it is both the one and the other
5. D: well because it is both white and black >sometimes it is PALE- or pale< ↑right
6. Ps: (1.0)
7. P: °°we[ll that i:s°°
8. D: [that is
9. Ps (1.6)
10. P: usually I have diarrhoea but ehm:
11. D: ↓mm
12. P: or a <u>bit</u> diarrhoea right (0.2) but ehm
13. D: do you have faeces every day
14. P: yes
15. ps: (1.6)
16. D: and tha:t okay
17. ps: (0.5)
18. D: but ha- d can it be °kind of p pale° sometimes
19. ps: (0.5)
20. P: °no pale° well what do you mean (0.3)
21. D: well it i:t is actually also s (.) a sign of that one can have that

something can be wrong with the liver and the gall(.)blad[der
22. P: [yes
23. ps: (0.5)
24. P: well i[t is not ehh it is not eh white or without colour or↓
25. D: [or do I remember it wrong
26. D: ↓mm but it can be black sometimes (0.3)
27. P: we:ll then it is a bit darker more or less well it can then [normally it is kind of dark yellow right (.) or I do not know [what (0.2) what is normal
28. D: [↓mm
[mm
29. D: DARK YELLOW (0.2)
30. P: well kind of yellowish or y[es
31. D: [yes okay
32. P: well
33. ps: (0.6)
34. D: so that is a bit paler
35. Ps: (0.8)
36. P: phh[h
37. D: [or kit coloured (.) kind of clay coloured maybe
38. Ps: (1.0)
39. P: °°no°° (.) [if it shou-
40. D: [?sticky
41. ps: (1.0)
42. P: I don't think so (0.2)
43. D: no okay (.) that is ps tha:t is eh a little (.) strange your doctor has written this I must admit that (xxx) [never heard of [before

In line 1, the doctor starts to summarise what she presumes the patient has told his GP. At the same time she creates an interaction with three interlocutors: herself, the present, hospitalised patient and a version of the patient that I term the distributed patient. Clark (2008) introduces the term *surrogate situations* to explain how real-world structures often are used to stand in for a potential or possible real event that serves as the decisive object of a certain cognitive undertaking (Clark 2008: 152–154). Inspired by this creative coupling, I use the term *distributed patient* to indicate how the doctor uses real-world structures as stand in for the present, local patient. The distributed patient represents the present living patient in the format of numbers and words in the medical record. Together, they indicate that a patient is a complex subject, a distributed person, consisting of many versions (numbers, narratives, symptoms etc.) brought forth at relevant times in interaction. The creation of the distributed patient is indicated in the linguistic construction of a second utterance as well as by the doctor's physical orientation within the distributed cognitive system. See Figure 4.2 below. In line 1, the doctor utters *you have told* as she gazes directly at the patient. Right after she introduces the distributed patient by saying that *you have some white faeces* as she simultaneously gazes in the record. The two deictics, in line 1, refer to two parties: the real patient and the distributed patient, respectively. The doctor subsequently turns to the real patient to see how he reacts. When the patient objects in line 2, *some <u>what</u>*, the doctor re-orients herself towards the narrative in the record *=NO let me see again* (line 3).

	D gazes at P	D gazes at the record	Comments
1 D:	and the you: have to (.) a:nd (o.1)	ld that you have some white faeces	"you" is a second person deictic that refers to the real patient. "you" is a second person deictic that refers to the distributed patient mediated by the record. Looking at P, the hesitation prompts the real patient to produce a turn (in line 2).
3 D:	=N	o (o.3) let me see again (.) some <u>BLACK</u> faeces	D turns from the real patient to the distributed patient; the information is attributed to the distributed patient's narrative to the GP.
5 D:	PALE or pale ↑right	we11 because it is both white and black >sometimes it is	D's logical connector, "because" recapulates the medical record, not the real patient's narrative to her in the situation. "↑right" functions as a discourse marker that prompts the real patient to confirm her utterance.

Figure 4.2 The real patient versus the distributed patient

In line 4, the patient recalls the conversation with his GP *oh yes [...] he asked what colour it was and then I say it is both the one and the other*. This answer leads to a paradox, since it is very unlikely that the patient's faeces have two colours simultaneously. Thus, the answer indicates several possibilities: (a) it could be the case that the patient merges several answers into one (if his faeces were different colours at different times), (b) he feels uncomfortable when taking the whole situation into consideration (the topic, his situation etc.) and thus just comes up with something to please the doctor or (c) he constructs a narrative that fits the proposals of the doctor: *the one and the other* (line 4) corresponds to her *white faeces ... BLACK faeces* (line 1–3). The doctor reacts by adding another category in line 5: *>sometimes it is PALE- or pale< ↑right*. In doing so, she seeks to bridge the gap between the distributed patient and the real patient, but the patient is unable to produce a meaningful response, which indicates that he is confused by her attempt to make him confirm the distributed patient's narrative in the medical record.

In medical distributed situations, there is often a need to compensate for human absence, for instance when heart rate and basic rhythm are represented in electrocardiograms. In this encounter, however, the patient is present and able to co-act with the doctor, but the doctor fails to see him as a cognitive resource. Instead of engaging with the patient, she produces the answers herself and seeks confirmation afterwards – to the great bewilderment of the patient.

In an emergency ward, the medical problem is often unknown and the relevant diagnostic variables are not given in advance. Under such conditions, practitioners are forced to engage in not merely problem-solving, but crucially in problem *finding*. In problem-solving activities, the problem is known and the doctor is the problem solver and hence the main cogniser within the distributed cognitive system. In problem finding, the diagnostic process is a non-linear mixture of procedural thinking, abductive hypothesis-testing, and solution probing (Steffensen 2013). The medical practitioner needs to rely on coaction between patient and doctor to generate valid hypotheses. This means that both cognisers are equally important, and successful diagnosing requires a focus on both medical measurements as well as engagement with the patient in a sensitive and dialogical way. The medical visual system is a result of how the novice doctor, in this case, takes refuge in the medical record where she looks for clues as to what the exact problem is. Thereby she reduces the problem finding process to one of problem-solving, and the situated cognitive dynamics do not match the patient's situation. In the words of the ecological time model, she has not developed sufficient professional experience on her autobiographical timescale, and she thus takes recourse in the institutional logic of using external authorities, here the patient's GP, as a resource for problem-solving.

3.2 The heterarchical roles of artefacts

In this section I investigate the function of sociocultural artefacts in the encounter between the novice doctor and the patient. In doing so, I plan to show that past events materialised as artefacts and tools, can affect the here-and-now interaction mediated by medical tools. Many tools increase the power and precision of human agency, just as they extend the peri-personal action space (cf. Kirsh 2013) in a way that is needed in order to complete a specific goal: A hammer is needed to hit a nail, and a racket is needed to hit a tennis ball. Many tools and artefacts in the medical ward facilitate communicative and cognitive actions, not by extending the action space, but by structuring it. Thus, where some tools by default secure a better outcome than if the tools were not used (for instance in tennis), many other tools have a facultative character in problem-solving and task performance. They may facilitate cognitive tasks and aid to maintain an overview in complex situations, but they can also have adhesive effects. An expert has learnt when tools constrain the action space, and when he is better off by not using the tool to perceive what to do. Maps are less used by experienced way finders, guidelines are less explicit in the world of experts, and training wheels are not needed when the rider becomes confident and brinkmanship reaches a certain level of expertise. The expert doctor thus knows when to rely on tools and when not to.

This insight is important and gives rise to a new understanding of perception, not as passive representation, but as a result of interaction in the environment over time. While tool-enabled actions allow for new affordances to emerge, they also narrow down the affordances of the non-tool agent system. As stated by Kirsh (2013) these new behavioural forms are not natural and innate, they are cultural and hence only natural in the artificial world that we inhabit today (Kirsh 2013: 3–9). Thus, we need to learn to handle tools and occasionally also to learn to abstain from handling tools. A visual system is continuously shaped and advanced through interactivity encompassing the environment, history, norms etc. In many professions, this interactivity is pre-organised in educational systems, which in themselves function as distributed situations where novice practitioners learn, not by doing, but by anticipating. Because the inherent intentions built into textbooks, guidelines and other medical artefacts by necessity are abstracted from reality, a crucial part of developing expertise is the ability to judge when such intentions do not fit real-life medical situations.

In the following, I turn our attention to how one such material artefact, the medical record, both constrains and facilitates problem-solving. As shown above, the doctor constantly holds on to the record during the conversation. The artefact serves as a cognitive resource: It enables the doctor to link information elicited by other practitioners to her own observations so she can generate hypotheses. However, the way she handles it also affects the interpersonal relation between the doctor and the patient negatively.

In the transcript above, the patient objects to the doctor's statement in line 2, *some what*. The doctor is thus forced to re-evaluate her utterance and come up with a new result. In line 3, she utters *=NO (0.3) let me see again (.) some BLACK faeces (0.3)*. From the verbal utterances alone, it seems as if the doctor looks in the medical record and spots the right answer, which enables her to generate a new category *BLACK faeces*. Nevertheless, a detailed analysis of this episode unveils another explanation. As the doctor utters *=NO (0.3) let me see again (.)*, she puts the medical record in front of her. At first glance, it looks as if the doctor searches for the right answer in the record, where she can *see* it. However, even before she has opened the medical record, she has started to produce the new answer, see Figure 4.3.

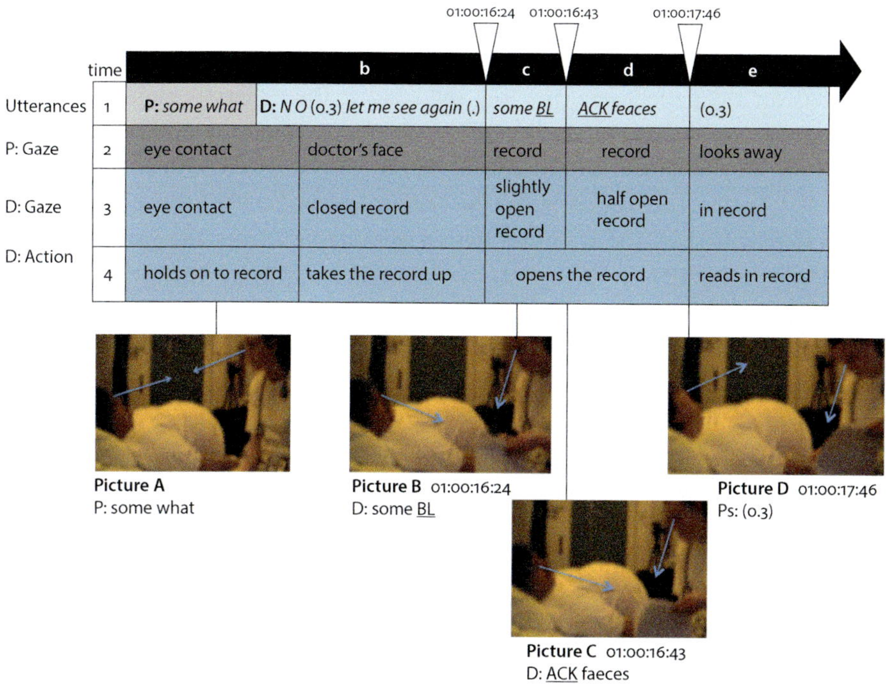

Figure 4.3 Gaze patterns and the opening of the medical record[3]

In picture A the doctor and the patient have eye contact. However, as the patient does not confirm the doctor's utterance, the doctor immediately assures the patient that she will have a second look (see Figure 4.3, box 2a and 2b). Hence in picture B, the doctor has already produced an alternative answer and the record has hardly been opened. Thus, she does not *see* the answer in the record. As the doctor utters *NO (0.3) let me see again (.)* the patient continues to gaze at the doctor, even though the doctor now orients herself to the record (see Figure 4.3, box 4b). The interaction has now changed from coaction to individual action, since the doctor interacts with the distributed patient rather than the real patient. In the pictures, the gaze pattern is indicated. As the eye contact in picture A is broken, the patient too gazes at the medical record, which has become the locus of interest (see picture B). In picture D, the patient gazes at the wall and the distributed cognitive system disintegrates. The doctor uses the artefact in a way that excludes the patient both cognitively and interpersonally. Because the patient has the answer, but is being excluded from the cognitive process, the problem finding activity is more complicated and time consuming than necessary.

3. Since I have no access to these data anymore, I cannot get hold of the exact time-code of picture A. If necessary, see Figure 4.3.

From an interpersonal or dialogical perspective, the way the doctor handles the record affects the interactivity negatively. The doctor's visual system serves as a display for the patient, and the way she handles the material artefact creates a boundary between the two. The boundary is both cognitive (the thinking becomes more individual and draws on personal experience rather than on coaction) and physical (the way the doctor holds the medical record makes it a physical barrier between the two and it guides her visual attention from the real patient to the distributed patient). The artefact serves as a constituent in several ways. It facilitates cognition and it affects interpersonal relations since it has a boundary constitutive effect. The doctor uses it to hold on to, to search for information in and to demarcate a distributed cognitive system for hypothesis generating. In this case, however, the artefact constrains the doctor's visual system. She is so keen to solve the problem that she neither sees nor feels the inter-bodily dynamics in real-time. It harms the dialogical relation with the patient, because he – a major cognitive resource – is being excluded.

The distributed cognitive system is dysfunctional since it only builds on the institutional timescales incarnated in the artefacts; it completely omits the autobiographical memory of the patient. The novice doctor relies on the symbolic properties of the record, and in doing so she ignores the fact that the record has concrete material properties too.

In this analysis I have shown how the material artefact – more than the symbolic representation incarnated in it – serves as an element in the distributed cognitive system by narrowing down the peri-personal sphere: It constrains the visual system of the doctor due to its structural affordances that force gaze, attention and sensitivity in a certain direction.

3.3 Semantic memory: Categories as constraints in diagnostic processes

The final analysis of this example scrutinises how abstract information structures (Baber et al. 2006) guide practitioners' perceptual processes via symbolic and semantic values established by a large and situation-transcendent, educational system. Thus, the doctor's education provides her with an intentionality that goes beyond what happens in local interaction. On a slow sociocultural timescale, the novice doctor's educational background has equipped her with perceptual categories that guide her real-life perception. In the educational system, practitioners are educated to solve problems (diagnose) on the basis of a given set of variables. The educational system thus provides practitioners with expertise by narrowing down what they pay attention to. When successful, this equips the novice with a pseudo-experience (i.e., she can rely on other persons' experiences as if they were her own); but at times novices face unexpected and irrational circumstances, and in such situations the educational visual system can almost blindfold them and limit their sensitivity to the real-time dynamics – to the danger of their patient and themselves. In other words, it can lead to human errors.

In this case, I will show how the novice doctor's vast categorical knowledge functions as a constraint as well as a necessity in diagnosing. Throughout the interaction the doctor seeks to determine the colour and the consistency of the patient's faeces. However, there is no sign of any clarification. On the contrary, while the doctor produces a cascade of colour categories, all of which are more or less fixed categories that stem from the educational system, the patient responds by producing fewer and vaguer categories, see Figure 4.4.

Figure 4.4 Semantic categories

FAECES CATEGORIES WITHIN THE SEQUENCE			
Line	**Doctor's fixed categories**	**Line**	**Patient's vague categories**
1.1	white	1.4	the one and the other
1.3	BLACK	1.20	no pale what do you mean
1.5	both white and black	1.24	not white or without colour
1.5	PALE- or pale	1.27	that darker more or less
1.18	°kind of p pale°	1.27	dark yellow
1.26	black	1.30	kind of yellowish or
1.34	a bite paler		
1.37	kit coloured		
1.37	clay coloured		
1.40	?sticky		
1.29	DARK YELLOW (patient's category)		

If one compares how these categories relate to well-known colour classifications, as the colour spectrum in Figure 4.5 below, the lack of conversational clarification is apparent from the categorical distance from the doctor's categories to the patient's. The two interlocutors simply seem to navigate semantically in different parts of the colour spectrum.

As the conversation proceeds, the doctor becomes increasingly frustrated. Her frustration is recognised, above all, in the cascade of categories fired at the patient. But her facial expressions also reveal a growing level of frustration, as illustrated below in Figure 4.6.

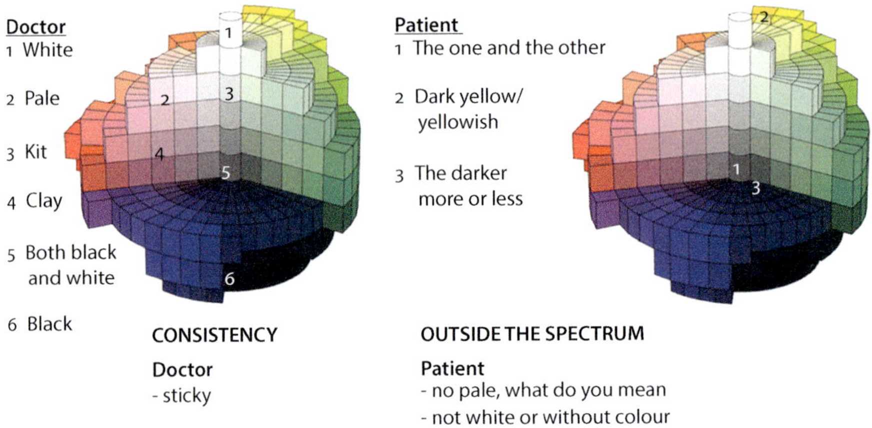

Figure 4.5 Colour spectrum

Her 'category firings' at the end of this diagnostic task show as a final attempt to match her categories derived from the educational system, with the ones of the patient. The doctor is fixated on verbal descriptions that almost sound like rote learning of colour names. However, by taking a closer look at the doctor's facial expressions as she proposes these categories, it becomes evident that she herself doubts their relevance. In Figure 4.6, picture A, the doctor furrows her eyebrows

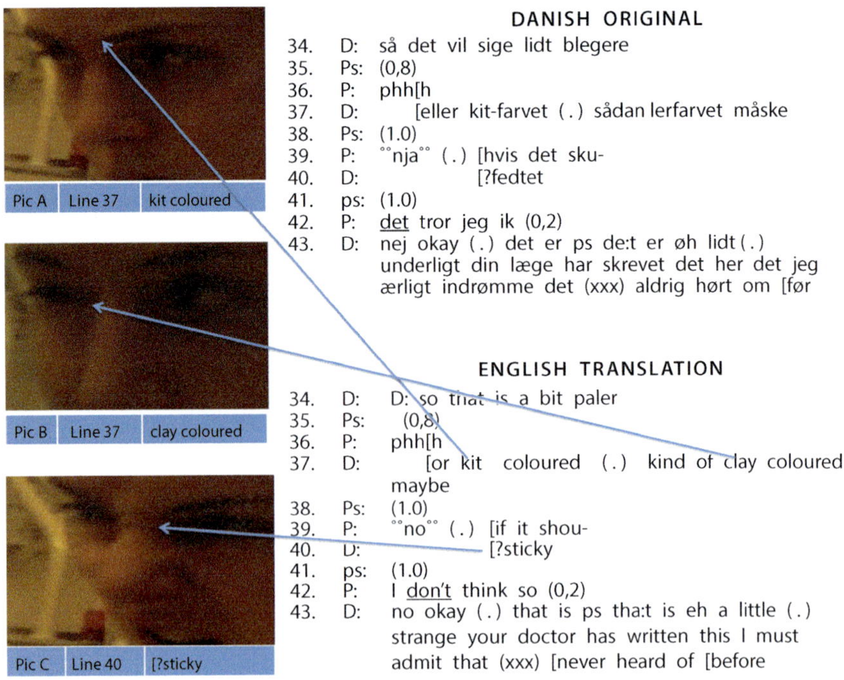

Figure 4.6 The doctor's category firings and facial expressions

when she utters *kit coloured*. In picture B she blinks with her right eye when proposing *clay coloured*. And finally, in picture C, she wrinkles her nose when uttering *sticky*. The doctor's facial expressions, and particularly their fine-grained synchrony with the semantic categories, are noteworthy since they mark a change in the flow of the interactivity: She produces a series of categories while facially marking them as non-conducive to reach her goal of categorical clarification.

Unsurprisingly, the result is frustration on her part and confusion on the part of the patient. The latter is visible in the still longer pauses in his turns: 0.8 seconds in line 35, 1.0 seconds in line 38 and 1.0 seconds again in line 41 and in his hesitating and desultory utterances: *phhh* (line 36), °°*no*°° *(.) if it shou-* (line 39) and *I don't think so* (line 42).

Being constrained by the sociocultural resources of medical school, the doctor fails to integrate her categorical knowledge with what happens in real-time. Her educational system is grounded in a 'word-world' (Pedersen 2010, 2012), and she thus relies on a diagnostic hierarchy with verbal categories in the top. Guided by this hierarchy she searches for the linguistically expressed 'truth' about the patient's faeces. The semantic categories from textbooks and the contradictory narratives of the real and the distributed patient confuse the doctor and prompt her to be insensitive to how the patient feels and what he expresses in situ. As shown, her strategy biases effective and dialogical diagnosing. The bottom line is that the doctor fails to establish a distributed cognitive system and to engage with the patient as a living being who is able to recall experience and provide reports of his experiences. The doctor sticks with a naïve view of what vision offers (e.g. memories of what colour names name), and it is striking how little use the doctor makes of the resources available. She almost exclusively focuses on abstract information structures. Thus, we witness a doctor who is blocked by cognitive economics, because her focus on colour names happens at the expense of her ability to feel the inter-bodily dynamics in real-time.

The doctor fails to initiate ways of seeing that might prompt her to deal with the situation in a more conducive way. She engages in dysfunctional cognitive work, which is biased by parameters established by other professionals. And as such her intention, attention and cognitive dynamics are not just guided and framed, but rather fixated by a larger system than her as an individual (cf. Goodwin 1994), in this case the educational system.

From a design perspective, much can be improved to enable the patient to be able to recall, identify and confirm shape, appearance and texture of his or her faeces. All the constraints we observe in the above examples may be facilitated through visualisation as done by the Bristol stool form scale, see Figure 4.7 below.

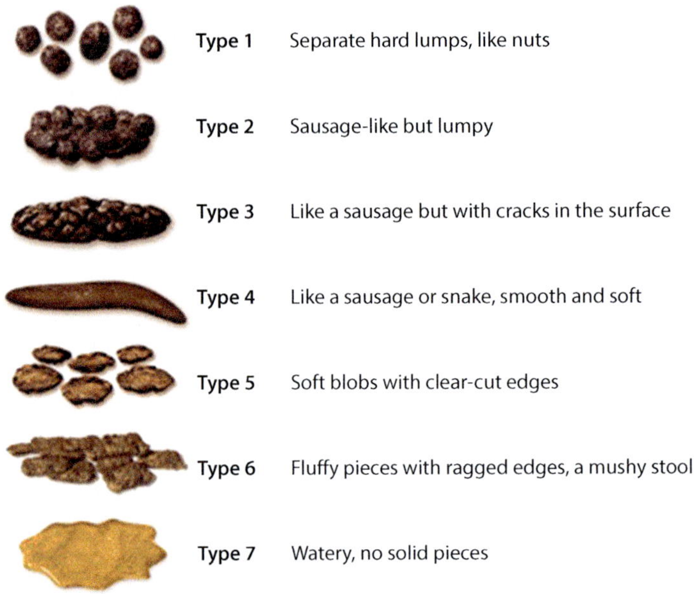

Figure 4.7 The Bristol stool form scale[4]

Such a material artefact might scaffold memory and facilitate situated cognition. The chart scaffolds memory as it uses both symbolic and visual distributed systems that trigger memory differently. The implementation of such tools in practice will enhance the dialogicality since it requires active cognitive work from the patient and the tool serves as a shared object, which all parties orient to and it will reduce the level of errors in information elicitation. Finally, it would be less time and energy consuming and would ease the interpersonal relations since the responsibility of the cognitive work would be distributed between the participants.

Overall, the analyses emphasised how multiple organising principles simultaneously constrain human interaction. I showed how a novice doctor's visual system both depends on local coaction and on non-local events (cf. Steffensen and Cowley 2010), such as the patient's prior visit to his GP, the doctor's experiences from medical school, and the sociocultural practice embedded and incarnated in the medical record as a tool and artefact. These non-local constraints became observable in how the doctor oriented herself to both the real-time patient and the distributed patient in order to manage multiple, causal frames simultaneously. They also showed in her fixation on categories, rules and procedures at the expense of situational awareness. Also, I identified the ambiguity and complexity of a distributed visual system encompassing historically given abstract information and

4. Lewis and Heaton (1997).

artefacts. For instance, a medical record is not just a paper with representational information that needs to be decoded; both its materiality and the trans-situational intentions built into its design affect its situated functionality. In a similar vein, Benne argues that literary materials are sociocultural material artefacts with a supra-individual and ecological ontology and function:

> Die Ontologie der Literatur ist nicht nur kulturabhängig, sondern überindividuell und distribuiert. Dies gilt im Unterschied zur Affordanz im Tierreich für alle kulturellen Affordanzen. Die Materialität der Literatur ist deshalb nie allein von einer ontologischen Analyse der Materie der Literatur als ihrer reinen Stofflichkeit herzuleiten, sondern muss bereits die Rolle dieser Stofflichkeit in ihrer kulturellen Signifikanz und Affordanz umfassen, die sich im Erlebnis manifestieren.
>
> (Benne 2015: 116)

As literary manuscripts, the function and intention of the medical record must be understood in relation to the intentions of design, the sociocultural and physical practice in which it is embedded and the situational circumstances in which it is being used. In this case, the medical record draws attention away from the patient and it frames perception and understanding through its inherent intentions, symbolic content and pre-designed purposes that are worked out by a situation-transcendent system that goes beyond the real-time dialogical system. Sometimes such framing is needed; at other times it fixates and blocks perception and understanding of important expressions in the local environment. As a consequence, such expressions are neutralised, or they might even become stress factors for the novice.

It is indeed a balance to know when the exclusion of supporting tools leads to a more dialogical behaviour and a richer affordance environment, and when such tools give rise to stress, cognitive overload and interpersonal frustration. In this case the doctor is stressed because she prioritises the educational system; her fixation bias becomes a positive feedback mechanism in the cognitive system that leads to a dysfunctional outcome: no shared sense-making, thus no precise categorisation. This activity trajectory includes a potential error cycle that can lead to a negative outcome if dialogue is not prioritised. Further, the materiality of artefacts always affects inter-bodily dynamics by their mere material properties. In this case the medical record becomes the locus of interest rather than the patient right next to the doctor. That artefacts can affect local sensitivity is a concern that needs to be understood when tools are embedded in the field of emergency medicine.

4. Case II: Sense-saturated visual systems, intentionality and tendencies in visual perception[5]

4.1 Moulding the optic array through sense-saturated locomotion

In the following case, a medical team moulds and recalibrates its optic array through joint inter-bodily coordination. It is not a case of direct manipulation of an external object, but rather an interaction within the environment where the system itself is being manipulated. With CEA (Steffensen 2013; Steffensen et al. 2016), the perspectives of dialogism (Linell 2009) and ecological psychology (Gibson 1979/86), I show how the team's movements constitute a shared intentionality that implies the maintenance of an optimal visual system which allows the team to keep focused on professional medical problem-solving without compromising the ability to keep track of what happens in the patient sphere. The following case involves a medical team consisting of a doctor, a nurse, a paramedic and a gastrointestinal surgeon from another ward. The surgeon brings with him a medical student, who observes from a distance. The following is a visualisation of the setting and an indication of the multiple elements within the cognitive system.

As we enter this interaction, the medical team is busy interpreting medical values on a computer screen. The patient lies in bed and is in pain. He arrived by 911 with massive stomach cramps and the two doctors explicitly evaluate the results of various tests that recently have appeared on the screen. They provide various hypotheses in order to make a coherent diagnosis and develop a strategy for further treatment. The nurse is occupied with medical measurements, reporting and following general procedure. The paramedic and the medical student observe from a distance and are loosely affiliated to the medical system organised around the two doctors and the computer screen. Figure 4.8 visualises to what extent diagnosing is concerned with dealing with the distributed patient, i.e., the medical team focuses on symbolic representations of the patient's medical condition on the screen as the real patient lies in bed, disconnected from the medical team next to him. This organisation is unavoidable since valuable test results, previous medically documented information etc. appear on the screen. However, the organisation is at the same time potentially critical for leaving the real patient alone at essential moments during diagnosing. Indeed, successful diagnosing is concerned with how sensitively a team is able to balance artefact-scaffolded

5. Sections 4.4–4.6 are an analysis which were originally published in the article "The Ecological Subject and Visual Perception" in a special issue of *RASK, the International Journal of Language and Communication*, 46, 2017. It is reused here with permission of RASK: https://www.sdu.dk/en/Om_SDU/Institutter_centre/Isk/Forskning/Forskningspublikationer/rask.

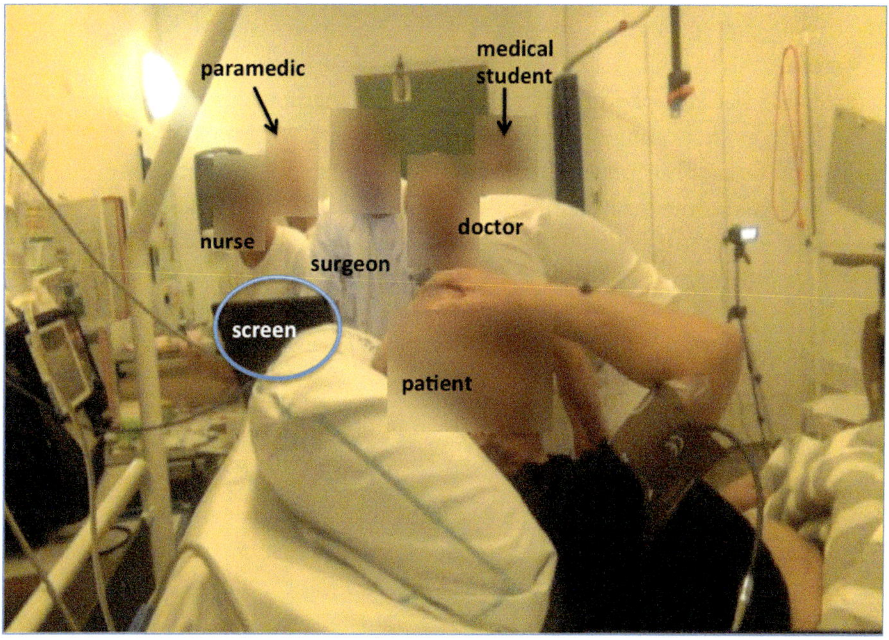

Figure 4.8 The layout and practitioner configurations in the cognitive system

medical reasoning and patient interaction. Such a balance requires that the team is able to focus on multiple concerns simultaneously in the diagnostic activity. This is exactly what the following investigates as it describes the mechanisms involved in whole-bodied visual perception in relation to the team's overall task, which concerns effective diagnostic interaction and the maintenance of a constant overview of the patient's local, medical condition.

The medical team focuses its attention on the distributed patient: They gaze at the screen and momentarily at each other as they remain focused on the medical discussion. While this task is crucial to successful task performance, the team members also need to be able to react to the slightest change in the real patient's condition. As his medical condition is critical, the team's focus will change with any negative changes in his medical condition. Within the team there are different dynamics that are characterised by more or less autonomous connections. For instance, the nurse is cognitively more loosely associated with the team than the two doctors. The nurse is primarily occupied with the completion of individual procedures and in this excerpt, we observe that she does not pay much attention to the task of the doctors and she focusses on the completion of individual sub tasks. Her sub-tasks involve patient contact, documentation and clinical tasks as preparing for tests etc., which means that she moves around in the location.

In this excerpt, I zoom in on the nurse's movements as they are crucial to changes in the overall system. During the medical interaction, the nurse walks towards the patient sphere, and by doing so she manipulates the doctor's visual array in a way that changes his environment and hence his possibility to perform functional tasks. Thus, the nurse's action initiates a series of interconnected actions within the medical team, which reorganises its position as a reaction to the changes in the layout of affordances, see Figure 4.9 below and the gallery A-L further below.

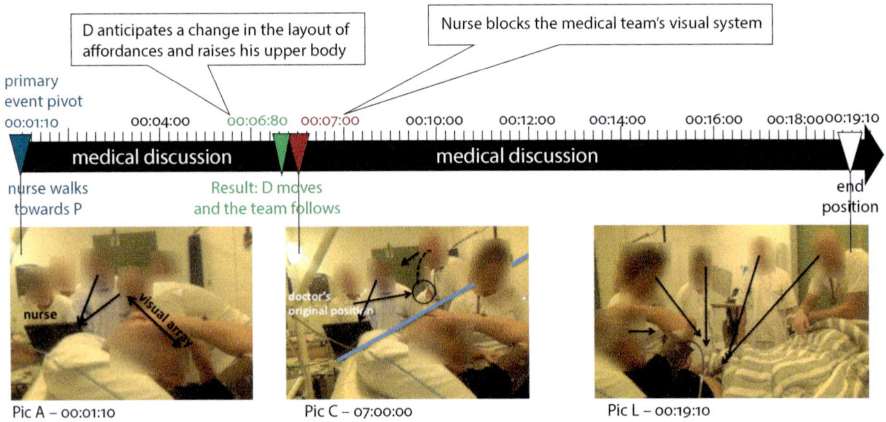

Figure 4.9 System reorganisation and cognitive focus
The blue line in picture C visualises the doctor's blocked visual access to the patient

Figure 4.9 illustrates how the nurse's movement prompts the team to move and recalibrate its boundaries without losing the cognitive overview: The medical team continues the medical discussion and hypothesis generating, and the doctor's movement is only functionally related to the movement of the nurse. The reorganisation takes 18 seconds and leaves the medical team with the best work conditions with a minimum of cognitive effort (see picture L). The remaining questions are: What does the doctor perceive that enables him to change position? And what are the mechanisms that enable him to perceive a change in the dynamical relation and to anticipate the consequences such changes in the layout of affordances entail? The first question serves as an organising principle for the analysis, which reveals important features of the second question, which is further elaborated in the discussion (Section 4.4.2). Methodologically, I zoom in on the small-scale dynamics of the doctor's adaptive behaviour, i.e., how he coordinates his movement with the changes in his environment. In the following detailed gallery, the overall flow of coordination is visualised. Because the nurse blocks the visual array between doctors and patient, the doctors are prompted to change position. Thus, the primary doctor initiates a move as a reaction to the change in the environment and to the potential future changes (Gibson 1979/86). The nurse's movement is defined as the primary event pivot in the figure, as this action initiates a dynamical physical change in the team constellation. The anticipatory action is shown in Figure 4.9 as the doctor moves before the nurse blocks the team's visual system. During this nested activity, the cognitive focus remains the same (see Figure 4.9). In the following detailed gallery the overall flow of coordination is visualised. It visualises the gaze, movement pattern and the visual array within the medical visual system.

The medical team discusses specific medical issues that are completely unrelated to the movement pattern indicated in the gallery above. The doctor summarises the patient's medical history, and as the nurse moves around the medical team, he utters: *well you just felt hi his pressure when he: arrived eh (xxx) eh when the ambulance arrives (xxx) it is 85 over 50 right*. The surgeon confirms, and as the doctor has reached the headboard, he continues: *and there has not been any (xxx).*[6] Again the surgeon confirms the doctor's utterance, and as they have both re-located to the end of the bed, (see picture K), they continue to evaluate the patient's medical situation.

In picture A-B, the team has full visual access to the real patient even though they bend forward and gaze at the computer screen. However, as the nurse needs to place herself next to the patient to complete her tasks, she will eventually block the visual array of the medical team (see picture D). She walks from the corner, around the team and towards the patient (picture A-C), and this changes the situation from a static, calm interaction to one characterised by movement. The nurse's movement (starting in picture A and ending in picture D) causes a corresponding movement pattern within the medical team, i.e., her action initiates a dynamical physical change in the team constellation (see Figure 4.9). However, movement in one sub-system does not necessarily afford movement in another sub-system. In the situations prior to this excerpt, the nurse has been moving in similar patterns: back and forth but without blocking the visual array between the patient and the team. The team, in those cases, did not respond to those actions; rather the team remained located around the screen. Therefore, the timing of the doctor's movement is crucial to understanding what prompts him to move in this particular case. First a detailed description of the doctor's and the team's movement pattern is outlined in order to generate an explanation of the mechanisms involved in it.

6. Danish original

```
D:  altså man mærker bare ha hans tryk da ha:n kommer øh (xxx) øh da
    [ambulancen kommer øh (xxx) det er 85 over 50 ik
    (…)
D:  og der har ikke været noget (xxx)
```

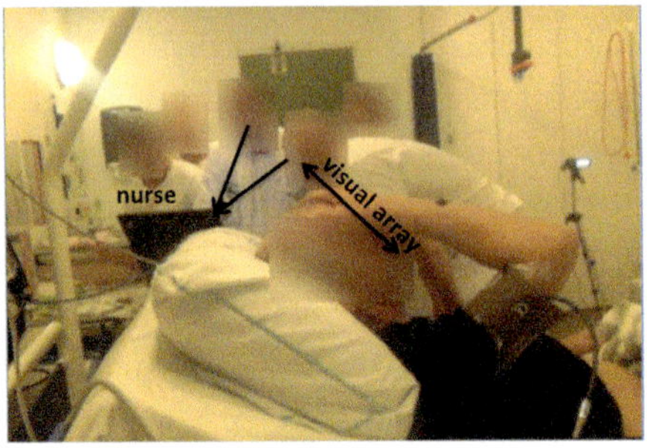

Pic A– 00:01:10

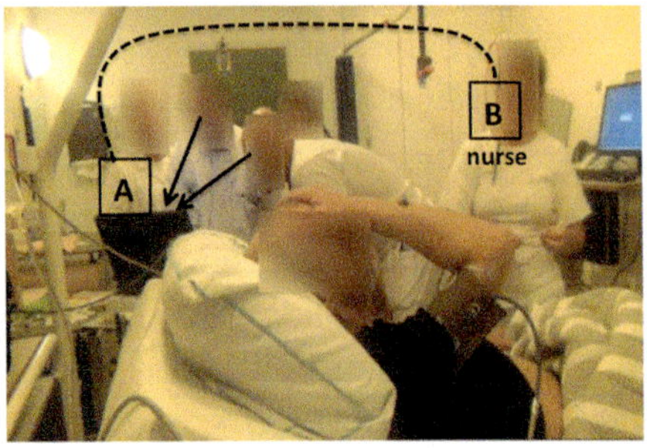

Pic B– 00:05:20

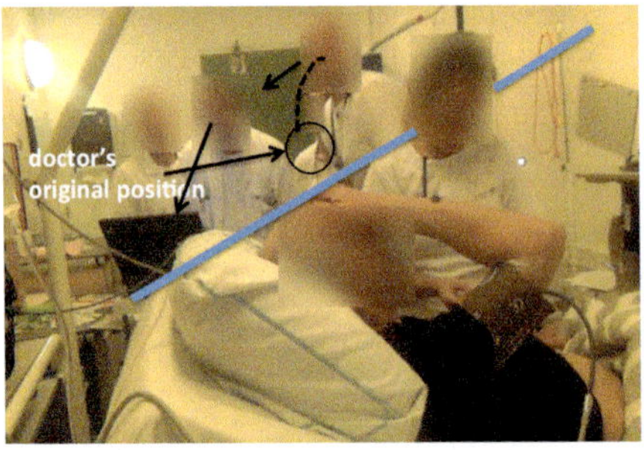

Pic C– 00:07:00

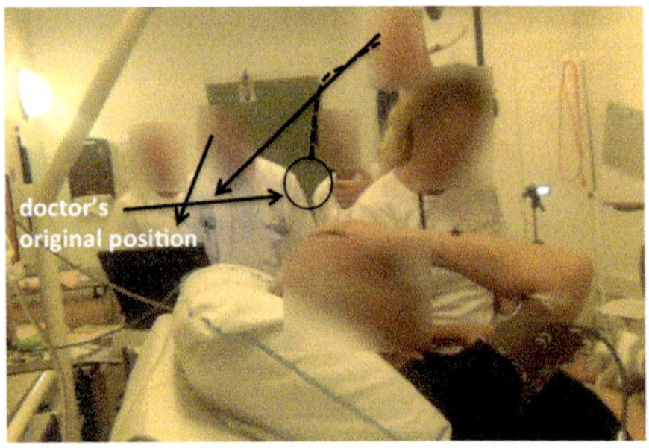

Pic D– 00:08:10

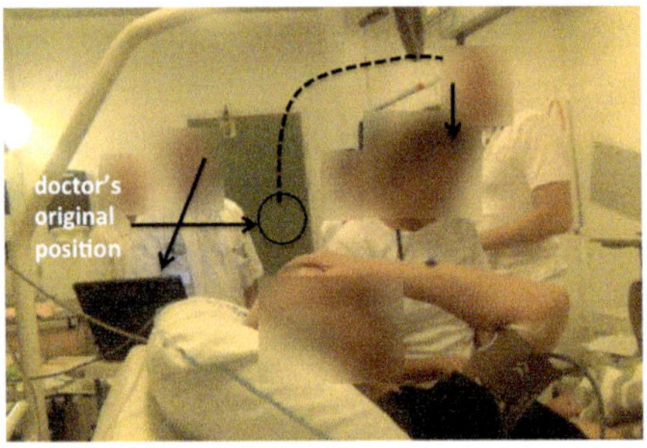

Pic E– 00:10:00

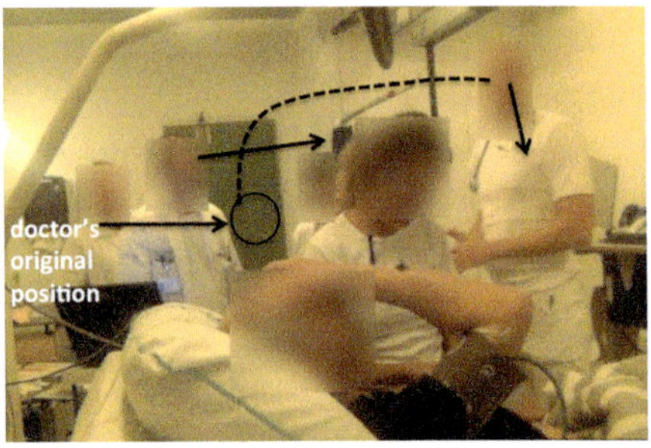

Pic F– 00:10:10

It is argued that the doctor initiates a move as a reaction to the change in the environment and as an anticipation of *potential future changes*. His movements are anticipatory because he moves (at 6.80) *before* the nurse actually blocks the team's visual array at 7:00 (see Figure 4.9). In picture C, the doctor is already moving and almost in an upright position, but the nurse is not yet blocking the visual access to the patient. However, as the nurse gets in the way and blocks the team's visual access to the patient (see picture D), the doctor has already anticipated this visual constraint, raised his upper body and started to move backwards away from the screen even though he has never gazed directly at the nurse. At no time during this movement does the team stop the verbal evaluation of the patient's situation

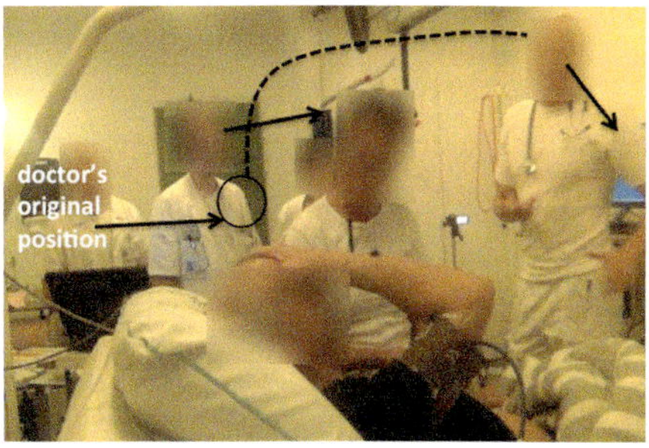

Pic G– 00:10:20

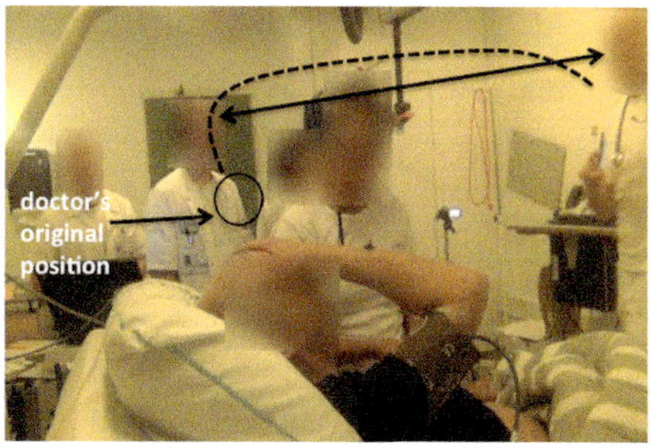

Pic H– 00:11:10

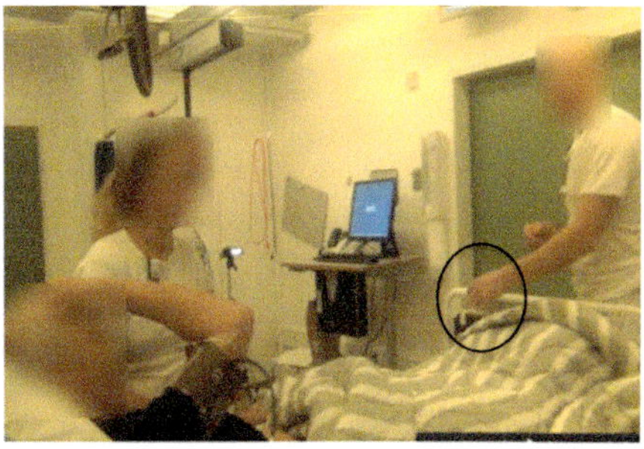

Pic I– 00:13:10

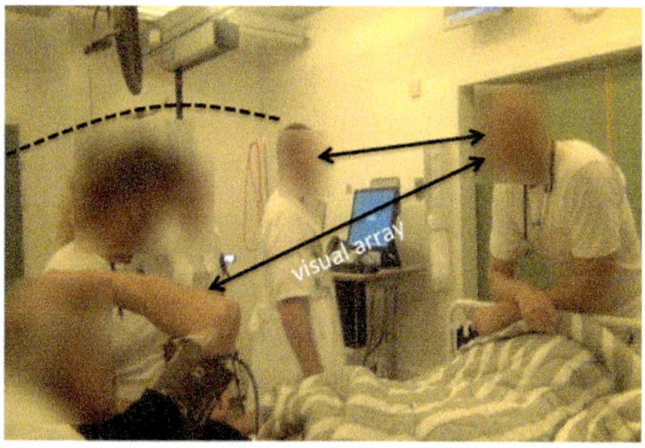

Pic J– 00:14:20

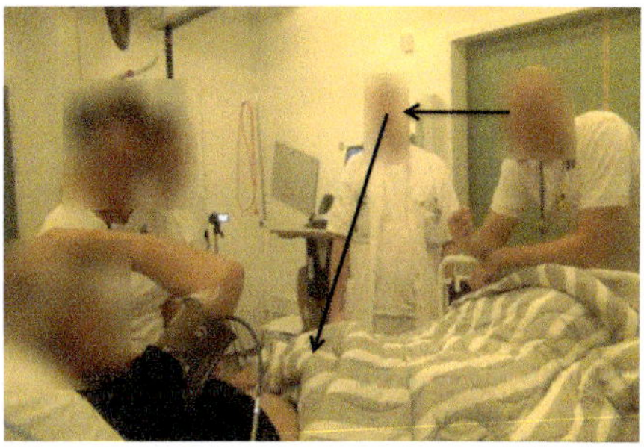

Pic K– 00:16:20

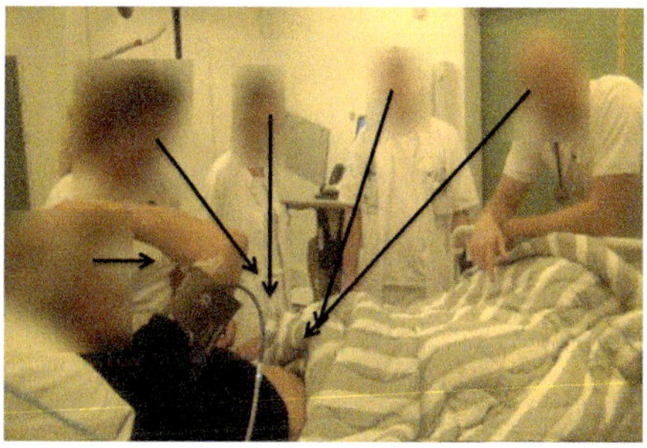

Pic L– 00:19:10

and the doctors continue to gaze at the computer screen as the main doctor moves backwards *without even looking in the direction of the nurse or the headboard* (see picture C-D). This means that the doctor does not *see* the nurse's blocking and he does not *see* the end point of his movements (the headboard); he simply starts moving. Without looking in the direction of the 'problem' (the nurse's itinerary) or the solution (the headboard), he anticipates a change in the interaction as a potential problem (blocking), which prompts him to act. His actions directly affect the team's working conditions. The surgeon shifts his visual attention from the screen to the doctor as the physical distance between them increases. The team then re-negotiates the best place to solve the medical problem, and the doctor marks the endpoint as he stops moving when he reaches the back of the headboard (see picture J). The whole medical team follows and relocates. The new position enables all team members to regain perfect visual access to the patient without interrupting their medical hypothesis activity (see picture L). During the 18 seconds the doctor has been summarising the medical history, and as they have both re-located to the end of the bed (see picture K), they continue to evaluate the patient's medical situation. This problem-solving activity was nested within the larger medical work of generating valid hypotheses about the patient's situation.

The team's re-organisation (from around the computer – to the end of the bed) affects the quality of the visual system positively. By anticipating not only the nurse's movement trajectory (her blocking) but also possible changes in the patient domain (severe changes in his medical condition), the team is continuously adapting to its environment in order to be in the best possible place at all times. *If* the patient's medical condition changes, the team will be able to pay attention to this immediately and they will furthermore be able to respond to it with a minimum of resources. The movements are nested within a cognitive problem-solving trajectory, and we observe how the doctor affects the locomotion of the whole team as the other team members have not perceived relevant changes in the environment: They remain at their initial location until the distance become too great between the doctors to continue the dialogue (see picture J).

This example does not describe a problem, but an anticipation that can be described as negative feedback mechanisms which prevent a potential problem from emerging. The feedback mechanisms reveal a case of meaningful locomotion probing rather than explicit goal-orientation (Steffensen 2013; Cowley 2014b). Because of the doctor's formal role as the main responsible staff in the team, he has different obligations to the surgeon. While the doctor is also responsible for patient interaction and general clinical tasks etc., the gastrointestinal surgeon's professional relationship with the patient is primarily characterised by a bio-medical focus on a specific body part (abdomen). The different roles in the medical team entail different foci. Institutionally the surgeon is not the main responsible person for identifying change in the broader environment. This is the job of the main doctor. On the other hand, the surgeon needs to and also does anticipate the movements of the doctor. Oganisational norms and procedures serve as constraints for their visual perceptions. The example points to how the same physical environment provides both shared and distinct affordances for actions for the medical team. The world at their feet is shared and meaningful only in relation to the task they attend to and to their specific roles and responsibilities. The doctor perceives the nurse's movements as an affordance for re-locating the team's position, and the surgeon also perceives the doctor's movements as an affordance for moving and in that way maintaining optimal conditions for problem-solving. In that way their qualifications and their competences built up over time saturate their local action-perception cycles and decision-making.

4.2 The historical body, the flow of perception, and timescales

By considering how longer, non-local timescales serve as a constraint for the local here-and-now, it becomes possible to investigate how inter-bodily dynamics mesh with social orderliness, and finally how perception is shaped by materiality and historical experiences as prerequisites for seeing useful action patterns and enacting intentions. Nothing in the data indicates that there exists a local plan or calculations that afford the doctor to think of how the visual system works most effectively. As mentioned in the analysis, he does not even *look* in the direction of the nurse or the headboard as he initiates the movement backwards (see picture C–D); rather, he *perceives* the reorganisation of the nurse as an important change in the layout of affordances that prompts him to move. In other words, his skilled, historical body functions as a visual detector of affordances, which enable certain actions. Thus, the whole act makes perfect sense since the re-orientation results in an optimally shared medical system in which the team's visual array works to its best effect.

The ease with which the main doctor anticipates the potential problem can be explained by the power of the subject's micro-social ecology, which transcends local interaction (Steffensen 2013, 2015; Pedersen and Steffensen 2014; Steffensen and Pedersen 2014). His repeated structural coupling with relatively stable medical teams equips him with an embodied professional history (Goodwin 1994, Noë 2004). We observe a case of anticipatory sense-making that is grounded in the bio-cognitive historical body. The notion of whole-bodied vision has been emphasised again and again, however, it still needs to be empirically tested and developed:

> The clinical gaze is not that of an intellectual eye that is able to perceive the unalterable purity of essences beneath phenomena. It is a gaze of the concrete sensibility, a gaze that travels from body to body, and whose trajectory is situated in the space of sensible manifestation. […] 'theory falls silent or almost always vanishes at the patient's bedside to be replaced by observation and experience; for on what are observation and experience based if not on the relation of our senses.'
> (Foucault 1973: 148)

Experts are able to adapt to pivotal changes immediately due to their developed professional vision. Therefore, as we observe in this example, visual perceptions are *not* explained as processes of representations or verbal embodiment with a gestural function; it is automatic and enabled by the developed ability to pick up relevant information in the world at their feet. Since the position is not pre-defined, the team members stop when they feel they are in the right place. The right place cannot be determined in advance, since the 'place' constantly moves simultaneously with the movement of the individuals (Anderson 2014). A successful movement is only successful in the case that the team's emergent capacity to interact as an emergent and self-organising system exists. The team's sensitivity towards environmental expressions allows it to anticipate potential problems without losing any cognitive power. Through detailed investigations of how a team interacts in a way that prompts the emergence of affordances, the analyses reveal that intentionality and problem-solving are shared activities that are maintained through the coordination of inter-bodily dynamics. From this perspective, explanation of individual agency is found beyond the individual agent. As mentioned in the introduction of Chapter 1, an understanding of human errors requires a focus on both negative and positive feedback mechanisms. This case example reveals how a potential error cycle is anticipated. As constraints emerge within the system, the system adapts flexibly to the changes in the environment. The system anticipates potential critical scenarios as a consequence of reduced visual access to the patient. As human error cycles are the main focus of interest, real-life examples of what inhibits error cycles are useful because they underline the importance of coordinated team performance and the function and possibilities of thinking in terms of distributed visual systems.

5. Case III: Random manipulation: Developing the visual system through probing-activities

5.1 Moving as seeing: An undeveloped visual system

> *The major difference between a thing that might go wrong and a thing that cannot possibly go wrong is that when a thing that cannot possibly go wrong goes wrong it usually turns out to be impossible to get at and repair.*
>
> \- Adams Douglas (2002: 720)

A medical problem never emerges in a vacuum and the complexity of finding and solving problems increases as multiple expressive features penetrate the environment. While multiple problems arise simultaneously in real life and while the order in which they should be dealt with or how they should be dealt with is a situational issue, in the medical books, a problem is often presented in isolation.

Unlike the previous example, the following interactivity trajectory reveals an inadequate approach to such a challenge. A doctor enacts an action pattern that constrains both cognitive problem-solving and interpersonal relations with the patient. The doctor is about to complete a simple task that in Adam's sense *cannot go wrong*: She needs to listen to the patient's lungs to clarify if there is a murmur, but that requires that the patient sits up and leans forward. However, the length of the tube attached to the oxygen mask that the patient is wearing prevents this simple standard task. As the patient cannot sit and keep on the oxygen mask at the same time, a dilemma emerges. What is easily completed in theory, becomes impossible due to practical issues, and it fixates the doctor, who needs to come up with alternative solutions. First, the emergence of the dilemma is illustrated in the gallery below. This dilemma leads to continuous cycles of probing and fixation, which are analysed in relation to the doctor's level of perceptual richness.

Red markings in the text indicate the verbal utterance articulated as the picture is taken

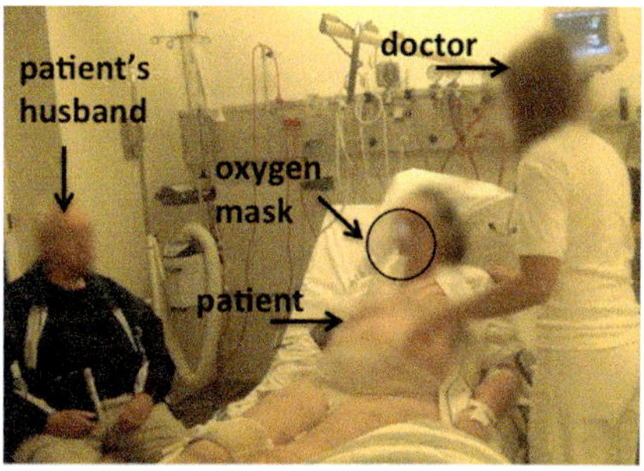

Pic A– 05:00:00
D: så skal vi lige
D: than we just need to

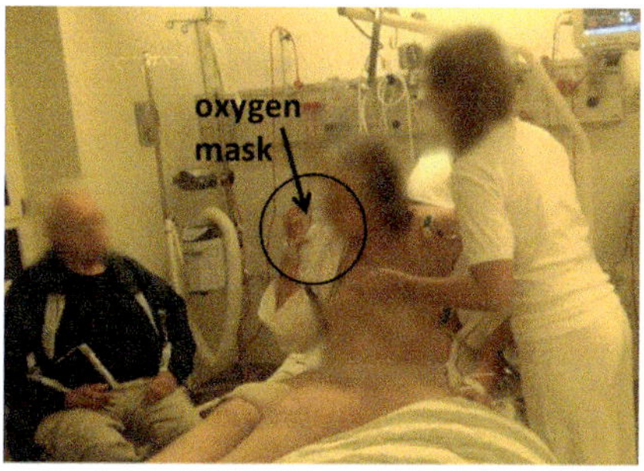

Pic B– 05:08:10
P: åh
P: oh

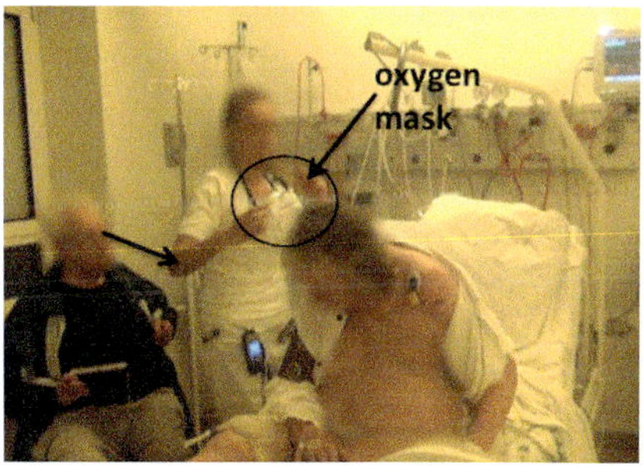

Pic C– 05:27:00

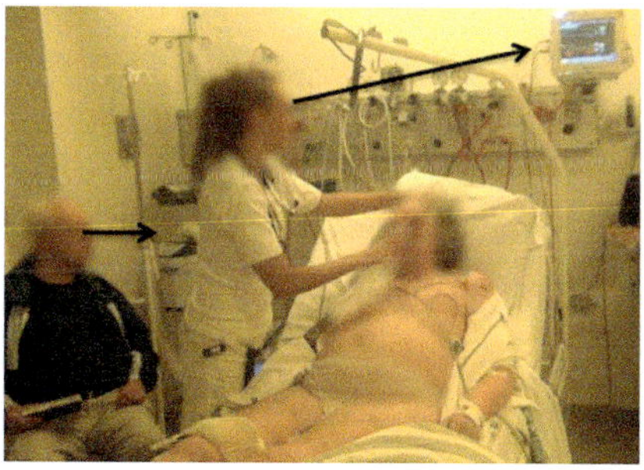

Pic D– 05:33:30

As the doctor helps the patient sit up in the bed in order to listen to her lungs, the oxygen mask falls off the patient (picture A–B). The doctor then walks around the bed to get the oxygen mask, which is indeed needed as the patient's oxygen saturation is low and causes her severe breathing difficulties. The doctor puts the mask back on the patient, who forcefully falls back in the bed again in exhaustion. The doctor then observes the medical measurements on the screen above the patient's head (picture C–D). The dilemma is now explicit for all parties involved: (a) the doctor freezes, (b) the patient appears exhausted and (c) the patient's husband is paying attention to the doctor's behaviour. The patient is in a critical and unstable condition, and the dilemma creates a series of activities that are unpleasant for the patient and which trouble the doctor.

From a rational point of view, one relevant reaction is to call for assistance so as to be able to listen to the patient's lungs. To get assistance to complete a very simple task is not usual in the ward, and the problem seems to be deferred by the doctor for a moment. Instead of calling for assistance immediately after the challenge is explicit, the doctor waits and walks around, doing what appears to be 'nothing', considering the context. She appears fixated and meets what Steffensen et al. (2016) describe as *suspended nexts*, or what Dewey (1910) characterises as a *forkedroad situation*.

While Steffensen et al. (2016) and Dewey (1910) describe cognitive challenges in problem-solving as constraining situations, Wittgenstein follows up on this idea by arguing that the solution to such cases is just to do *something*: "If I have exhausted the justifications, I have reached bedrock and my spade is turned. Then I am inclined to say: "This is simply what I do"" (Wittgenstein 1963: 85e, §217).

The following emphasises the complexities that follow a situation in which a suspended next inhibits the doctor from solving the problem (listen to the patient's lungs). Thus, working from the hypothesis that perception is dynamic and altered by an individual's interaction with the environment, a rational approach in order to expand the visual system seems to be related to action, or rather moving around within the environment. Theoretically, the situated environment in which the problem appears can be described as a spatial problem-zone in which one moves around to perceive the problem from as many new angles as possible and to contain embodied frustration in order to overcome the suspended next. This is what we observe the doctor doing.

When the suspended next overwhelms the doctor, she fixates on procedures that do not contribute to the solution of how to overcome the fixation. As a consequence of reaching cognitive bedrock, she literally moves around and changes the visual array of the cognitive system. This is illustrated in the following event trajectory below:

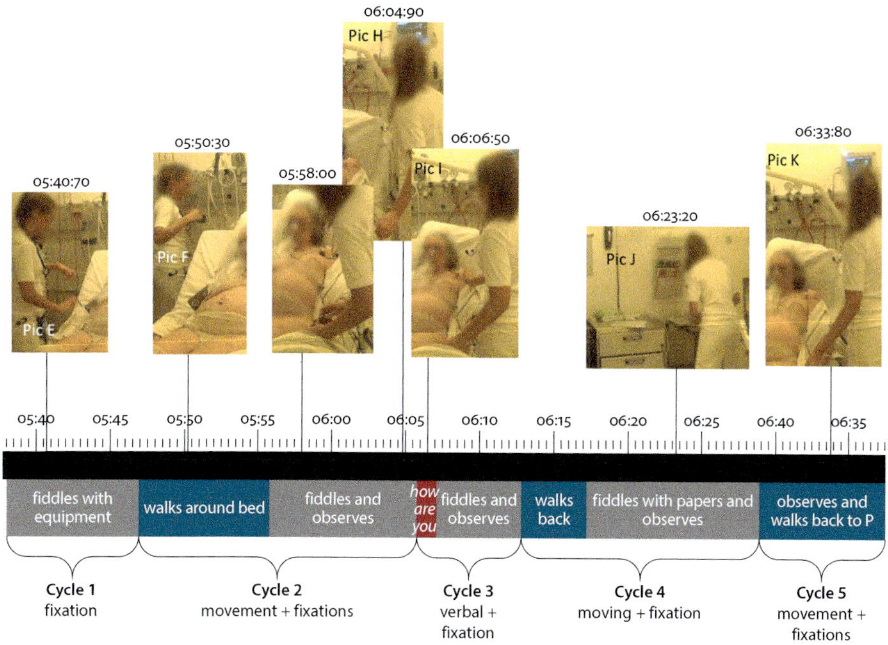

Figure 4.10 Moving in-and-out of a problem-zone as cognitive manipulation

After the doctor has realised that she is unable to listen to the patient's lungs, she initiates various behavioural contortions and procrastinations when time becomes a limited resource. In Figure 4.10 it is visualised how the doctor employs five action cycles in order to manage the increasing frustration within the cognitive system.

The first cycle involves the doctor's fiddling with the tubes and attempt to arrange them nicely (see picture E). As the tubes are the problem, this aesthetical organising does not contribute directly to the problem-solving. In another study, Steffensen et al. (2016) identify:

> a *general* tendency to impose an aesthetic order onto the physical layout of her surroundings [...] To account for this dimension of [the participant's] cognitive trajectory, we define an aesthetic action as an action that (a) transforms the physical layout of the environment in order to make it more ordered, and (b) has no task-related, cognitive function. (Steffensen et al. 2016: 93)

In this context the neat reordering does not provide the doctor with a useful overview and she is prompted to do something to contain her frustration. She walks away and initiates a second cycle that involves a new combination of moving and fixed-procedure following: She checks if the equipment works and gains information about the patient's medical condition. Specifically, the doctor walks behind the bed. Apparently, her behaviour displays no specific intention (see picture F) and she walks back to the other side of the bed. As she moves, the visual system changes its perceptual array, but as the emerging properties of the system have not yet provided her with any functional affordances for proper action, she becomes fixated on procedures. She fiddles with the medical equipment attached to the patient's finger (see picture G) and observes the values on the screen (see picture H). Nothing appears to provide the doctor with decisive information and she fixates on the measurements for 5.5 seconds (see Figure 4.10). The third cycle differs from the previous attempts to gain information. The doctor asks a verbal question: *how are you feeling* as she touches the patient's shoulder (see picture I). The patient utters: >*oho* and the incomprehensive answer further indicates that her condition is critical. Thus, the response does not contribute to the process of figuring out what to do next. The doctor then resumes the fiddling with the equipment. The husband and the patient gaze momentarily at the doctor (see picture F–G) as they do not know what strategy the doctor is working on. The doctor has not yet been successful in exiting the negative loop, and a fourth cycle of moving and fixation in order to manage the problem space is initiated. The doctor continues to seek a solution on her own. She turns away and walks to another corner of the room where she fiddles with a paper record without looking further into its content (see picture J). Once again she stops, removes some papers, puts them back on the table and observes medical measurements on the electronic display. Time elapses and although she paces around the ward, the doctor fails to resolve the situation. So far, her actions have not led to new insights and she moves away from the corner again. As she returns to the bedside, she hesitates before she once again observes the medical values on the screen (see picture K).

Every time the doctor gets back to the patient the challenge remains the same. Paradoxically, the doctor knows exactly what the local goal is (listen to the patient's lungs), but she is unable to attain it. After the oxygen mask falls off, the doctor spends a minute on walking around and repeating nested tasks: checking oxygen saturation etc. (see Figure 4.10). Essentially, there are only three solutions to the problem: (a) to call for assistance, (b) to get a longer tube or (c) to reorganise the position of the bed so that the tube will reach. The doctor initiates none of these solutions and moving in-and-out of the problem-space seems to be an escape strategy. Her moving around is identified as loops of fixation patterns, which can be interpreted as a strategy of getting out of a literal problem zone. Moving around within the room allows for different perceptual possibilities. One way of developing a visual system is by trying to manipulate the situation in order to connect phenomena in new ways, to perceive the world from different angles, to understand alternative perspectives etc. In this case, intuition and frustration guide the doctor's actions, but the functional result remains absent and she wastes important time in a critical situation. The doctor's actions indicate an undeveloped medical visual system that is biased by local constraints (the length of the tube and the patient's unresolved medical condition) and non-local expectations of individual problem-solving. Even though the doctor clearly perceives the problem, identification of functional solutions is inhibited within these constraints .

On the one hand there is no good reason for the doctor to pace around the room (behind the bed, around the bed and to the corner of the room), and yet on the other hand it makes sense to do something when bedrock is reached. When challenges emerge, frustration and stress often co-emerge. Logical and abstract reasoning (trying to think of a solution) requires stillness and a hierarchy with one isolated problem after the other: if/then sequences. In this situation the doctor needs to balance the heterarchy of multiple nested activities: taking care of the patient's emotional and medical condition, completing certain procedures (physical examination) and figuring out how to deal with a sudden dilemma (completing a task that cannot be completed within the actual setting). The working hypothesis emphasised that moving around leads to an alteration of the visual system. Moreover, her moving around can indicate that she is trying to reduce complexity. When stress and frustration emerge as a result of incomprehensive initiatives, a natural bodily response to such emotional chaos is movement, an escape-pattern that gives the doctor time to contain the unbearable: not knowing what to do. Hence, the doctor's retrying-moving strategy is interpreted as a strategy for dealing with complexity (emotional, medical and interpersonal) and a strategy for manipulating the visual system to become able to perceive new affordances in a way that yields solutions. However, in this case the moving around does not expand her visual perception in a functional way. Fixation wins.

As the doctor does not call for assistance at an earlier stage, she enacts an activity pattern that allows error cycles to emerge. Her actions serve as positive feedback mechanisms, and as she gets no closer to any solution, time elapses and the patient suffers from pain and anxiety.

6. Understanding visual systems

I have discussed how perception is altered by an individual's ability to adapt flexibly to changes in the layout of affordances (Gibson 1979/86; Noë 2004). Thus, purposeful movement becomes an important strategy for manipulating the organism-environment system. In emergency medicine, moving in, out and around in problem-zones becomes an important strategy for exploring new solutions, solving problems and dealing with challenges and dilemmas. When challenges and hard problems emerge, roughly two interaction patterns are possible, (a) active, purposeful and anticipative manipulation of the organism-environment system or (b) fixation identified as either paralysis or random movement.

Learning includes an exploration phase, an exhibition phase where various strategies are tried out and finally the skill is learned and the activity becomes more fluid, automatic and effortless (Merlaeu-Ponty 2012, Dewey 1910). When practitioners have different cognitive resources for diagnosing and treating patients, they use the pre-designed medical artefacts differently. Their professional visual systems operate on the basis of experience, personality and situational factors and this leads to very different processes of behaviour. Also, as analysed in the first case, artefacts are not only used intentionally. Their mere object properties make a difference: They can serve as boundary markers, change the visual sensitivity and afford actions that are both functional and dysfunctional to the overall goal in these kinds of settings. I emphasised how the environment matters as regards visual perceptions and cognitive outcome. The materiality of the environment either constrains or expands a professional visual system. Some artefacts are tools that expand the peri-personal action space or enable certain tasks to be completed that could not be completed without the tool.

The analyses indicate how perception is a result of a sense-saturated visual system. The three cases revealed the diversity of medical visual systems in diagnostic situations that were caused by the practitioners' various level of expertise and adaptive flexibilities. Thus, perception depends on a visual system that is a spatio-temporally constituted ability to perceive and prioritise certain solutions over others. In similar task-based situations (cases where error cycles are present) various strategies are implied. In case 1, the erroneous actions penetrate the cheese (cf. Reason's Swiss cheese model, Chapter 1) in a way that results in human error (without anyone recognising them as such).

From a dialogical perspective, the team in the second case makes sense in a way that allows different individuals to co-act. An analysis of fine-scaled coordination and attunement of whole-bodied interaction through reciprocal adaptation reveals the core dynamics of human coaction. By emphasising the spatio-temporal, dialogical and embodied aspect of sense-making, I argued that the medical team constitutes a shared intentionality through dialogical sense-making based on the doctor's developed visual system in particular. Specifically, the doctor is a skilled and experienced doctor, and his professional visual system is shaped by experience, knowledge and real-time dynamics. As he initiates his movements, he actively manipulates the organism-environment system to sustain the best visual system. Due to his embodied historicity, he knows how (Ryle 1949) to be in the right place without consciously considering where the right place is. His actions are not explained as accidental and random but rather as sense-saturated. Merleau-Ponty argues that perception is less about explicit calculation than understanding movement:

> If I possess the habit of driving a car, then I enter into the lane and see that "I can pass" without comparing the width of the lane to that of the fender, just as I go through a door without comparing the width of the door to that of my body [...] Places in space are not defined as objective positions in relation to the objective position of our body, but rather they inscribe around us the variable reach of our intentions and our gestures. To habituate oneself to a hat, an automobile, or a cane is to take up residence in them, or inversely, to make them participate within the voluminosity of one's own body [...] One can know how to type without knowing how to indicate where on the keyboard the letters that compose the words are located. (Merleau-Ponty 2012: 144ff)

If perception is action, then moving towards something is a continuous process of being in the right place. The nature of medical vision is explained as a visual system that not only deals with the embodied experience, but a distributed experience, that transgresses individual, embodied, 'tacit' knowledge. Seeing is a whole-bodied sensorimotor skill that enables the doctor to adapt flexibly to the changes in the environment. An average person perceives a situation differently than the medical expert and hence he would move differently, placing himself in different position etc.

The excerpt above supports Noë's (2004) hypothesis based on the critique that conventional literature on perception has mistakenly assumed that phenomenology is about structures in the visual field. Instead he proposes: "We experience the world as unbounded and densely detailed because we do not inhabit a domain of visual snapshot-like fixations. [...] Vision is active; it is an active exploration of the world" (Noë 2004: 72). The doctor is able to apply his clinical abilities in a social practice of medical problem-solving. Sense-making is brought to life *in situ* (Linell 2009: 222), but it has often been explained retrospectively as a logical and mechanistic process as if it happens in a vacuum with clear boundaries and a beginning and an end:

> Of course, when the road has been travelled, we can glance over it, mark its direction [...] as if there had been pursuit of an end. [...] But, of the road which was going to be travelled, the human mind could have nothing to say, for the road has been created pari passu with the act of travelling over it, being nothing but the direction of this act itself. (Bergson 1911: 51)

According to Bergson, linear causation is behind us, and the creative nature of human life is in front of us. Following Dewey (1910) a cognitive system is enabled to act functionally according to the changes in its environment due to the information the system has gained over time. In other words, the team's coordination is sense-saturated (Steffensen 2013) and different from random movements. Random action does not necessarily manipulate anything. Thus timing, coordination and coaction are fundamental criteria for successful and purposive manipulation and recalibration. Such criteria require that we investigate the adaptive flexibility of a cognitive system rather than the behaviour of individuals. Knowing what to do, where to be, where to look and what to look for can be related to a degree of automaticity and fluidity of actions of the system. Ryle (1949) argues against the idea that there is a causal dependency between knowing *that* and knowing *how*. He argues that for an individual to know how to do something and to do it, has nothing to do with knowing the facts about how to accomplish it (Ryle 1949. Thus, the team's movement is an embodied, tacit and skilled knowledge.

As emphasised in the beginning of this chapter, visual systems are shaped by historically repeated interactions. By engaging in situations with repetitive features, the visual system is enhanced and primed to see certain actions and situations as affordances for problem-solving (Goodwin 1994; Gibson 1979/86). The enabling conditions are grounded in *repetition without repetition* as Bernstein famously said (Bernstein 1996: 204). This statement refers to a system's ability to see proper solutions in a wide range of task conditions of which a basic activity is repeated while the actions are adjusted and adapted to the situation. In this perspective, the goal is not to slavishly train stable and nearly identical stimuli, muscle forces, movements and other actions. Rather, the aim of training and education is successful realisation of values that is solved in ecologically real environments, in this case diagnostic processes in emergency settings where practitioners are subject to unpredictable changes (Ito 2011). The doctor's embodied historicity of being alert provides him with an ability to see small-scale changes that reduce his visual array no matter how different such small-scale changes might appear. Though each particular situation varies in many respects, the task (and momentarily the constraints) often takes on a similar contour. Repetition without repetition is sense-saturated (Steffensen 2013) and allows for flexible behaviour in goal realisation processes. If the movements were not sense-saturated, the goal would not be achieved in such a smooth and coordinated way. The team moulds the optic array and their joint movement serves as a negative feedback mechanism, the successfulness of which is defined by its anticipatory intentions, which facilitate fluid and smooth task performance. The successfulness of this team relates to its cognitive abilities to align its verbal utterances (a cognitive agenda of hypothesis generating) with movement (to secure visual contact with the patient). Much seems to be encountered and anticipated in a way that feeds back on the interaction so it never appears to be a problem. The claim that the doctor's successful, highly coordinated, anticipatory actions are based on repetitions without repetitions, is supported with a counterexample where a novice doctor moves without any purposive or convincing strategy, and where fixation and frustration prompt her to do merely *something*. The final case emphasises the operations of an undeveloped visual system in which the ability to solve a problem does not match the perceptual complexity of the situation. Thus, dilemmas arise, problems emerge, and the practitioner finds herself in a *forkedroad situation* (Dewey 1910), which prompts her to anticipate a possible change of plan. Frustration emerges as a result of positive feedback mechanisms in the cognitive system. However, although with an unsuccessful result, the doctor's moving-strategy is an embodied way of trying to manipulate the situation and move out of a problem-zone.

Understanding the processes of becoming a master within a discipline is key to facilitating and scaffolding learning. If repetitive situations and task performances reshape our perception and make professionals revise their concepts and thinking in general (Kirsh 2013; Noë 2010), we need to describe *how* this happens. Importantly, a visual system can be developed in many ways: through intuition-based probing, as in the latter case, but also by letting an experienced practitioner guide a novice (facilitation). In the latter proposal, the visual system is efficiently informed and developed. Finally, visual perception has less to do with processes of representation than being aware of how and what can be manipulated (Gibson 1979/86; Noë 2004, 2010; Pedersen and Steffensen 2014).

CHAPTER 5

The function of procedures in the diagnostic process

Anamnesis and physical examination

1. The function of procedures

This chapter investigates how the role and use of procedures are related to the prevention or emergence of human error cycles. By so doing, it investigates how doctors manage to balance multiple expectations during history taking and physical examination by relying on procedures, guidelines and medical protocols. The chapter further questions the systemic function of such tools and it scrutinises what makes them vital in some diagnostic processes and dysfunctional in others. Understanding how procedures on the one hand scaffold medical decision-making and on the other constrain such processes, is crucial to enhance patient safety and to develop suitable educational practices.

Coming up with a valid diagnosis in the emergency ward involves an assessment process where various clinical methods, procedures and protocols are used. Overall, the medical team needs to balance both medical and interpersonal aspects in interaction. Specifically, they are required to (a) collect data about the patient's medical history, real-time problems and experienced symptoms (anamnesis), (b) to examine the patient via palpation and/or auscultation, (c) to come up with a diagnosis and a plan for further treatment and (d) to register and document relevant information in the electronic medical record (Miller and Sim 2004). This chapter zooms in on the initial part of the diagnostic process and focuses on how doctors manage anamnesis and in one case also physical examination by relying on procedures in various ways.

During anamnesis the practitioner is expected to cover specific areas of the patient's general situation and document the results in the electronic record. The procedures in anamnesis cover information about: reason for hospitalisation, the patient's actual situation, circumstances related to infectious diseases, work situation, travels abroad, allergies, previous medical history, actual medical issues, information about organ systems and related medical issues (dizziness, headaches etc.), tobacco, drug and alcohol intake, social circumstances and functional level. Besides the anamnesis (the patient's narrative) the practitioner needs to document information based on objective examination. Such information covers the practitioner's interpretation of the patient's general health condition (state of nutrition, age appropriate condition, skin colour, temperature, level of consciousness etc.). Multiple clinical conditions must be documented in the record. Some of the conditions are based on observation and others are based on measurements and physical examination.[1]

During anamnesis there are several nested tasks the doctor must attend to in order to accomplish the task efficiently and dialogically. First, the doctor needs to make the patient feel as comfortable as possible and establish trust, which enables him to generate links between the perceived medical situation, objective measurements and the patient's narrative. Second, as resources are limited, the healthcare practitioner must continuously prioritise and guide the patient towards the medical relevant points in the interaction. Third, the information must be interpreted in relation to the real-time medical measurements and further translated into medical categories that can be shared with other healthcare professionals. As will be shown in the analyses, it is crucial that the practitioner picks up relevant information in a way that guides action and yields cognitive results. Within the emergency ward multiple written protocols are developed to structure the respective clinical tasks in the overall diagnostic process. Such protocols need to be followed in practice and their functions have been discussed in various studies. For instance, Angeli (2015) emphasises: "Participants memorized protocols and guidelines and drew on this memorized, professional knowledge to treat patients [...] Protocols allowed participants to reduce cognitive workload and focus on the patient" (Angeli 2015: 28). Based on an ethnographic study Angeli emphasises that without protocols the organisation would break down. While acknowledging the importance and necessity of procedures and protocols I also challenge the profound positive and simplistic understanding of such performance aids and I discuss the consequences of relying on such procedures in various contexts. Finally, I discuss procedures in relation to conventional understandings of interaction and I emphasise the importance of dealing with embodied resources in procedure following situations.

In this context procedures encompass standards originating from protocols and clinical and communicative guidelines. Protocols and medical guidelines have been defined within the literature as "official standardized treatment plans" (Angeli 2015: 3). Further, each patient condition has its own protocol, e.g. cardiac arrest, respiratory arrest, sprained ankle (cf. Angeli 2015). Communicative guidelines refer to procedures often learned outside the classroom and they are

1. This information is based on internal instructions. I am not allowed to attach the original written instructions for internal use at the ward.

not regulated in the same way as medical protocols. However, they function in the same way and provide a set of fixed expectations about proper performance. Angeli (2015) argues that such expectations facilitate communication as script and protocol structure responses.

During these activities, skilled doctors ensure that the patient is aware of the direction, intention and results of the nested tasks. Accomplishing the cognitive task (anamnesis) and at the same time balancing nested tasks, depend on procedures. Again, the way procedures are embedded and relied upon relates to medical expertise and general experience. In emergency settings, a great deal of prior experience is distilled in action procedures that are constructed ahead of time in that they serve to structure future situations. In a similar vein Hutchins (1995a: 165ff) discusses how "precomputations are saved representational structures that transform the nature of the task performance [...] Each of these precomputations is a way of building local invariants into the structure of the tools that are used in the performance of the navigation task." Similarly, at the emergency ward, expectations and rules for behaviour serve as local invariants intended for structuring the clinical encounter. For instance, doctors and nurses are trained in structured medical history taking and they are taught consultation skills, communication strategies and related standard operating procedures such as ISBAR[2] and ABC-procedures.[3] Angeli (2015) argues that within emergency medical services communication (EMS), healthcare professionals collaborate by relying on non-situational professional memory "which is comprised of textbook knowledge and protocols that EMS professionals learn during training. Collaborative memory refers to the process of individuals working together on the same task, remembering pieces of information, and gathering that information together to complete an activity" (Angeli 2015: 10ff). Such memory aiding protocols are designed to release cognitive powers and to automatise action and perception with a minimum of cognitive effort in situations where cognitive resources are scarce, for instance due to a high level of stress or time pressure. Further, the aim is to standardise and automatise outputs to narrow the risk of human errors. Thus, inherent in the procedures is a set of pre-made decisions and action plans that leave minimal room for reflection, but a huge responsibility for rule following. Procedures, just as tools and abstract information structures, serve many purposes depending on how they are managed (Klein 2008). While the use of such aids releases cognitive power and guides

2. ISBAR is an abbreviation for: Identification, Situation, Background, Analysis, Advice (*Råd* in Danish). The protocol has been developed by the Danish Society for Patient Safety.

3. ABC is an abbreviation for: Airways, Breathing, Circulation. This protocol serves as a memory aid when dealing with the unresponsive patient. The three functions are vital to the maintenance for the patient's life and they constitute a priority for assessment, diagnosis and treatment.

practitioners to achieve their goals, analysis reveals that they also constrain situational sensitivity and paralyse practitioners in situations where the unexpected happens – and at worst, increase the risk of human error.

Overall, the current chapter pivots on challenges in anamnesis and physical examination that relate to competing requirements to balance (a) efficient problem-solving with a dialogical and caring approach, (b) invariant procedures with adaptive flexible behaviour and (c) system expectations with patient requirements. The chapter uses two cases to investigate how the use of procedures results in functional or dysfunctional outcomes and how they relate to the emergence or prevention of error cycles. Specifically, the cases describe how cognitive events emerge and are managed as practitioners use procedures, tools and their bodies (a) to organise and structure the patient narratives, (b) to gain precise information, (c) to structure memory processes, and (d) as a means to reduce patient insecurity.

The first case is an example of best practice. It underlines how an experienced doctor manages procedure following in a flexible way that allows for creative and dynamic decision-making as he uses his body as a dynamic tool for adapted and situated procedure following. The second case, in contrast, illustrates how a novice doctor is forced to replace a task heterarchy with a rule-following hierarchy by prioritising standard procedures over local demands for interaction. Altogether, the chapter investigates how the practitioners rely on non-local procedures and norms to extend and scaffold decision-making in situated and artefact-rich interaction. Furthermore, dialogical approaches afford elaboration of micro-sociological findings as for instance how patient and practitioner are unable to coordinate turn-takings.

2. Case I: Enacting and discarding procedures

This case emphasises how procedures can be secondary to patients and modulated to fit the overall situation. That means that standard and fixed procedures are always latent in the professional's mind and discarded or adjusted as a result of an experienced practitioner's flexible behaviour. Because procedures relate to standard situations, their general applicability inhibits sensitivity to situational particularities and deviances if they are followed slavishly and function as a fixed hierarchy for actions. The following case demonstrates how an experienced doctor is able to balance procedures, medical knowledge and emerging affordances all at once. Attention is given to the points in the cognitive trajectory where the doctor realises that the working hypothesis is insufficient, and a new strategy is needed; these points are characterised as insights or breakthroughs that have consequences for what happens next. Specifically, attention is given to (a) how the doctor gets information that enables a diagnostic outcome as he meshes anamnesis with physical examination, (b) how he tests hypotheses by linking the patient's knowledge to medical procedures and perceptual insights achieved through whole-bodied interaction, (c) how he guides the patient's narrative by indicating what is irrelevant in order to reach a diagnosis efficiently and professionally, (d) how he uses the patient as an important cognitive resource as he relies on his own body as a dynamical tool for adapted procedure following and, finally, (e) how procedures are part of his automatised, skilled behaviour in a way that releases cognitive powers for situational cognition leading to functional task performance. Below is an illustration of the setting.

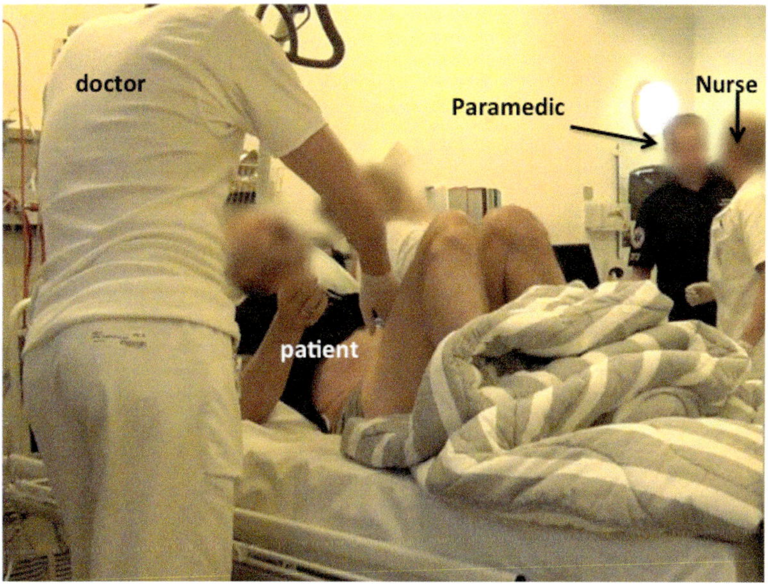

Figure 5.1 Overview of the layout: The abdominal patient

2.1 Beyond fixed procedures: Meshing anamnesis with physical examination

As we enter this conversation, the doctor has just received information from the ambulance team who handed the patient over to the medical team. The doctor is an experienced young man and the patient is a middle-aged man with no significant medical history. Under transportation to the hospital he has complained about severe stomach ache and diarrhoea and he has had several intense stomach cramps. The patient has a very low pulse rate, which is discussed several times during his stay in the ward. When he arrives, he is still in great pain and he has difficulties breathing, which impedes his speech and his power of concentration. The medical team initiates the diagnostic task and works with an abdominal patient hypothesis.

Transcript 5.1[4]
Danish original

```
1. 03:55:80, D:    KAN DU PRØVE AT PEGE PÅ MAVEN HVOR DET GØR ONDT HENNE
2. 03:57:80, P:    °°.h°°
3. 03:58:90, D:    ER DET HER ↑OPPE
4. 04:00:00, P:    ja (.) det der der det er det (.) det er ikke dernede det er fint
                   (.) min min (xxx) det er fint (.)
5. 04:06:60, D:    °°det er fint°°
6. 04:07:60, ps.   (3.3)
7. 04:10:90, D:    ER DET OPPE I BRYSTET ELLER ER DET NEDE I MAVEN DU HAR ONDT=
8. 04:12:90, P:    =det er oppe i brystet
9. 04:13:90, D:    DET ER OPPE I BRYSTET (.) HAR DU SLET IKKE ONDT HER NEDE I MAVEN
10. 04:17:70, P:   ne:j .h (.) jeg er holdt op med at ta:ge (.) medicin (.) øh (.)
                   søndag middag (.) de de:r øh Pinex
11. 04:26:50, D:   ↓ja
12. 04:27:00, P:   og de f. (x[xx)
13. 04:29:60, D:             [DU HAR HAFT MASSER AF DIARRÉ ik os
14. 04:30:90, P:   ja: øh ja
15. 04:32:20, D:   gennem det sidste døgn
16. 04:33:10, P:   narj (.) siden klokken to i nat (.) der har jeg men det har ikke
                   været det har ikke været sådan noget (.) vandligt
17. 04:39:20, D:   nej
18. 04:40:00, P:   men det (.) det er gået nemt .h
19. 04:42:90, D:   men det er jo maven ik
20. 04:44:00, P:   jo
21. 04:44:50, D:   nu siger du du har ondt i brystet
22. 04:46:30, P:   det (.) kramper heroppe
23. 04:47:60, D:   det kramper her
24. 04:48:70, P:   ja
25. 04:48:90, D:   og her
26. 04:49:60, P:   ja og den ene skulder også
27. 04:51:60, D:   og den ene skulder (.)↓o:kay
28. 04:52:90, ps.  (1.0)
29. 04:53:90, D:   har du ondt heroppe i brystet (touching)
30. 04:55:50, ps.  (1.0)
31. 04:56:50, P:   ne:j .h
32. 04:57:20, D:   nej (.) har du udstråling til armen (touching)
33. 04:59:00, P:   ne:j det synes jeg ik[ke
34. 04:59:70, D:   [har du åndenød (.)
```

4. *PM* is an abbreviation for paramedic; ges is an abbreviation for gesture.

35. 05:01:50, P: når det kramper så øh (.) [så øh så har jeg svært ved at trække vejret i bund

36. 05:02:80, D: [så kramper det

37. 05:05:10, D: ja (.) og så stråler det op ud til skulderen herومme bagpå

38. 05:08:20, P: ja

39. 05:08:80, D: okay (.) så prøv at peg med fingeren hvor det det gør mest ondt

40. 05:12:70, ges: (P points)

41. 05:14:80, D: der tværs over o:kay (.) ja men vi bestiller et EKG for en sikkerheds skyld men mit umiddelbare indtryk er at det i:kke er noget kardionalt (.) men nu må vi jo lige se

42. 05:22:60, PM: ja

43. 05:23:00, D: der er også visse point må man sige til noget abdominalt

44. 05:26:00, PM: (xxx)

45. 05:28:10, D: ja

46. 05:29:00, P: der er pissekoldt mand (.)

47. 05:31:50, D: ja (.) vi skal nok få varmet dig op

48. 05:33:10, ps. (2.1) (D covers P with the duvet)

49. 05:35:20, D: prøv at lægge benene ned

50. 05:36:30, ps. (2.5)

51. 05:38:80, D: har du haft feber derhjemme (.)

52. 05:40:30, P: ja:eh lige f jeg sad og sf ja (.) jeg svedte af helvede til

English translation

1. 03:55:80, D: PLEASE POINT AT YOUR STOMACH WHERE IT HURTS

2. 03:57:80, P: °°.h°°

3. 03:58:90, D: IS IT UP ↑HERE

4. 04:00:00, P: yes (.) that there that that is (.) it is not down there that is fine (.) my my (xxx) that is fine (.)

5. 04:06:60, D: °°that is fine°°

6. 04:07:60, ps. (3.3)

7. 04:10:90, D: IS IT UP IN THE CHEST OR IS IT DOWN IN THE STOMACH YOU FEEL PAIN=

8. 04:12:90, P: =it is up in the chest

9. 04:13:90, D: IT IS UP IN THE CHEST (.) YOU DO NOT FEEL ANY PAIN DOWN HERE IN THE STOMACH

10. 04:17:70, P: no: .h (.) I just stopped taki:ng (.) medication (.) eh Sunday midday (.) tho:se eh Pinex

11. 04:26:50, D: ↓yes

12. 04:27:00, P: and they f. (x[xx)

13. 04:29:60, D: [YOU HAVE HAD A LOT OF DIARRHOEA right

14. 04:30:90, P: ye:s eh yes

15. 04:32:20, D: over the last 24 hours

16. 04:33:10, P: no: (.) since 2 am this night (.) then I have but it has not been it has not been kind of (.) watery

17. 04:39:20, D: no

```
18. 04:40:00, P:   but it (.) has been coming easily .h
19. 04:42:90, D:   but that is the stomach right
20. 04:44:00, P:   yes
21. 04:44:50, D:   now you are saying that you have pains in the chest
22. 04:46:30, P:   it (.) cramps up here
23. 04:47:60, D:   it cramps up here
24. 04:48:70, P:   yes
25. 04:48:90, D:   and here
26. 04:49:60, P:   yes and the one shoulder as well
27. 04:51:60, D:   and the one shoulder (.)↓o:kay
28. 04:52:90, ps.  (1.0)
29. 04:53:90, D:   do you have any pain up here in the chest (touching)
30. 04:55:50, ps.  (1.0)
31. 04:56:50, P:   no: .h
32. 04:57:20, D:   no (.) do you have any pain radiating to the arm (touching)
33. 04:59:00, P:   no: I do not think [so
34. 04:59:70, D:                      [any difficulty breathing (.)
35. 05:01:50, P:   when it cramps then eh (.) [then eh I have difficulty breathing
                   fully
36. 05:02:80, D:                              [when it cramps
37. 05:05:10, D:   yes (.) and then it spreads up out to the shoulder here at the back
38. 05:08:20, P:   yes
39. 05:08:80, D:   okay (.) try to point with your finger where it hurts the most
40. 05:12:70, ges: (P points)
41. 05:14:80, D:   across there o:kay (.) yes but we will order an EKG just to be sure
but
                   my immediate impression is that this is no:t something cardiologic
                   (.) but now we will wait and see
42. 05:22:60, PM:  ves
43. 05:23:00, D:   there are also certain points one may say to something abdominal
44. 05:26:00, PM:  (xxx)
45. 05:28:10, D:   yes
46. 05:29:00, P:   it is freezing man (.)
47. 05:31:50, D:   yes (.) we will get you warm again
48. 05:33:10, ps.  (2.1) (D covers P with the duvet)
49. 05:35:20, D:   please put your legs down
50. 05:36:30, ps.  (2.5)
51. 05:38:80, D:   did you have any fever at home (.)
52. 05:40:30, P:   yea:eh just f I sat and sf yes (.) I was sweating like hell
```

Right after the doctor has greeted the patient, he asks him to *show* specifically where it hurts: *PLEASE POINT AT YOUR STOMACH WHERE IT HURTS*, line 1. The history taking is immediately initiated in a way that requires the patient to use a whole-bodied approach, which enables precise identification of the current medical problem. As the patient locates his pain with his hand, he responds with an embodied deictic rather than with a linguistic category such as "the chest", "breast", "upper body" or "the right side". The answer turns out to be tricky as the original starting point (abdominal medical issues) is now expanded to incorporate further symptoms and hence even more possible and complex cause-effect relationships. Thus, the moment the patient touches his chest is identified as an event pivot that prompts the doctor to clarify, re-evaluate and determine whether the patient suffers from one or the other medical condition. Specifically, he tests the two hypotheses six times during the next excerpt (see Figure 5.2)

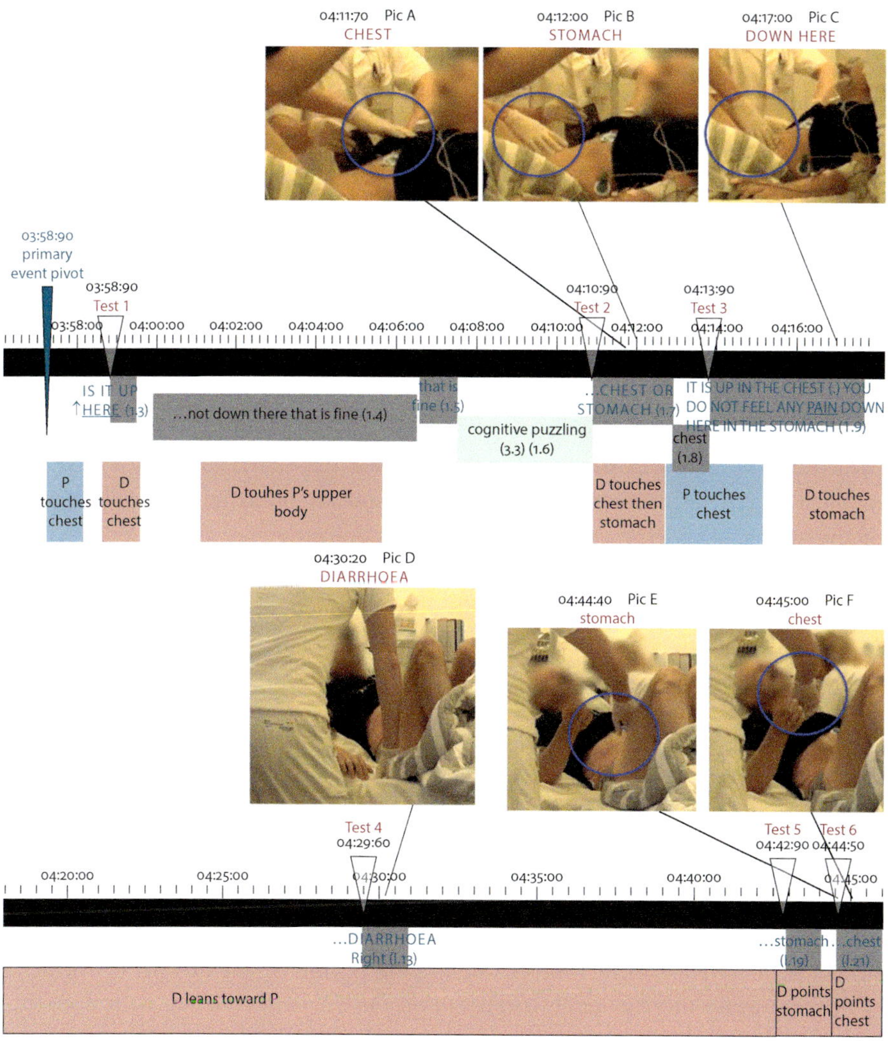

Figure 5.2 Embodied procedures in hypothesis generation

The figure illustrates how the doctor tests two competing hypotheses as he relies on embodied expertise. As he re-evaluates the medical situation, he meshes physical examination and history taking. This process is defined as a clarification task, methodologically identified as a breakthrough phase in which the doctor links new insight with non-local information, real-time perceptions and medical expertise.

First, the doctor double-checks that the patient is certain about the location. He poses a counter question *IS IT UP ↑HERE* (line 3). The emphasis on the ↑*HERE*, and the rising intonation indicate an element of surprise. As the patient confirms, the doctor acknowledges this new information, and a lapse of 3.3 seconds emerges (line 6) and the doctor freezes. The remarkably long lapse indicates a cognitive puzzling and marks a transition phase in the interactivity trajectory. Before the lapse, the patient and the doctor engaged in history taking. However, as the doctor after a first validation test (see Figure 5.2), realises that the situation is not as straightforward as anticipated the realisation serves as an affordance for re-evaluation. During the 3.3 seconds the doctor's cognitive puzzling has significance for how he continues the task performance. After the lapse a different strategy is enacted, and the doctor meshes history taking with physical examination to validate and generate hypotheses about medical issues. As the doctor meshes the two tasks, he is able to contrast the patient's narrative with perceived information achieved through physical examination.

The doctor tests the patient's localisation of pain a second time by giving him the choice to articulate which body part (the chest or the stomach) is related to his pain (line 7). When the doctor asks the question explicitly, he also uses his own medical expertise to identify and locate the specific areas that define the areas of the stomach and the chest respectively by pointing specifically to each area with his fingers (see picture A and B above). When the doctor selects concrete areas of the body and demarcates them through touch, he also allows the patient to relate the area of touch to the area of pain in real time rather than relying on pure memory.

The doctor relies just as much on the information he sees and senses as what he hears. To paraphrase Foucault (1973), he uses 'the ear of his finger' in direct perception of the patient's symptoms. The information he perceives by gazing at the patient's deictic gestures and locations of touch, prompts him to work with two competing hypotheses concerning two medical scenarios, with two different patient categories: the abdominal patient as initially hypothesised, and the cardiologic patient as hypothesised through the interaction with the patient. As the doctor now works with two competing hypotheses, he systematically investigates which one seems more evident than the other. As will be shown below, he does this by (a) using the patient as a cognitive resource, (b) using his own body encompassing touch, gesture, voice, gaze and posture to gain comprehensive information about the patient's medical condition, (c) meshing examination and anamnesis and (d) explicating reasoning during the task performance.

General procedures in the diagnostic process dictate structural steps, for instance to complete anamnesis before examination, and to follow general guidelines for information retrieval. According to this procedure, the first step is to welcome the patient. However, this doctor barely introduces himself before he meshes anamnesis with examination. Picture C illustrates how the doctor examines the patient's stomach as he tests the medical claim a third time: *YOU DO NOT FEEL ANY PAIN DOWN HERE IN THE STOMACH*. He examines the abdominal wall with his fingertips in order to identify possible abdominal tenderness. The patient is encouraged to explicate his experience as the doctor compares it to medical measurements (the result of the palpation). The doctor's experience is identified in his adaptive behaviour. First, he relies on what he perceives *in situ*, and he is able to adapt to the situation by meshing two tasks as this proves useful according to the situation. However, no procedure in the ward accounts for the function of meshing tasks; rather they dictate an action hierarchy, for instance following protocols and procedures for the abdominal patient and the cardiac patient, respectively. Further, such procedures are saturated with what Linell (2005) defines as the written language bias. Communicative procedures within the anamnesis process are developed with an exclusive focus on verbal information retrieval, for instance which questions to ask in a pre-defined sequential order. In the following, it is exemplified how the doctor both relies on standard medical procedures as he asks standard questions and guides the patient's narrative, and how he also relies on inter-bodily dynamics as he uses gaze, touch and gestures as crucial means in anamnesis. While the doctor's embodied task performance is functional and effective, it is rarely discussed comprehensively in educational programmes or protocols.

As the doctor is not yet convinced of which of the working hypotheses should be excluded, the highest priority in the diagnostic task is to clarify which body part the medical condition relates to. This prioritisation is seen in the way the doctor balances multiple constraints in the situation and specifically in (a) the way he guides the patient's narrative, (b) how he relies on standard procedures to clarify cause-effect relations and (c) how he circumvents fixed procedures by relying on embodied resources and inter-bodily dynamics. By so doing, the doctor adapts to the situation by initiating what appears to be the most efficient move in order to achieve the goal as efficiently and precisely as possible without losing sensitivity and without performing in a recipe-like fashion.

When the patient embarks upon a narrative concerning his intake of Pinex, (line 10 and 12), the doctor interrupts, changes the subject and tests the medical symptoms in relation to previous medical conditions: *YOU HAVE HAD A LOT OF*

DIARRHOEA right. And again later on: *but that is the stomach right* as he touches the domain of the stomach with his fingers to relate his question to a physical area that can be felt immediately by the patient (picture E). The patient confirms that his diarrhoea relates to problems with the stomach. And the doctor then explicates what appears to be a medical inconsistency as he comments: *now you are saying that you have pains in the chest* (line 21) (Figure 5.2, Picture F).

Again, the patient uses his hand to locate where it hurts as he utters: *it (.) cramps up here*, (line 22). In what follows, the doctor repeats and puts emphasis on the: <u>here</u>, (line 23). Rather than referring to a distinct part of the patient's body

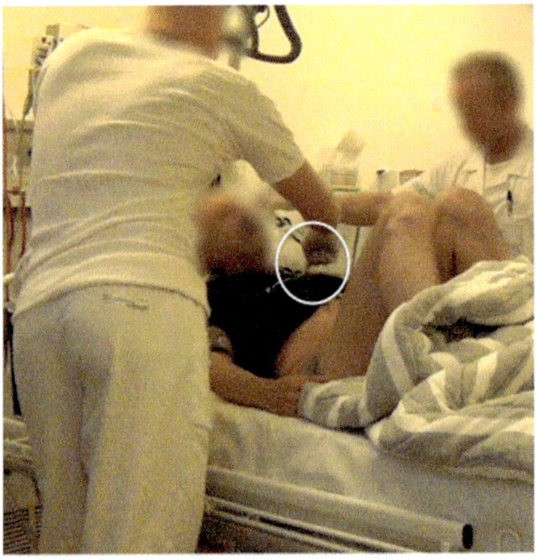

Picture G– time: 04:58:10
l. 32, D: no (.) do you have any pain

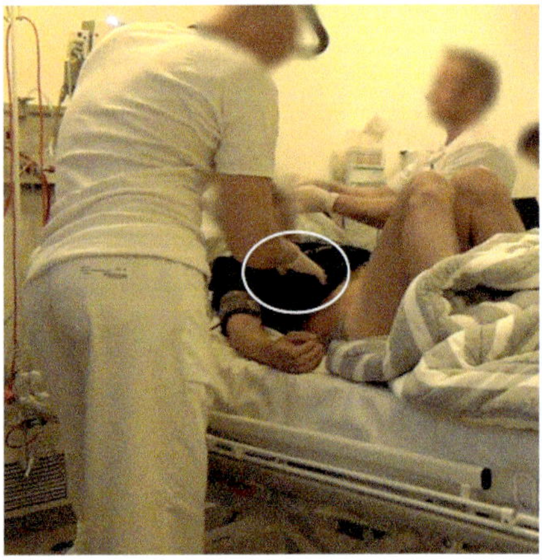

Picture H – time: 05:00:00
l. 34, D: [any difficulty breathing (.) radiating to the arm

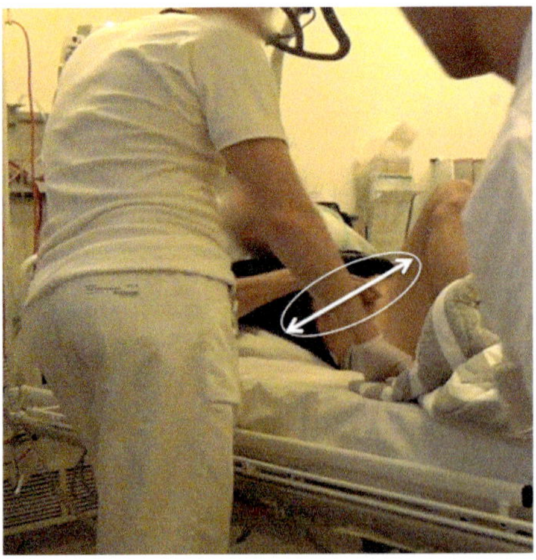

Picture I – time: 05:14:10
l. 40, (P locates the area with his hand)

(*there*), the doctor puts himself in the position of the patient. By touching the patient's chest as he utters here he minimises the distance between them, because he meshes the patient's explanations with his own perceptions through touch. Finally, the doctor validates the seriousness of the patient's chest pain symptoms by asking a few standard questions as he touches the physical body areas to underline the movement of pain, the directions of pain and the precise location within the body part (see picture G, H and I).

This embodied strategy affords a dynamic, interactive and participatory behaviour from the patient as the doctor asks the patient, not to tell, but to *show* where it hurts (line 1 and 39).

It is complicated to articulate the feeling of pain and its exact location; thus other strategies – such as pointing and touching – can turn out to be helpful.[5] Interestingly, the patient does not immediately recall the location and it takes him a moment to identify the right location (see picture I). For 8.5 seconds the patient moves the tip of his fingers back and forth on his stomach to narrow down the area. Because he is able to use his body actively in the diagnostic process, the relevant location is prompted through actions (a felt place) rather than through pure mental simulation. Touching is a means for enacting non-local experience as real-time perception is linked with bodily experience (Noë 2004, 2010). The patient identifies not only the area of pain, but also the direction and movement of the pain he perceives. This approach equips the doctor with valuable information, since horizontal pain movements are related to some cases of illnesses and not to others. The approach is useful and provides the doctor with vital information that makes him change his current hypothesis once again. Initially the abdominal hypothesis that originated from background information from the paramedical team was replaced with the cardiac patient hypothesis which was generated on the basis of the patient's localisation of the pain in his chest. Finally, after gaining further insight into the patient's narrative combined with physical examination, the symptoms point in the direction of an abdominal medical condition (see line 41). Rather than being an unreliable patient, it is common that the average patient is not aware of the exact boundary between physiologically defined body parts, as for instance the exact domain of the stomach and the chest, the sternum and the ribs etc. Thus, rather than relying on verbal language as the only means for history taking, the doctor draws on his experience and uses his body as a coordinating

5. There are examples of guidelines that include the use of gestures, for instance in a chapter on palpation: "Ask patients with abdominal pain to point to the area of greatest pain. Then reassure them that you will try to minimize their discomfort and examine that point last" (Ferguson 1990: 474). However, in such interpretations gestures are used as a means of sequential information gathering rather than dynamical possibilities for coaction.

tool. Such a whole-bodied approach is useful in reaching efficient and relevant information about the patient's medical situation. However, standard procedures in diagnostic tasks are biased by the view that language is the primary tool for representing information. This doctor actively searches for answers by relying on inter-bodily dynamics. As the patient is an integral part of the cognitive system, the diagnostic process is characterised by joint interactivity rather than individuals engaging in question-answer sequences. This approach enhances efficiency and coordination in the diagnostic process, and it leads to a useful result: as the patient locates the pain across the stomach, the doctor perceives just enough information to reach a preliminary decision and move on, (line 41). The doctor orders an

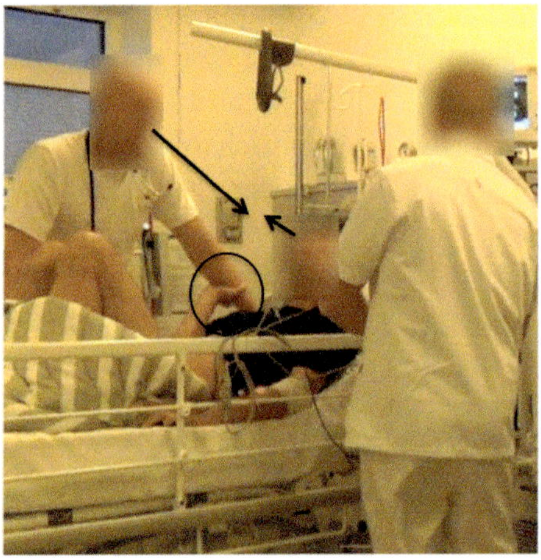

Picture L – time: 05:31:40
l. 46, P: it is freezing man (.)

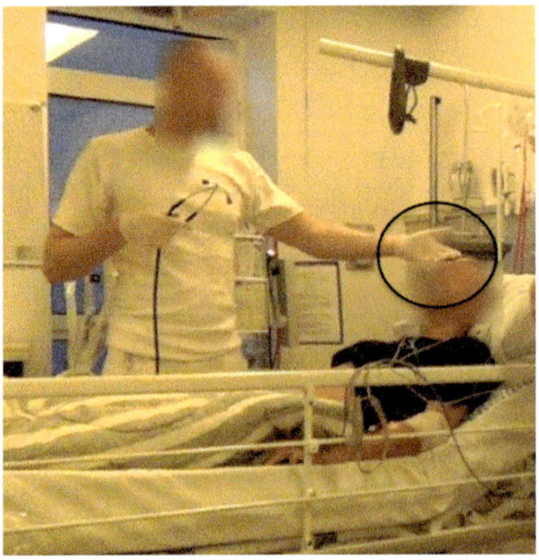

Picture M – time: 05:39:50
l. 51, D: did you have any fever at home (.)

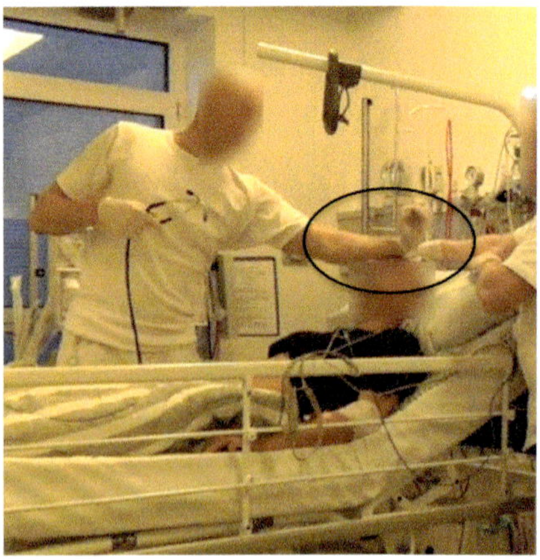

Picture N – time: 05:41:10
l. 52, P: yeah just f I sat and

EKG, as he has not been able to eliminate the possibility of cardiac problems even though he is convinced that the medical condition relates to abdominal issues. The breakthrough leads to a new, broader cognitive focus. The doctor asks general questions and initiates obligatory examination procedures.

However, as there are standard procedures that must be followed – some information is always needed – other procedures are optional. When the patient grabs the doctor's arm as he utters that he is freezing (see picture L), the doctor is prompted to check the patient's temperature. He relies on his own body temperature to decide if the patient's temperature is critical. However, his first attempt is constrained by the latex gloves he wears (see picture M), and he immediately uses the backside of his wrist to perceive the warmth directly (see picture N).

In standard cases, healthcare practitioners rely on material equipment when measuring medical values. Indeed, a thermometer is, in principle, more precise than a wrist, but this doctor uses a less precise, yet less time-consuming approach as he uses the temperature of his own body to gauge the temperature of the patient's body. By doing this, he avoids wasting time on getting hold of a thermometer and can instead continue the flow of interaction without interruption. The doctor's behaviour indicates an efficient prioritisation of the relevance and function of medical, nested tasks in relation to the overall goal. In this case, it seems important at first to state whether the patient has a fever or not. However, immediately after this activity, the doctor needs to listen to the patient's lungs, which involves the use of his stethoscope. During this task, he starts thinking aloud and he rephrases the medical puzzle related to the patient's low pulse rate in a way that leads to valuable results.

2.2 Think-aloud strategics: Verbal utterances as material anchors[6]

A final example of how best practice involves activities that are not accounted for in protocols and guidelines relates to how a think-aloud strategy and overt cognitive puzzling can lead to valuable insights in task accomplishment (van Someren et al. 1994). In particular, the following excerpt involves a situation in which the same doctor from the situation before listens to the patient's lungs when the electronic equipment above the patient's head starts beeping. Apparently the beeping alerts the medical team about the patient's pulse rate, which has been low during the whole episode, and even in the ambulance. The reason for the

6. Sections 5.2.2–5.2.3 were originally published as "Insights and their Emergence in Everyday Practices: The Interplay between Problems and Solutions in emergency medicine" in *Pragmatics & Cognition* 24, 2017. It is reused here with permission of John Benjamins: https://www.benjamins.com/catalog/pc and the co-author, Per Linell.

low pulse is unknown at the time, but as the doctor uses a think-aloud-approach, he solves the problem.

It is hypothesised that thinking aloud when challenges and problems emerge, increases the chances for problem-solving due to the transitory structural and quasi-stabilising qualities of verbal articulation. Compared to abstract reasoning (Clark 2008), verbal articulation has a local materiality, whichincreases the ability to engage in cognitive manipulation as utterances are activities, and activities change the world. To support this hypothesis, I draw on Hutchins' (2005) idea of material anchors, Kirsh and Maglio's (1994) notion of epistemic actions and Clark's (2008) notion of linguaform thinking.

Hutchins defines material anchors in relation to external cues such as annotations and material artefacts: "I call an input space from which material structure is projected into a blend a 'material anchor' for the blend. The term material anchor is meant to emphasize the stabilizing role of the material structure" (Hutchins 2005: 1555). I refer to thinking aloud as a strategy for creating material anchor points that facilitate complex cognitive problem-solving. Utterances are locally perceivable in interaction and as we do things with words, we change situations and perceive them in a way that can be useful for task accomplishment. Torre (2014) characterises written annotations as material anchors for future action, and Fauconnier and Turner (2002) similarly investigate verbal and written language as material anchors. Hutchins (2005) hesitates to define written and verbal language as material anchors, but the crucial point, in my view, is not to mistake words as material anchors for the concepts they represent. It is the physical act of articulating wordings that functions as a material anchor.

In a similar vein, Kirsh and Maglio (1994) describe how skilled Tetris players move a Tetrazoid before they have decided where to place it. They describe such moves as having an epistemic function: "These actions are not used to implement a plan [...] or reaction; they are used to change the world in order to simplify the problem-solving task" (Kirsh and Maglio 1994: 513). Finally, Clark (2008) hypothesises that "in addition to the important cognitive-affective role of inner dialogue, there may also be cases in which verbal rehearsal supports a kind of perceptual restructuring via the controlled disposition of attention" (Clark 2008: 48).

In what follows, I show how a think-aloud strategy serves as cognitive scaffolding rather than as a communicative purpose as the doctor suddenly links a problem with a solution. This situation pivots on the cognitive benefit from thinking aloud when cognitive challenges emerge, and that much is gained by investigating what practitioners do beyond procedure-following. As we enter this interaction, the doctor is being reminded about the unsolved problem as the equipment warns the team about the critical medical values.

Transcript 5.2
Danish original Excerpt 2

94. 06:29:80, ps. (7.6) (D examines P with the stethoscope and the surveillance monitor bibs)
95. 06:37:40, D: altså selvom han har en hå han har en pu øh en puls på 46 han er altså også i (xxx)behandling som sænker hans puls
96. 06:43:30, ps. (0.4)
97. 06:43:70, D: så det er formentligt derfor
98. 06:44:70, ps. (1.8) (D listens to P's lungs)

English translation Excerpt 2

94. 06:29:80, ps. (7.6) (D examines P with the stethoscope and the surveillance monitor bibs)
95. 06:37:40, D: well even if he has a ho he has a pu eh a pulse rate at 46 he is also in (xxx) treatment right which lowers his pulse
96. 06:43:30, ps. (0.4)
97. 06:43:70, D: so that is presumably the reason why
98. 06:44:70, ps. (1.8) (D listens to P's lungs)

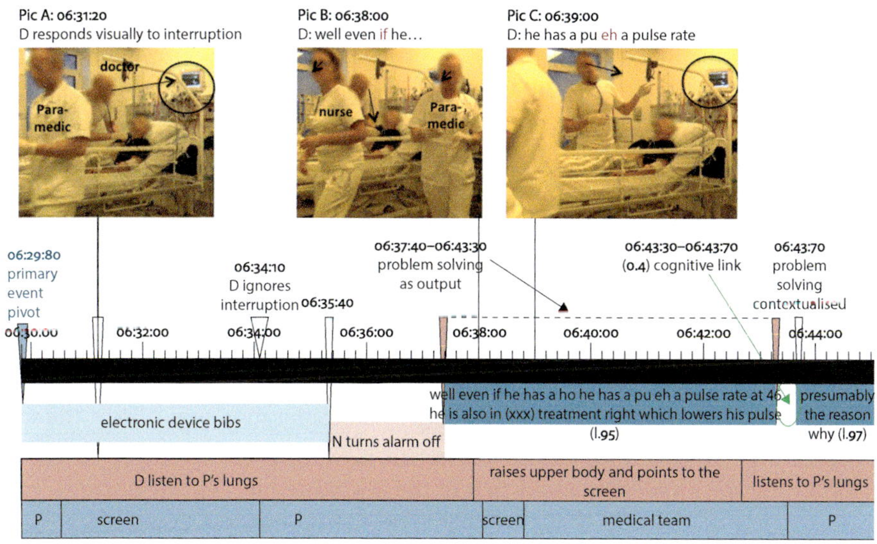

Figure 5.3 Thinking aloud as a cognitive strategy
The dark blue layer indicates the doctor's vocal utterances; the pink layer indicates the doctor's actions; the light blue layer indicates the doctor's gaze.

Figure 5.3 visualises how the doctor balances task performance (patient examination) with emergent information about the patient's unclear condition (the values appearing on the screen). As he engages in task performance, he combines procedure following with a thinking-aloud strategy that affords new perceptions with consequences for how a locally nested problem (the patient's low pulse rate) is understood. As the doctor initiates the examination, he gazes at the patient's chest. The surveillance equipment starts to beep, and it continues for 5.60 seconds. The doctor responds to the interruption through gaze 0.8 seconds after the equipment starts beeping (see Figure 5.3, picture A). The beeping serves as an event pivot and it guides the doctor's attention towards the screen even though he continues to listen to the patient's lungs. He gazes in the direction of the screen for 3.5 seconds, perceives the values on the screen and then gazes back at the patient's chest. The doctor contains the demanding disturbance and 5.60 seconds after the beeping started, the nurse responds and stops it. The doctor does not switch tasks but prioritises the continuation of what he is doing (see Figure 5.3, picture B). However, with a delay he does orient to the previous beeping – the event pivot that is crucial for the changes in the interactivity trajectory – and he begins to utter: *well even if he has a ho- he has a pu- eh pulse rate at 46 he is also in (xxx) treatment right which lowers his pulse* (line 2). Just as he initiates this utterance, he raises his upper body, stops examining the patient and continues to talk as he gazes briefly at the screen and then towards the medical team for several seconds (see Figure 5.3, picture C). Cognitively, he interrupts his own examination task and he shifts from listening to the lungs to explicating a hypothesis before he resumes the examination. As he finalises his utterances, he resumes the examining task.

If we scrutinise the doctor's utterances futher, they seem to indicate a cognitive aspect of dealing with a medical puzzle. His utterance in line 2 is in many ways different from his utterances beyond this sequence. It lacks coherence and clarity as his sentences are non-grammatical and contain self-interruptions. Initially, the doctor's utterance, which was in fact punctuated with internal pauses, indicates a concern about the consequences of the low pulse rate: *well even if he has a ho- he has a pu- eh pulse rate at 46*, but he then ends up concluding: *he is also in (xxx) treatment right which lowers his pulse*, which takes the form of an explanation. The segment *(xxx) treatment* is followed up by an elaboration topicalising the side effects of the treatment. In this case, one side effect appears to contribute to understanding the problem, namely that of the low pulse rate. Yet the doctor seems unaware that he has solved the problem, and he resumes the examination task. However, by framing the problem verbally, he provides public (though evanescent) material anchors that scaffold cognitive understanding. Thus, as his utterances materialise in the cognitive system, they become perceivable affordances for sense-making. The pause of 0.4 seconds is a sign of a realisation phase in which the doctor experiences his observation as an insight, which is expressed immediately afterwards: *so that is presumably the reason why* (Figure 5.3, line 4). Hence, the problem is solved during his utterance in line 2, but it is only afterwards perceived as a result or solution. Cowley (2014b) has shown this reverse, or non-linear, order in problem-solving in an experimental study, and he underlines that solutions are perceived as solutions due to the act of perceiving verbal utterances and linking them to a specific problem or task: "Far from speaking because he has found a solution, it is because he says [a task-relevant utterance] that he finds the solution." (Cowley 2014b: 61)

Even though the doctor verbally articulates situated cognition, he is not communicating with the team in a traditional sense. No one responds to his utterances, and he has no eye contact with any of the team members, who are occupied with other tasks. Nonetheless, he chooses an alternative to silent reasoning: the think-aloud strategy. His verbal articulation is the final event pivot, which makes him both develop an argument and realise it as a solution. The claim is that due to the local material attributes of verbal utterances, it becomes easier to structure and alter chaotic thinking, just as when intermediate results are written on a blackboard during complicated calculations. Rather than articulating hypotheses to achieve a goal (a pragmatic action), verbal articulation is perceived in action in a way that can yield cognitive results (because of its epistemic function). Verbal utterances thus enable the doctor to either sculpt or mould processes of valuable attention (Clark 2008) as the chaotic wordings suddenly become manifest in a perceivable order. Clark (2008: 48) further discusses how experts to a higher degree than novices benefit from uttering 'small strings of words' and 'simple maxims', as they:

> [...] can use them to tune and modulate highly learned forms of embodied performance [...] Linguaform reason, if this is correct, is not just a tool for the novice [...] Instead, it emerges as a key cognitive tool by means of which we are able to objectify, reflect upon, and hence knowingly engage with our own thoughts, trains of reasoning, and cognitive and personal characters. This positions language to act as a kind of cognitive superniche: a cognitive niche, one of whose greatest virtues is to allow us to construct [...] an open-ended sequence of new cognitive niches.
> (Clark 2008: 59)

Put simply, the doctor is able to engage in interactivity as he relies on his own expertise and the qualities of verbal articulation. He comes to understand the patient's situation in a new light as he creatively animates the material resources for thinking in the local interaction. The example illustrates how speaking (aloud) and cognition are part of the same activity in complex cognitive reasoning. While his expertise affords him with the opportunity to work calmly and professionally on multiple tasks simultaneously, sense-making emerges as he exploits multiple conditions for problem-solving locally: speaking out loud, focusing on information (the screen) and linking perceived symptoms to information about the patient's history, as Figure 5.3 visualises. Finally, the problem emerges locally as the beeping reminds him of important medical problems.

2.3 Embodied procedures

Overall in this case, the doctor knows the procedures backwards, which enables him to balance expectations *in situ*. Indeed, the doctor relies on procedures, but he is not constrained by their inherent sequential order and he is able to perform beyond what procedures prescribe when the unexpected occurs and when it enhances performance. For instance, the doctor meshes nested tasks in the overall diagnostic process: anamnesis and physical examination. This approach saves time and enhances task efficiency and the dialogical relationship between the patient and the doctor.

The procedures emerge as an underlying function in his adaptive skilled behaviour. Gibson describes how embodied skills afford automatic behaviour: "The sailor can feel the rope and tie the knot even in darkness. […] The man with a walking stick can even feel stones, mud, or grass at the end of his stick. Yet all these perceptions come from the contact between the adjacent surfaces and the contacts of bones upon another" (Gibson 1966: 112). The doctor's historical body becomes a functional procedure-tool that empowers diagnostic processes. While the doctor integrates the patient as an important cognitive resource in the anamnesis and examination process, the risk of misunderstandings is minimised remarkably. When co-acting, the patient and the doctor jointly achieve their goal by relying just as much on touch as on verbal narratives. The doctor applies an alternative think-aloud strategy that makes possible cognitive work that yields results due to its quasi-material quality. Finally, we observe how medical decision-making is a synthesis of understanding the patient's narrative through whole-bodied interaction and relying on experience to the extent the procedures prove functional in the situation. This analysis is a counterexample of human error cycles. Yet such examples are important for understanding how error cycles can be anticipated. While it underlines the negative feedback mechanisms that characterise best practice, it helps identifying absence of such mechanisms in situations where practitioners follow protocol but, because they do so, struggle to adapt flexibly to changes in the situation.

These insights open for alternative approaches to be applied in education programmes, which can shape sociocultural dynamics eventually and lead to a more dialogical and less error-prone practice. The importance of gestures, procedure biases and cognitive strategies could profitably be discussed in the preparation of educational programmes. Thus, if doctors are not fully versed in the procedures, following them requires a lot of cognitive effort as the following case demonstrates. The procedures become so important that more cognitive power is allocated to the process of following them than to critically relying on them.

3. Case II: Procedure following: Cognitive complexity and simplicity

This case presents common obstacles related to novices' use of procedures in emergency medicine. The case emphasises how a novice male doctor is constrained by multiple, diverging expectations during history taking. As he relies on procedures, his focus is on getting sufficient information that he can document in the electronic medical record at a later stage.

The case involves an elderly female patient with no previous medical history. She woke up the same morning feeling unwell. She went to see her GP who referred her to the hospital as he detected some irregularities in her EKG. In the meantime, the woman's condition has improved, and as she arrives at the ward, her medical condition is normalised, and no symptoms are immediately detected as she is introduced to the doctor. However, she is nevertheless shaken by the heart conditions she experienced earlier. Below is an illustration of the layout.

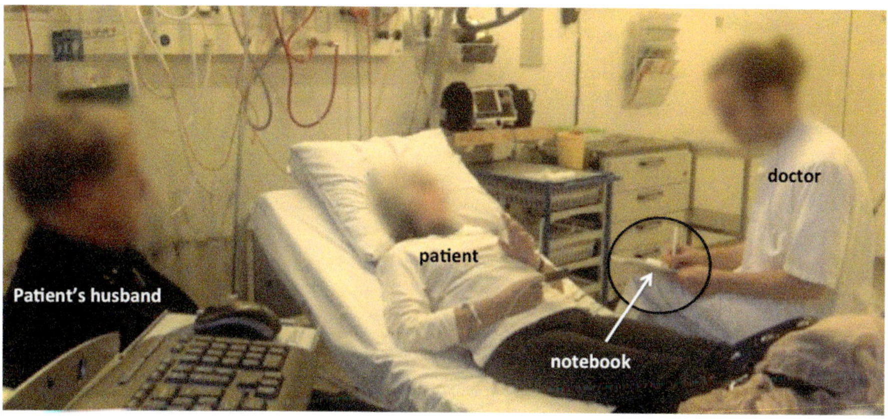

Figure 5.4 Overview of the layout: Anamnesis

3.1 The use of notebooks in anamnesis: Managing the complexity of writing and interacting at the same time

The doctor has been working at the department for only a week or two at the time the recordings took place. A crucial work procedure involves documentation of specific information in the electronic medical record after anamnesis and physical examination. All relevant information needs to be documented so other healthcare staff can check and follow up on what has been done and decided by whom. Thus, to structure and ensure detailed memory, novice doctors often use notebooks.

As we enter the conversation, the novice doctor has just initiated the anamnesis to determine what has caused the patient's condition and has just asked her the broad question: *what has happened?* The patient begins her narrative by referring to two conversations she has had with her husband and GP respectively:[7]

Transcript 5.3
Danish original

```
1.  00:02:00, P:   Jeg synes jeg har ondt i hjertet siger jeg så til ham [GP]
2.  00:04:20, D:   okay
3.  00:04:80, P:   så siger han (.) nå men det var jo ikke så godt vel
4.  00:07:00, D:   nej
5.  00:07:30, P:   og så øh (.) så slog vi det lidt hen (.) men så synes jeg at jeg
                   har haft det nogen gange siden
6.  00:13:50, D:   okay
7.  00:14:20, P:   Og så tænker jeg (.) er det så fordi det gør ondt (.) eller er det
                   fordi man er fokuseret på det eller hvad er det for noget
8.  00:20:00, D:   ja
9.  00:20:10, P:   og det vil så fordi min mor hun havde dårligt hjerte
10. 00:23:00, D:   ja
11. 00:23:60, P:   og min far han er død af en blodprop
12. 00:25:60, D:   okay
13. 00:26:00, P:   og så så så tænkte jeg [pl
14. 00:27:40, D:                           [er din mor død os?
15. 00:28:50, P:   ja ja
16. 00:29:30, D:   ja
17. 00:29:50, P:   men det er mange år siden
18. 00:30:40, D:   ja
19. 00:31:40, P:   og så øhm (.) men så i går så siger jeg til [husband's name] det
                   gør altså ondt (.)
20. 00:36:80, D:   mm
21. 00:37:40, P:   så var vi blevet enige om at jeg skulle gå op hos lægen i dag
22. 00:40:20, D:   ja
23. 00:41:50, P:   og så (.) øhm blev der taget sådan et (.) kordiogram eller hvad
                   det hedder
24. 00:46:20, D:   ja
25. 00:46:80, P:   og så øhm var der sådan noget han sagde der var forkert i det
26. 00:50:40, D:   okay
```

English translation

```
1.  00:02:00, P:   I think that I have some pains in my heart I then tell him [GP]
2.  00:04:20, D:   okay
3.  00:04:80, P:   then he says (.) well that is not a good thing, is it
```

7. An invariant communicative pattern is registered. Variations of *and, and then, then* utterances (yellow) are responded to with variations of minimal responses as *okay, no, yes, mm* (green). This pattern is discussed in the analysis.

4.	00:07:00, D:	no
5.	00:07:30, P:	and then eh (.) then we shrugged it off (.) but then I think I have had it a couple of times since then
6.	00:13:50, D:	okay
7.	00:14:20, P:	and then I start thinking (.) is it because it does hurt (.) or is it because one becomes too focused on it or what is it
8.	00:20:00, D:	yes
9.	00:20:10, P:	and that will then because my mother she had a heart condition
10.	00:23:00, D:	yes
11.	00:23:60, P:	and my father died of a blood clot
12.	00:25:60, D:	okay
13.	00:26:00, P:	and then then then I thought [pl
14.	00:27:40, D:	[is your mother dead as well
15.	00:28:50, P:	yes yes
16.	00:29:30, D:	yes
17.	00:29:50, P:	but that is a long time ago
18.	00:30:40, D:	yes
19.	00:31:40, P:	and then eh (.) but then yesterday I tell [husband's name] it does really hurt (.)
20.	00:36:80, D:	mm
21.	00:37:40, P:	then we agreed that I should see my GP today
22.	00:40:20, D:	yes
23.	00:41:50, P:	and then (.) eh he did a kind of a (.) cordiogram or what you call it
24.	00:46:20, D:	yes
25.	00:46:80, P:	and then eh there was something he said was wrong in it
26.	00:50:40, D:	okay

The local goal is to get sufficient information from the patient in order to compare the narrative with medical measurements, which finally leads to successful diagnosis and a plan for further treatment. The task is history taking and the starting point is the patient who has arrived due to previously experienced chest pain. The task is constrained by the doctor's dual orientation to the material artefact (the notebook) and the patient.

During the 48.9-second-long excerpt, the novice doctor uses pen and paper to document every detail of the conversation as he gets hold of the narrative. His visual attention is on the documentation activity, and in total, he gazes in the notebook for 27 seconds.

Apart from line 1, 8 and 10, all the patient's utterances start with a variation of *and, then* or *and then*. The doctor confirms with continuers (*yes, no, okay* and *mm*) as co-constitutive devices in the interaction (Hutchby and Wooffitt 2011). In this way, the doctor treats all information as factual, equally important and this prompts the patient to continue her narrative. As a result of this structural organisation, the patient provides the doctor with subjective descriptions of what she finds relevant to bring into the anamnesis process. The doctor's minimal responses, invariance in voice dynamics, his gazing into the notebook and his primary attention to the writing task altogether leave the patient with no ability to judge how her utterances are interpreted and whether they are sanctioned or not. To keep the dialogue going, the patient continues to elaborate the narrative by interactively adding new information: *and then*. Furthermore, she constantly seeks eye contact with the doctor, who only gazes at her when he is not documenting.

According to Goffman, (1983: 5ff) a "game's rules" determine a set of roles and unequal rights that afford a certain distribution of turn-taking sequences. This can be investigated specifically in the pattern of question-answer distributions. A question is seen as a powerful device where the questioner possesses the powerful role in interaction (Goffman 1983). Ample research on doctor-patient interaction has investigated the question-answer distribution as the key mechanism to constitute power asymmetries (Fairclough 1992; Liddicoat 2011; Goffman 1983). For example, Fairclough (1992) underlines how doctors direct the interaction by engaging in a three-part cycle, in which a doctor is the one to decide the initial question the patient needs to respond to, and to which the doctor utters a specific acknowledgement (Fairclough 1992: 149). However, in this case, the three-part cycle is not completed by new questions. The doctor uses minimal responses, which affords the patient to continue and elaborate endlessly.

During the overall conversation, this pattern is only paused by relatively small interruptions, for instance when the doctor realises that he needs extra information. These answer-response cycles are visualised in the Transcription 5.3 and they indicate the default interactivity pattern in this sequence. However, an event pivot causes changes in the interaction pattern for a short moment. Prompted by particular, relevant medical information, the doctor tests a hypothesis, but with a minimum of engagement. This is illustrated below:

Figure 5.5 indicates the event pivots that lead to the doctor's medical hypothesis testing. As he follows protocol, he responds to relevant information, but as he is primarily concerned with documentation his interpretations are delayed which consequently affects both the emotional alliance and the interaction pattern.

While the patient tells the doctor that her mother had a heart condition (line 9) and adds that her father died of a blood clot (line 11), she reveals medically relevant information, which is potentially relevant for the diagnostic process. The information (line 11) is defined as a secondary event pivot as the doctor reacts to the information after he has documented it in his notebook. Thus, it is hypothesised that as he perceives the represented narrative in the notebook, it serves as a primary event pivot prompting him to interrupt (line 14) 2 seconds after the patient has uttered the information. As he follows procedures strictly and documents

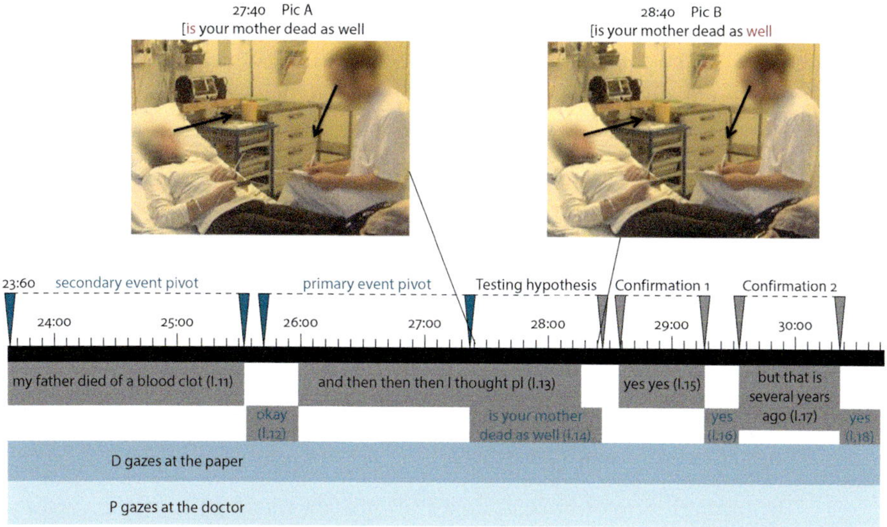

Figure 5.5 Delayed hypothesis testing

every detail on paper, the doctor-patient relationship is indeed constrained by the doctor's primary attention to the documentation task and it reduces sensitivity. Moreover, this reduced sensitivity reveals itself in the doctor's interruption. The *as well* (line 14) underlines the factual aspect of the question *is your mother dead as well?* and as he seeks clarification, the doctor gazes in the notebook rather than at the patient, see picture A and B in Figure 5.5.

Balancing multiple tasks to achieve the overall goal increases cognitive complexity. Writing and interacting with the patient requires a strict focus on what is being said, how this is interrelated and causes relevant medical associations, and what is being represented in the notebook. Evidently, such procedures complicate another nested activity in the anamnesis task: situated sensitivity. As mentioned in the beginning of this chapter, an important aspect in the diagnostic process is to make the patient feel comfortable. In this case, the interaction is affected by the way the notebook and pen are immersed into the doctor's working body. Following Kirsh (2013), the added effort of using material artefacts affects one's perceptual array:

> Perception is altered by our skill in using tools. This is the next implication of extending the embodiment paradigm to include tools. Hills look steeper than normal to subjects wearing a heavy backpack. When a tool is absorbed into our body schema, our perception of height, distance, and related magnitudes changes. The added effort of carrying around weight affects perception. (Kirsh 2013: 3–9)

Analogously, the doctor's use of the notebook affects his perception. First, he uses it as an aid to free cognitive power from remembering, but as the doctor-artefact cognitive system becomes centred on writing, this activity draws attention away from other elements that are important in the diagnostic process. He does not perceive the patient's embodied dynamics, and the artefact-rich interaction makes him at risk of losing overview of the narrative since he is constrained by the delay that interpretation and writing cause. To understand why the doctor is so fixated on procedure-following, the function and effect of procedures need to be compared to staff's expectations and consequences of missing relevant information. For instance, Angeli (2015) explains how a medical director, during a staff meeting at an emergency service unit, pointed out the importance of protocols and procedures because a lack of solid communication and recall entailed misunderstandings about a patient's treatment:

> The medical director brought up a PCR [patient care report] on the overhead projector and verbalized the information written on it. He said, "Based on this patient's status, he should have been given two IV lines and not one. The PCR states that he had one IV line, which could have caused many complications for the patient. This treatment doesn't follow protocol." A paramedic sitting across from me raised his hand: "That was my patient. I started two IV lines following protocol." The medical director responded, "Well, you didn't write it down, so you didn't do it. We have to get better a documenting our work, folks. Patients' lives depend on it." (Angeli 2015: 34)

As the doctor lacks embodied experience with procedures and how this work practice emerges, he relies on rules and medical protocols for proper behaviour – and he does so by the book. However, healthcare professionals have mentioned that knowing how to act efficiently and smoothly comes from experience (Angeli 2015).

While material aids enable comprehensive documentation at a future point, they also inhibit the dialogical flow of anamnesis due to the complexity that follows in managing verbal interaction *and* writing as well as a focus on which procedures follow next. The act of writing itself requires cognitive power and time that delays his situational sensitivity. He cannot pay equal attention to two cognitively different tasks at the same time. By maintaining an action hierarchy, the doctor prioritises the documentation activity, which reduces the chances for negative feedback mechanisms in interactivity. The doctor enacts no signs of frustration and he does not take control of the anamnesis process, which exacerbates the process. The patient's continually varied use of *and then* establishes an interactivity trajectory where the doctor continues to document the patient's narrative and he continues to be a step behind in the process.

As the local outcome is functional and acceptable according to medical standards, the doctor gets medical information by a circuitous route and he uses multiple cognitive resources and time on the anamnesis task. The amount of resources spent means less resources to other diagnosis situations at the ward. As resources already are low, priorities are crucial for maintaining a good work and patient flow in the ward. However, when left alone and unaware of the positive feedback mechanisms in interactivity, potential error cycles are only perceived by the observer and momentarily by patients. In such situations, becoming an expert depends solely on repetition that *eventually* releases cognitive power to accomplish other tasks and adapt to situational changes.

4. Understanding the status and function of procedures and expertise

Angeli (2015) argues that professional memory, which is distilled in textbooks, protocols and other procedural guidelines have "to structure a response, but it needs to be flexible enough to account for all types of unpredicted situations. In short, protocols need to prepare [...] EMS professionals to care for a patient but allow them freedom to adapt the protocol according to the patient's needs" (Angeli 2015: 31). In this work, inflexibility appears to be the main problem with the working procedures, and inexperience is a challenge in relation to how procedures are managed *in situ*.

Procedures are important, necessary and useful, and they must be followed to sustain the organisation (Angeli 2015). Understanding the invariant nature of task performance is crucial to adapt procedures successfully and for future coordination to be managed effectively. The problem with procedures is thus not a question of their raison d'être; rather it is related to the status and understanding of the function of the procedures in the ward. First, procedures work like models for proper behaviour and they have been developed with a focus on what to ask in a sequential order. The procedures are formed with a written language bias as interaction tasks are described as static, autonomous and structure-like information steps in treatment (Linell 2005). Second – and related to the written-language bias – the procedures do not embrace the qualities of whole-bodied coaction. As focus is on what to say (and only on what to do in relation to physical examination), the interpersonal relationship and the dialogue between healthcare practitioner and the patient are reduced to information exchange sequences. However, as the first case underlines, functional task performance can be accomplished efficiently when the healthcare practitioner meshes procedures and relies on inter-bodily dynamics in task performance. When protocols have built in a step-by-step procedure with specific questions to ask in a specific logical order, flexible adaptive behaviour is difficult to manage without violating procedures. Education programmes could benefit from the insight that procedures are in themselves neither good nor bad. Their functionality depends on how they are managed. The management of procedures in situated interaction depends on the practitioner's level of expertise and experience, which again equips the practitioner with the ability to adapt flexibly and maintain an overview of the situation. Such flexibility is exemplified in the first case, where the expert creatively develops alternative strategies: (a) he meshes tasks, (b) he relies on inter-bodily dynamics in coaction and (c) he uses a think-aloud strategy that materialises as material anchor points, which become affordances for sense-making.

In this analysis, procedures prove functional for the cognitive system when the expert applies them to expand the perceptual system. The expert is able to embody the procedures and avoid getting overwhelmed as he moulds them creatively to fit situations where the unexpected occurs. To the novice doctor, procedures are functional as their guiding action steps *afford certain decisions* of how and what to do, but to the cognitive system in general, they are dysfunctional as they entail reduced sensitivity. Moreover, procedures prompt the novices to rely on artefacts in order to scaffold and enhance memory. By documenting the anamnesis in a notebook, the practitioner is capable of following protocols *in situ* and at a future point. Knowing that procedures can be followed during the whole process is a way of avoiding being overwhelmed.

The suggestion of "procedure ambiguity" supports the hypothesis that novices in general adopt and follow explicit standard procedures and guidelines in a rigid way. Experienced practitioners rely on embodied expertise and situational features that equip them with an anticipatory understanding of which procedures and tools are useful, and most importantly, which procedures and tools constrain decision-making and thus afford dysfunctional results. This is important in order to understand how error cycles are anticipated or not as practitioners disobey or follow the logic of the organisation to achieve the overall successful output: optimum treatment for the patient. Indeed, it is a balance to know when the exclusion of aiding tools leads to more dialogical behaviour and a richer layout of affordance environment, or alternatively leads to stress and cognitive and interpersonal overload.

CHAPTER 6

Interruptions and multitask tolerance in emergency medicine

1. Interruptions and values realisation in emergency medicine

Coding revealed that interruptions appear regularly during task performance. Interruptions count as any situation in which a practitioner is required to change his or her orientation to the interrupting source, either briefly or for a longer period of time. Thus, sometimes the interruption leads to a task switch before resuming the original task; at other times they just cause a few moments of pause before the practitioner resumes the work. In my data several kinds of interruptions occurred during diagnostic processes and pre-treatment. Overall, two types of interruption patterns emerged. On the one hand, the more responsibility and expertise a practitioner has, the more frequently he or she is interrupted for advice, permissions and overview reports. Thus, primary doctors were frequently interrupted.[1] As part of their job, they need to maintain the overview of the patient flow at the ward, and they need to facilitate the junior doctors when difficult decisions need to be made. Consequently, they spend considerable time and effort to get back into the workflow. On the other hand, the less experienced a practitioner is, the more frequently he or she is interrupted for other work-related aspects such as clarifications, explanations etc. When comparing doctors and nurses, the nurses are the less interrupted group in the dataset.

Based on coding I enlist a heuristics of interruption types. However, the list is not a suggestion of a general interruption typology or taxonomy, but merely a list of the interruptions identified within this dataset. Thus, the practitioners were interrupted by (a) phone calls to which they are required to respond immediately, (b) other local team members who need information to get on with their

1. The primary doctors are the most experienced doctors in the ward. They serve as flow masters and team coordinators as they delegate assignments to the medical teams and manage the patient flow. They also supervise the junior doctors in medical and clinical issues. This primarily happens backstage (Goffman 1959) in a coordination room, but sometimes a situation requires the primary doctor to check up on the patient to supervise the novice doctor. When needed, the primary doctor visits patients, and in highly acute situations he is always present from the beginning. The primary doctor refers directly to the physician on call.

individual tasks and procedures,[2] (c) colleagues outside the local team who enter the room and interrupt for various reasons, for instance with questions regarding other patients whom the practitioner has been involved with (at other times they need advice, status reports etc.), (d) the patient or his relatives who ask for elaboration, for instance on previously given information that leads to task switch and (e) alarms and other electronic surveillance equipment or monitoring displays that disturb the current workflow. The most frequent and distracting interruption types identified in the dataset are phone interruptions. Further, the nature of phone interruptions is distinctive: Their complete lack of timing compared to verbal interruptions for instance and their demand of immediate response is distinctly palpable.

Several studies on interruptions in emergency medicine conclude that (a) the number and frequency of interruptions are staggering and should lead to serious concerns about intervention strategies amongst healthcare educators and providers (Chisholm et al. 2000, 2001; Clark 2011), (b) that interruptions often lead to task switch or cause practitioners to leave tasks unfinished (Clark 2011), (c) that interruptions have a negative impact on patient satisfaction (Jeanmonod et al. 2010), (d) that interruptions often disrupt working memory (Coiera et al. 2002) and, finally, (e) that interruptions predispose healthcare practitioners to making human errors (Clark 2011).

Chisholm et al. (2001) label emergency practitioners as "interrupt-driven" and underline that even though we have extensive knowledge about interruptions from other fields – e.g. aviation – we have not yet gained a comprehensive understanding of interruptions in the emergency ward. Though the amount of studies within this field has increased, the studies primarily provide evidence of the amount of interruptions faced in healthcare emergency settings (Berg et al. 2013).The consequences of interruptions, in such cases, are at best elaborated in relation to specific outcomes. While such insights are important, these studies lack qualitative investigations of how interruptions emerge and are countered in situated interaction. Thus, whether such studies cover the amount of interruptions, how interruptions are distributed across various departments (Chisholm et al. 2001), or what kind of tasks or which groups are interrupted most frequently, the studies lack an understanding of the particular interactive dynamics before, during and after interruptions occur. Advancing the understanding of interruption cycles depends on investigations of how a cognitive system deals with disturbances rather than assumes that interruptions are something which is being imposed on the individual.

2. This kind of interruption is often more *timed* as the local team members know what and when they interrupt contrary to when a colleague interrupts by calling on the phone.

By turning to how individuals attend to typical interruptions, the most common intervention programmes point to implementation of electronic coordinating tools, general team training and more education about what interruptions can do to the working memory of the individual. For instance, recent studies have investigated interruption resumption amongst nurses in intensive care units (Rajkomar and Blandford 2012; Grundgeiger et al. 2010). They show how nurses keep track of which step of a task remains or is to be completed by employing artefacts as reminders (Rajkomar and Blandford 2012). While these studies focus on how nurses distribute the cognitive task in space as they rely on material artefacts as useful cognitive anchor points, they maintain an understanding of interruptions as local cognitive obstacles. Interruptions unquestionably have a negative effect on outcomes. However, studies need to expand the scope to investigations of the cultural dimension of interruptions. Why are interruptions, in some situations, rather harmless, when, in other situations they eventually lead to human error? According to the ecological perspective on human error, it is not an interruption in itself that causes human error; it is interactivity in which interruptions are embedded which guides what happens. Thus, while conventional observational studies (including studies with retrospective interviews) tend to focus on medical tasks and content, a richer understanding is gained by scrutinising how a cognitive system draws on interactivity (Steffensen 2013), and situational and cultural affordances for actions (Pedersen 2010).

To explain how interactivity, including cultural and material affordances for action, leads to different outcomes in different contexts, Hodges and Baron's theory of values realisation is applied on two different cases. Hodges and Baron provide an ecological account of values that propose thinking in terms of a value heterarchy (Hodges and Baron 1992). It is argued that this theoretical concept can clarify how cognitive systems make sense and deal with interruptions in situated interaction characterised by multiple diverging constraints on action. A few comments on the theory are added prior to the analysis.

With Gibson and Crooks (1938), Hodges argues that task performance "is a skill of perceiving and acting within a *field*" (Hodges 2007a: 154). A field is defined as a continuously changing set of potential pathways. With the example of driving, Gibson and Crooks emphasise how the field of safe travel constitutes an ecosystem defined by values. Safety is an important value (Hodges 2007a), but as other values also constitute the ecosystem, the field is constrained by multiple values. Thus, as an ecosystem, driving is at the same time bounded and dynamical for instance. Physical laws and social rules are, according to Hodges, constraints that serve as resources for performing a task, but Hodges defines the actual task as: "a moral task that requires steering a vehicle through a cluttered environment safely and accurately. The use of the term moral in this context means motivated by goods (i.e., values), including those that are epistemic (e.g., accuracy) and ethical (e.g., justice)" (Hodges 2007a: 155). Thus, driving is defined by multiple constraining values, for instance safety, efficiency and tolerance (Hodges 2007a). Hodges presents a radical claim about the obligatory status of values:

> Thus far, I have claimed that the physical field identified by Gibson and Crooks (1938) is an ontologically real dynamic (i.e., it is continuously evolving) that is defined by its potentials for realizing values. Because values define the field, they are obligatory. Driving, as such, cannot exist unless values such as safety, accuracy, tolerance, comprehensiveness, and efficiency are properly acknowledged in the recruitment of physical laws and the construction and use of social rules. Driving became possible for humans when they discovered enough about physical laws to organize them comprehensively enough to build vehicles. As soon as the number of vehicles increased enough for collisions to happen, social constraints were added to the physical constraints. However, the motivation for engaging in physics and engineering, as well as the development of regulations about how vehicles could be constructed and used, emerged from moral obligations to realize values. The development of goals (e.g., building an automobile) and the development of rules (e.g., supervising a traffic system) are motivated by and answer to the ecosystem and the values that provide its constitutive standards."
>
> (Hodges 2007a: 156)

Hodges argues that recent studies on driving, for instance, tend to isolate single values when considering how the task is accomplished, and this reduced view leads to incomplete and faulty conclusions about what happens in driving. In a similar vein, Dunbar and Garud have investigated how the inability to balance two different assessment criteria (safety and a concern for meeting schedules) caused the Columbia Shuttle Flight STS-107 to disintegrate (Dunbar and Garud 2007). Dunbar and Garud argue that the majority of studies of the Columbia Flight disaster have built their interpretations on a traditional conceptualisation of organisations as information-processing systems "that are somehow subject to the objective control and direction of responsible individual decision makers" (Dunbar and Garud 2007: 417). Thus, when systems break down, individuals are blamed for irresponsible and inattentive behaviour (cf. Chapter 1). Dunbar and Garud propose to think in terms of distributed knowledge to underline that a single individual "cannot know all of the relevant information that it requires to categorise an event in real time and, consequently, investigations will be forced to consider a wider range of explanatory factors" (Dunbar and Garud 2007: 417). By combining Dunbar and Garud's proposal of distributed knowledge with Hodges' values heterarchy, the following two cases are investigated as diagnostic fields – or systems – with a cognitive agenda constrained by multiple values. When interruptions occur, the system needs to adapt to the changes without violating its boundary conditions by balancing the field's constitutive values. One way of balancing the values is by relying on distributed resources and managing nested tasks through joint coordination as the case examples demonstrate.

Specifically, this chapter investigates the overall cognitive systems in which interruptions emerge. Interruptions are inevitable in the ward, but they are not anticipated and managed in the same way amongst practitioners. As interruptions are local demands for immediate action that stress and disturb real-time cognition, it is hypothesised that practitioners prioritise interruptions over the ongoing task (often dialogue with the patient) to reduce the immediate stress and pressure. If an interruption is not responded to, it often continues to demand a response (incoming phone calls, electronic alarms etc.), and few people can cope with such pressure even though they are occupied with other important tasks. Consequently, a fixed task hierarchy dominates interruption management and local interaction is at risk of breaking down. The hypothesis was investigated in two cases. The first case presents how a novice doctor handles information coming from multiple sources: (a) the patient, (b) a team member and (c) a colleague on the phone. He is interrupted several times during a sequence of 54 seconds when he tries to get hold of the patient's narrative. Multiple expectations – inherent in the organisational system of which he is part – prompt him to move in and out of different modes of interaction. He becomes overloaded and prioritises some expectations over others. The second case investigates how a medical team successfully handles a telephone interruption during history taking. While an interruption always affects the flow of interactivity, it does not necessarily have to be a significant or problematic disturbance that violates the boundaries of the cognitive system. By exploiting the qualities of team collaboration this example emphasises how an interruption is managed functionally through a highly coordinated team performance initiated by an experienced nurse.

2. Case I: Treating interruptions as what?

This example emphasises how challenging it can be for doctors to act dialogically and in a caring manner towards the patient in an interruption-driven workplace. Repeated interruptions increase the level of complexity, stress and cognitive effort in otherwise simple tasks. The focus is on how a young novice doctor acts to satisfy multiple demands of attention simultaneously in a rather critical situation.

At the moment we enter the conversation, the patient, an elderly woman, has just arrived through a 911 call. Earlier the same day she felt dizzy and she suddenly fainted shortly after she went to the lavatory where she had lost a large amount of blood. The patient now updates the novice doctor about her concerns and thoughts up until the moment she fainted. Below is an illustration of the situation.

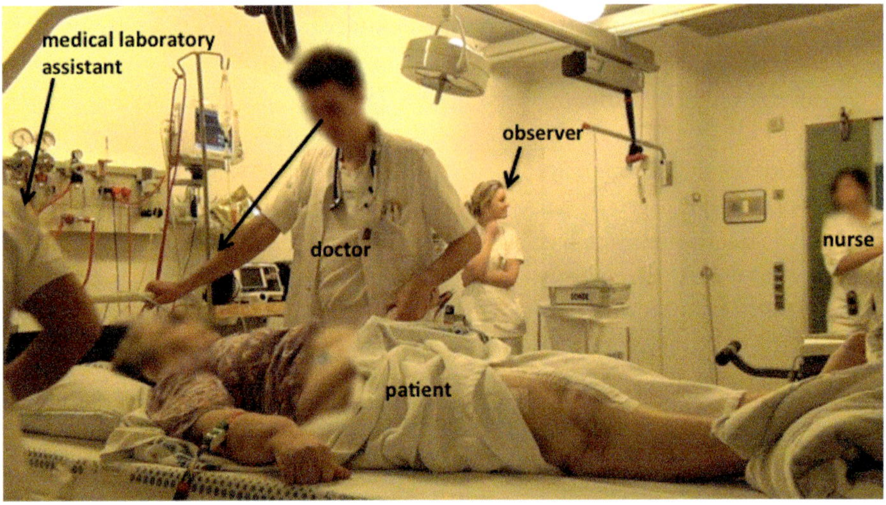

Figure 6.1 Overview of the layout: An interruption-driven practice

2.1 Low multitask tolerance

In this 54-second excerpt below, seven interruptions occur. First, attention is paid to each of these interruptions. Second, it is investigated in detail what the interruptions do to the dynamics in the cognitive system as a whole.

Transcript 6.1[3]
Danish original

```
1. 01:06:30, P:    så blev jeg jo bange for jeg var alene hjemme ik (nurse enters)
2. 01:08:40, D:    ja
3. 01:09:10, ps.   (0,5)
4. 01:09:60, P:    og så ringede jeg til (xxx) og de var ikke hjemme og så ringede
                   jeg til [xxx] og de var heller ikke hjemme=
5. 01:13:00, D:    =tak
6. 01:13:40, ps.   (1.1)
7. 01:14,50, P:    og vagtlægen havde lukket og det det hele [det (.) ramlede for mig
                   (.) så tænkte jeg om jeg skulle ringe til 112
8. 01:16:80, D:                                              [NÅ
9. 01:20:60, ps.   (0.6)
10. 01:21:20, P:   s så slemt var det heller ikke vel
11. 01:23:10, ps.  (2.1)
12. 01:25.20, D:   nej=
13. 01:25:90, P:   =men så [her (xxx[x) jeg tror fredag, så skulle jeg på toilettet
                   i[k
```

3. Interruptions are marked in. *Ph* is an abbreviation for phone.

14. 01:26:40, N: [var der en (xxx) på hende derovre
15. 01:27:70, Ph [ring ring=
16. 01:32:00, Ph ring ri[ng
17. 01:32:30, D: [ja
18. 01:33:50, P: og så måtte jeg jo kalde på min datter som siger mor det er ikke (.) det er ikke [(xxx) det er blod=
19. 01:36:40, Ph [ring ring
20. 01:37:00, D: =det er blod [jeg skal lige tage den her (D talks on the phone for 15,8 seconds)
21. 01:38:40, P: [(xxx)
22. 01:56:00, D: er det okay (.) jeg li:ge går u:d o:g giver en besked
23. 01:57:60, N: ja selvfølgelig
24. 01:58:30, D: ja (D leaves the room)

English translation

1. 01:06:30, P: then I got scared because I was home alone right (nurse enters)
2. 01:08:40, D: yes
3. 01:09:10, ps. (0,5)
4. 01:09:60, P: and then I called (xxx) and they were not home and then I called (xxx) and they were not home <u>either</u>=
5. 01:12:80, D: =thanks
6. 01:13:40, ps. (1.1)
7. 01:14,50, P: and the duty doctor was closed and and [it all (.) fell apart (.) so I thought about calling 911
8. 01:16:80, D: [OH
9. 01:20:60, ps. (0.6)
10. 01:21:20, P: i- it was not so bad after all was it
11. 01:23:10, ps. (2.1)
12. 01:25.20, D: no=
13. 01:25:90, P: =but then [this (xxx[x) Friday I think then I had to go to the toilet ri[ght
14. 01:26:40, N: [did we have a (xxx) on her over there
15. 01:27:70, Ph [ring ring=
16. 01:32:00, Ph ring ri[ng
17. 01:32:50, D: [yes
18. 01:33:50, P: and then I had to call my daugther who says to me mum this is not (.) this is not [(xxx) it is blood=
19. 01:36:40, Ph [ring ring
20. 01:37:00, D: =it is blood [I have to answer this one (D talks on the phone for 15,8 seconds)
21. 01:38:40, P: [(xxx)
22. 01:56:00, D: is it okay (.) if I ju:st lea:ve a:nd give a message
23. 01:57:60, N: yes of course
24. 01:58:30, D: yes (D leaves the room)

During the initial part of the anamnesis seven interruptions are detected. The doctor is interrupted five times: twice by the nurse and three times by the phone. Further, the nurse interrupts both doctor and patient, and finally, the doctor interrupts the patient. In Figure 6.2 below, each interruption is highlighted, and the precise timing of the interruptions is marked in relation to the cognitive undertaking. The doctor's gaze, pace and the interlocutors' verbal utterances are analysed in relation to the interruptions. Finally, the relationship between the interruption, the task being performed, and the interaction type is discussed in relation to the communicative and cognitive consequences interruptions can have on the general flow of interactivity.

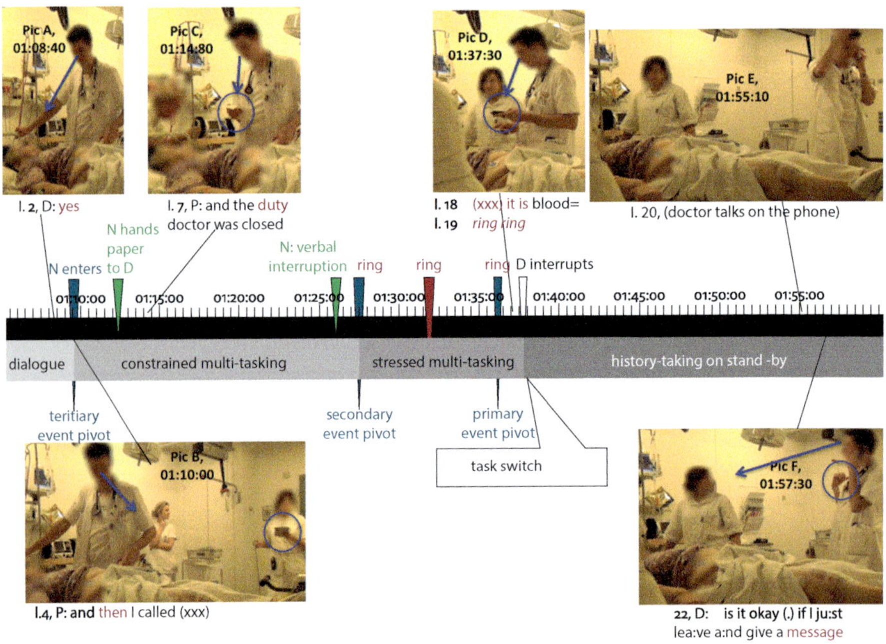

Figure 6.2 The effect of interruptions' on cognitive task performance
The green triangles indicate nurse interruptions; the red one indicates phone interruptions; the white one indicates doctor interruptions. Red markings in the text indicate the verbal utterance articulated as the picture is taken. The blue triangles are event pivots in the trajectory.

The figure illustrates how interruptions permeate and disturb simple task performance. Practitioners have constrained conditions for dialogical diagnostic task performances as sensitive interaction requires a high, multitask tolerance in a stressful and unpredictable environment. Most importantly it emphasises the feedback mechanisms *in the process* and how the stress level in interaction increases in line with the number of interruptions. The figure finally indicates how the enabling conditions for task performance are constrained and lead to task switch.

In the following, each interruption is elaborated on and discussed in relation to the context in which it appears. The analyses focus on how multiple values are balanced. An interruption requires that the (members of a) medical team live(s) up to multiple expectations simultaneously.

This doctor is engaged in history taking. He and the patient constitute a cognitive system, which is defined by the task and their interpersonal relationship. There is an implicit agreement that to solve this task, they need to coordinate and establish a trustful relationship. Hodges argues that: "coordination among humans involves two or more intentional agents synchronizing their activities; cooperation requires their working together to achieve a common goal. It is the thesis [...] that caring is the larger context that makes social cooperation and coordination possible" (Hodges 2007a: 154). Thus, as a human socio-cognitive system, caring and understanding are intrinsic, dynamic and moral constraints (Hodges 2007a). Such moral obligations are obligatory for the system to uphold its boundaries. The doctor is under pressure as demands and expectations coming from outside the cognitive system conflict with activities within the system. A dilemma emerges and forces the doctor to make decisions.

To begin with, the doctor engages in dialogue with the patient. She provides him with information about what happened when she discovered her rectal bleeding at home. At the beginning, the two have eye contact and the doctor leans towards the patient and holds on to the bed headboard (see picture A). At 01:08:40, the nurse enters the room. She carries a medical sheet in her hand, and she approaches the doctor. An event pivot indicates the moment when the doctor responds to her entry as an interruption (see Figure 6.2). At 01:10:00 he turns his upper body around to learn about the nurse's errand even though the patient continues: *and then I called (xxx)* (see picture B). From that moment the doctor does not gaze at the patient for 21.3 seconds. The doctor notices the sheet which the nurse holds in her hands as she approaches him, and right after he receives the sheet he utters: *=thanks*, overlapping the patient's utterance. The interruption immediately leads to a change in the interactivity trajectory. In Figure 6.2 this is indicated as a transition phase form *dialogue* to *constrained multitasking* as the conditions for fulfilling both activities effectively decrease. As the doctor responds to the nurse's action, he also shifts his attention from the patient to the artefact and the nurse. In this way he interrupts his own task and increases the stress level in the cognitive system between him and the patient. The boundary conditions of the system are vulnerable as caring for the patient becomes secondary to responding to a colleague's request and to scrutinising the newly received information further. The doctor gazes at the sheet and his responses are late. In the following nine lines from the transcript it appears how the doctor's prioritisation stands out through his late or absent minimal responses.

```
4. 01:09:60,  P:   and then I called (xxx) and they were not home and then I called
(xxx)
                   and they were not home either=
5. 01:12:80,  D:   =thanks
6. 01:13:40,  ps.                                       (1.1)
7. 01:14,50,  P:   and the duty doctor was closed and and [it all (.) fell apart (.) so
I
                   thought about calling 911
8. 01:16:80,  D:                                        [OH
9. 01:20:60,  ps.                                       (0.6)
10. 01:21:20, P:   i- it was not so bad anyway right
11. 01:23:10, ps.                                       (2.1)
12. 01:25.20, D:                                        no=
```

To the patient's utterance: *and they were not home either=* (line 4), the doctor does not respond and 1.1 seconds elapse (line 6). The lapse marks a break in the interactivity flow. The interactional fluidity and the interdependency between the two are constrained. However, the patient continues: *and the duty doctor was closed and and,* (line 7), and the doctor produces a late response *[OH,* (line 8), remarkably higher than his normal volume. After the patient has uttered *it all (.) fell apart* (line 7) she holds a brief pause before continuing. This pause is in an obvious, transition-relevant place (Sacks et al. 1974) at which the doctor could comment with a continuer or express an understanding of the uncomfortable situation the patient has been – and still is – in, but the doctor responds neither verbally nor non-verbally. The patient then uses a logical connector: *so* (line 7) and concludes that she was thinking about calling 911. The whole utterance (line 7) reveals the serious and intimate concerns the patient has had about her own medical and mental condition, but the doctor barely responds to it. Instead, he continues to gaze at the sheet. After a pause of 0.6 second, the patient finally explains that: *i- it was not so bad anyway right* (line 10). The patient now explicitly seeks confirmation from the doctor, who does not respond. A lapse of 2.1 seconds emerges (line 11) and finally the doctor confirms. from the result of this interaction, the doctor appears offhand inattentive and preoccupied with other stuff. Thus, the main question is: Why did the doctor change his orientation from the patient to the nurse and the sheet he received? The answer seems to be related to temporal dynamics (Steffensen and Pedersen 2014) beyond the enchronic timescale of interaction.

The sheet contains medical information about various measurements that have been provided by the paramedics who handed the patient over. Nevertheless, this information is important just as the patient's narrative is. When scrutinising his actions further, it becomes clear that the doctor does not choose to do A or B; rather, as he reads, he also maintains a dialogue with the patient. He stays close to her and even though his responses are delayed, he does respond – momentarily. However, as both history taking and interpretation of medical measurements on the sheet require cognitive effort, his attention and sensitivity are constrained by the nested tasks he engages in simultaneously. However, as the situation evolves, the doctor engages more and more in the reading task than in history taking.

The initial interruptions do not only have an immediate effect on the interaction; they change the interactivity flow from dialogical and caring to monological and constrained. As the number of interruptions and expectations to act in a specific way increases, the doctor becomes cognitively overloaded and the situation deteriorates. Eventually, this dilemma leads to a task switch and communicative breakdowns.

2.2 When caring for more than the patient becomes a constraint for task performance

In what follows, the way in which five interruptions affect the interactivity further is scrutinised. First, the nurse interrupts the doctor-patient interaction as she makes herself heard above their conversation and second, an incoming call interrupts several times which eventually prompts the doctor to abruptly drop the conversation. Despite the two previous interruptions, the patient continues her narrative even though the doctor only reads the sheet (see picture E). The patient is interrupted three times in just one sentence (line 14, 15 and 16).

Almost immediately after the patient resumes her narrative (line 13), the nurse interrupts as she asks the medical laboratory assistant for specific information (line 14). The distance between the nurse and the medical laboratory assistant prompts the nurse to speak *over* the patient. No one is paying direct attention to the patient, but each team member (the medical laboratory assistant, the nurse and the doctor) is occupied with individual tasks that are valued higher than the dialogue with the patient. The patient, however, does not stop talking, but mumbles something unrecognisable into empty space when the phone rings and interrupts her verbal utterance. The patient appears oblivious to the interruptions, and she continues her narrative in direct continuation with the ringing and as she finalises her utterance: *to the toilet ri[ght*, she is interrupted for the third time by a second ringing. At 01:32:50 there is an overlap of interruptions. The patient seeks confirmation: *ri[ght* as the phone rings and the doctor utters *[yes*, (line 17). The doctor has gazed at the sheet for 17.70 seconds and as he responds to the patient's statement in line 13, he does not gaze at the patient. Instead he briefly gazes at the phone's display on which the incoming number appears (see picture D), but he still does not respond to the call even though its ringing prompts his orientation to a third element in the diagnostic event. The phone interruption is thus defined as a secondary event pivot leading to a second change in the interactivity as the stress level increases further: The doctor needs to engage in dialogue, comprehend the information on the sheet, interpret the relevance of the incoming call and perceive the situation as a whole in order to decide how he should respond to the multiple disturbances. In Figure 6.2 this is indicated as: *stressed multitasking*.

At that moment the doctor struggles to balance multiple activities simultaneously: taking the patient's history, reading the sheet and containing the interruptions. The patient is persistent and continues to ignore the ringing and completes a point in her narrative: *and then I had to call my daughter who says to me mum this is not (.)* (line 18). As she starts her utterance, the doctor gazes at the phone, but as the patient holds her breath for a short moment *(.)*, the doctor again gazes at the patient, who continues: *this is not [(xxx)*. As the patient utters something unrecognisable, she is interrupted for the third time by the ringing phone, which still does not prevent the patient from finalising her utterance: *it is blood=* (line 18). The doctor immediately follows up on this utterance and repeats the patient's last three words: *=it is blood*, and continues: *I have to take this one* (line 20). He then responds to the call, walks away from the patient and gazes out in the room as he speaks on the phone (see picture E).

The final ringing is identified as the primary event pivot that leads to a task switch. In Figure 6.2 its consequences are defined as changes in the interactivity trajectory and the change is characterised as: *history taking on standby*. As the doctor finally responds to the incoming call and leaves the room, he re-enacts a value hierarchy, which leads to the breakdown of the cognitive system, both functionally (goal orientation) and interpersonally (seeking good prospects). In my data, dysfunctional interactions often emerge as a person has low multitask tolerance. In this case, the cognitive event is characterised by multiple event pivots, which finally lead to a task switch (see Figure 6.2). As this doctor is forced to respond to multiple demands within the cognitive system, he loses overview of the situation. The interesting questions are why the doctor chooses to answer the phone call during another task and secondly why it takes him such a long time to respond to the incoming call – when he finally chooses to do so. The cognitive patient-doctor system is constituted by moral values such as caring and trust, and it is a dialogical and situational system that only exists for a limited time. However, the doctor is also morally and socially obligated to maintain a relationship to non-local, though long-lasting social systems, for instance systems that include other colleagues and management staff. Such systems consist of values that guide healthcare professionals' behaviour even though they are not physically present (Bang and Døør 2007). "Humans are always interdependent with others, although the degree and kinds of interdependencies will of course vary with individuals, cultures and situations" (Linell 2009: 13).

For him to maintain a good reputation, the doctor is dependent on organisational credibility, which he achieves by being sensitive to social systems and responding to the phone call interruption. As non-local relationships matter in local interaction, it is of consequence whether team members follow protocols and orders or not. The phone call symbolises an anonymous 'other' (Linell 2009), and depending on how the abstract and trans-situational other is managed, it guides the local actions in a certain direction. In this context it means that the doctor is expected to respond when a superior seeks contact. If he chooses not to do so, he can be reprimanded. Answering the call thus realises important values within the social system. As caring within the social system is achieved by responding to the call, caring within the dialogical system is realised by not-responding to the call. As the doctor is unable to engage in dialogue and respond to the interruption at the same time, a dilemma emerges. As the doctor sees no other solutions to the dilemma, he needs to choose between caring for the dialogical system or for the social system. The doctor hesitates and postpones answering the call, which indicates a double sensitivity towards both local interaction and non-local expectations. However, the stress level increases: The phone has rung three times and will soon stop ringing. If he does not respond in time, his behaviour could be categorised as inattentive from a social systemic perspective. Further, while the patient might have felt the interruptions as constraints for dialogical interaction, her 'ignorance strategy' enables her to treat the first six interruptions as non-interruptive. Her strategy complicates the doctor's options for managing the interruptions as interruptive as this strategy requires that he interrupts the patient and undermines her strategy. If the patient had oriented herself towards the interruptions as such, conditions for dialogical coordination were better as there would be a shared agreement about the complexity of the situation. That the doctor does not respond immediately to the call is thus interpreted as a sign of caring for the patient even though his behaviour appears hesitant and non-engaging. When he becomes stressed by the pressure of time (the third and last ringing), the main problem with the doctor's behaviour is that he is forced to find the first possible completion point and interrupt the patient by announcing that he is going to respond to the call (line 20). The second problem relates to the way he manages the phone call. Before he leaves the room, the doctor orients himself towards the nurse and asks for permission to leave for a short moment as he points towards the door (see picture F). The nurse agrees and the doctor leaves without informing the patient, without looking at her and without letting her know what is happening and for how long he will be gone.

Together the number of interruptions adds up and results in a task switch (see Figure 6.2), and it attests to how the doctor in the end prioritises the organisational system and its authorities at the expense of dialogue with the patient. The situation changes as disturbances within the interactivity trajectory disintegrate the cognitive system and reorganise its boundaries; in this case consequently with a dysfunctional outcome. While the doctor is cognitively overloaded by the disintegration, the patient is emotionally affected: She withdraws, and she does not respond to the doctor's explanation: *I have to take this one* (line 20). In fact, she stares vacantly into space without gazing at the doctor or responding to his announcement.

From the moment the patient arrives, the medical team does not know what caused the severe rectal bleeding, and it is a serious medical condition. Thus, from a patient perspective, the interaction with the doctor does not reflect much understanding and the logic of the system is not immediately transparent, explicit or caring: "all doctors and health systems purport to put patients first, but ample evidence tells that it often doesn't feel that way to patients. They regularly feel like cases rather than people, and what is important to patients is often different from what is important to doctors" (Smith 2003: 1433). The doctor's performance appears irrational and insensitive since the patient, in the end, is valued lowest in a diagnostic situation. Paradoxically, the negative outcome overshadows the multiple failed attempts to maintain a dialogical relation with the patient.

2.3 Seeking good prospects

The multiple interruptions do not only disturb cognitive activity, but they also affect the interpersonal relation between the doctor and the patient and the flow of interactivity in a way that impedes the completion of a shared task. Thus, even though the underlying intentions behind interruptions are only addressed to one person, the interruption itself often disrupts the current undertaking of a cognitive system.

Analysis demonstrates how interruptions affect the flow of interactivity as change in gaze, the handling of artefacts and values-realisation within multiple fields lead to local disturbances in the cognitive system. The system appears to have reached a peak level of cognitive load and consequently the boundary of the dialogical system between the doctor and the patient dissolves and he switches from history taking to another task. The doctor's actions are thus caused by stress rather than cognitive prioritisation. When they manage interruptions, the practitioners' strategy is decisive for how they bounce back from the interruption. Rather than arguing that doctors should always prioritise completion of ongoing local tasks and ignore interruptions, I argue that they should be equipped with the ability to manage interruptions efficiently and in a caring way. Hence a functional and dialogical approach to interruptions is based on an evaluation of the situation. The doctor's attempt to care for the patient by postponing the task switch entails a hectic situation in which he is forced to act. He could have distributed the responsibility across the team (this is what the following case explores), responded immediately to the interruptions to avoid a stressful interaction situation or briefly explicated why he needs to respond to the call.

Hodges argues that caring in the long run depends on realising multiple values over time. To exemplify, he argues that in an experiment where people should tell the truth, they tend to both tell the truth (truth-telling), and sometimes the adverse happens as they honour other people's understanding of truth (caring) (Hodges 2009). In the medical ward interruptions are not dysfunctional *per se*. Responding to interruptions only becomes problematic, if it indicates a fixed attention-hierarchy and it happens repeatedly without prioritising the patient. Patients are aware that much goes on in the ward and the healthcare practitioners are busy. However, when they feel overlooked and valued lowest *by default*, the boundary conditions are challenged. Thus, the healthcare practitioner must treat interruptions situationally, and in the long run a heterarchy of attention tasks will emerge.

In contrast, in another case a primary doctor interrupts history taking as she is needed outside the ward. As she leaves the ward, she explicates that part of her job description involves her presence at multiple locations at unpredictable times, but that she will be back as soon as possible. She further excuses this interruption-practice, so the patient is left with the feeling that it is not the doctor's decision or prioritisation but the work procedures which make her respond to interruptions during conversation.

As we have seen, interruptions do more than distress working memory; they also affect sensitivity and inter-bodily dynamics in a way that impairs the interpersonal relationship between healthcare practitioner and patient. In the next section, it is shown how interruptions can be managed to avoid pivotal disturbances.

3. Case II: Team coordination as values realisation: Managing interruptions so they do not interrupt

This case focuses on how a telephone interruption is successfully dealt with during history taking. A novice doctor talks to a female patient, who presumably has a serious infection causing her to have breathing problems and a bad cough. She is weak, dizzy and exhausted. The nurse observes the interaction and she is ready to assist in getting the measurements they need. The layout is visualised below and followed by a transcript that indicates what happens before, during and immediately after the interruption occurs.

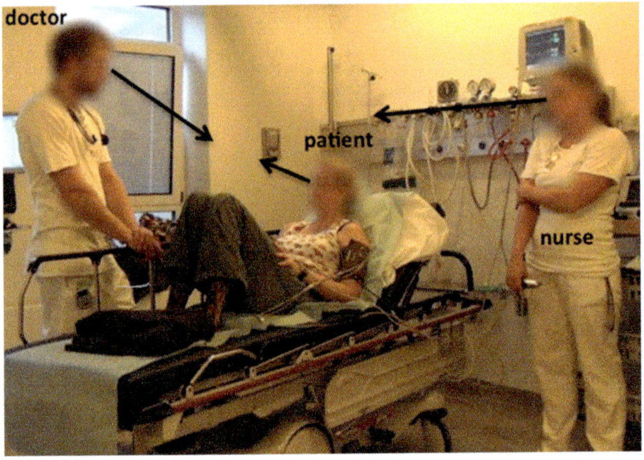

Figure 6.3 Overview of the layout: Interruptions in teams

Transcript 6.2[4]

Danish original

```
1. 00:00:00, D:   har du noget åndenød synes du
2. 00:01:10, ps.  (0.8)
3. 00:01:90, P:   altså jeg trækker vejret overfladisk
4. 00:03:90, D:   ja (.) okay
5. 00:05:10, P:   og det er for ikke at komme til at hoste
6. 00:06:80, D:   for ikke at komme til at hoste (.) okay godt føler du at du sådan
                  har hjertebanken kører det hurtigt hele tiden eller (.)
7. 00:11:90, P:   altså efter jeg fik det der (.) sulfid i går
8. 00:14:60, D:   mm
9. 00:15:00, ph   ri[ng ring
10. 00:15:70, P:    [der [s:ynes jeg at (.) der nogen gange er sådan
11. 00:16:10, D:         [hov (nurse takes phone in her hand)
12. 00:17:80, ps. (1.3)
13. 00:19:10, P:  m[en det har jeg haft (hoster)
14. 00:19:20, ph   [ring ring
15. 00:21:20, ps. (0,5)
16. 00:21:70, P:  d[et har jeg haft før (.) (xxx) føler jeg at (.) det lige slår
17. 00:21:80, N:   [det er [nurse's name] (.) det er bare lige [doctor's name]
                  telefon
18. 00:25:50, D:  at det li:ge slår en lille kolbøtte
19. 00:27:30, P:  en enkelt gang i[k
20. 00:28:20, D:                   [men det er ikke sådan noget der bliver ved (.)
                  [(xxx) op og ned (.) nej [godt
21. 00:29:30, P:  [(P nods 'no' with her head as she coughs)
22. 00:31:50, N:                           [super
```

4. Interruptions are marked in red. *Ph* is an abbreviation for phone.

```
23. 00:31:70, ps.  (1.9)
24. 00:33:60, D:   var det noget (rækker ud efter telefonen)
25. 00:34:00, ps.  (0.9)
26. 00:34:90, N:   det var bare om stue seks var kørt
27. 00:36:20, D:   nå
28. 00:36:60, ps.  (2.9)
29. 00:39:50, D:   godt (.) nogen smerter mere noget kvalme
```

English translation

```
1. 00:00:00, D:    Do you feel as if you have difficulty breathing?
2. 00:01:10, ps.   (0.8)
3. 00:01:90, P:    I do in fact breathe shallowly.
4. 00:03:90, D:    yes (.) okay
5. 00:05:10, P:    and that is just to avoid coughing
6. 00:06:80, D:    to avoid coughing (.) ok fine do you feel that you have heart
palpitations constanly, or (.)
7. 00:11:90, P:    well after I have got this (.) sulphide Yesterday (.)
8. 00:14:60, D:    mm
9. 00:15:00, ph    ri[ng ring
10. 00:15:70, P:     [then I [thi:nk that (.) sometimes there is a kind of a
11. 00:16:10, D:             [oops (nurse takes phone in her hand)
12. 00:17:80, ps.  (1.3)
13. 00:19:10, P:   b[ut I have had this (coughs)
14. 00:19:20, ph    [ring ring
15. 00:21:20, ps.  (0,5)
16. 00:21:70, P:   I [have had this before (.) (xxx) feel that (.) it just somer
17. 00:21:80, N:     [[nurse's name] speaking (.) it is [doctor' name] phone
18. 00:25:50, D:   that it ju:st somersaulted
19. 00:27:30, P:   just once ri[ght
20. 00:28:20, D:               [but it is not something that continues (.) [(xxx) up
                   and down (.) no [okay
21. 00:29:30, P:                                                               [(P nods
                   'no' with her head as she coughs)
22. 00:31:50, N:                  [super
23. 00:31:70, ps.  (1.9)
24. 00:33:60, D:   was it something important (reaches for the phone)
25. 00:34:00, ps.  (0.9)
26. 00:34:90, N:   just checking if ward six was cleared
27. 00:36:20, D:   oh
28. 00:36:60, ps.  (2.9)
29. 00:39:50, D:   well (.) any pains anymore any nausea
```

When we enter this conversation, the doctor has just greeted the patient and informed her about what he is going to do next: ask for information that enables him to reach a diagnosis. From line 1–7 the doctor and patient engage in history taking. The doctor is a novice and he has only been working at the ward for less than a week at the time of the recording. Rather unusually, he does not rely on any aiding tools during this task performance. He leans towards the patient and gazes at her as he asks for specific information. The patient gazes momentarily at the doctor and straight ahead when she is going to recall memory. As the patient utters: *b[ut I have had this* (line 13), the doctor's phone rings (line 14). Figure 6.4 and 6.5 illustrate how the interruption affects the current undertaking and how the medical team acts to prevent the interruption from leading to task switch and from harming the current dialogue. This efficient team performance is initiated by the nurse's anticipatory actions, which will be investigated in detail in the following.

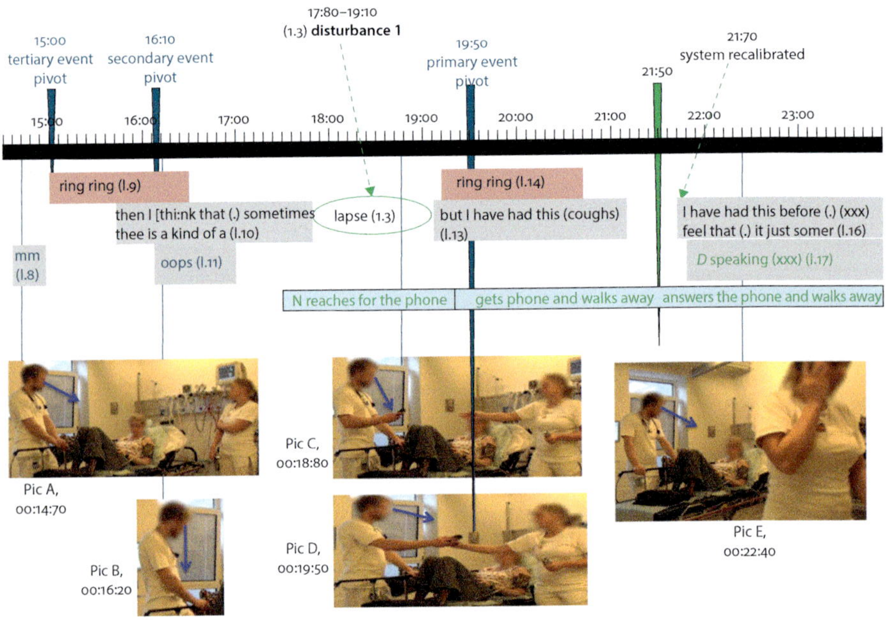

Figure 6.4 Anticipatory dynamics in interruptive practices
The black text indicates the patient's utterances, the blue text indicates the doctor's utterances, the green text indicates the nurse's utterances.

The telephone rings at 15:00 just in the patient's breathing (line 7). The ringing leads to several anticipatory actions (tertiary event pivot). The doctor immediately treats the interruption as relevant. Until the interruption occurs, the doctor gazes at the patient (see picture A), but at 15:70, he pays attention to the interruption as he gazes at his pocket in which his phone is located (see picture B). However, the patient overlaps the loud ringing and finishes her explanation at the same time as the doctor changes his visual orientation from her to the phone: *[then I thi:nk that (.) sometimes there is a kind of a* (line 10).

Like in the previous case, a dilemma emerges as the doctor is expected to realise values in two systems simultaneously. First, he engages in a dialogical system where history taking is managed together with the patient. Second, he is also part of a larger, socio-cultural and organisational system that prompts a professional, standardised behaviour: immediate response, as delayed response can lead to bad outcomes in other locations. Thus, the doctor is expected to balance caring for the patient and smooth work procedure in the ward, which means caring for colleagues and other patients. Values realisation in such two different systems is constrained and enabled by different dynamics. In the former system, inter-bodily dynamics affect decision-making directly, and this was a major explanation for why the doctor in the previous case postponed his interruptive behaviour. In the latter system, rules and norms constrain the moral obligations that affect real-time decisions.

Thus, in case II, the doctor explicitly orients himself to the interruption as unfortunate: *[oops* (line 11), as he takes the phone out of his pocket. Altogether, this course of events prompts the nurse to interfere. The nurse's subsequent actions can be characterised as negative feedback mechanisms within the system that prevent latent breakdowns to emerge, prompted by the tertiary and secondary event pivots (the ringing and the doctor's response to the disturbing source). The doctor's visual orientation towards the phone and his verbal utterance *oops* thus mark the secondary event pivot in the cognitive event trajectory, and this utterance affords a series of anticipatory actions (see Figure 6.4). The patient does not treat the ringing and the doctor's behaviour as a reason to stop her narrative. The doctor himself seems annoyed by the interruption and as he picks up his phone, he gazes at the patient, who continues to speak. Just as the phone stops at 16:50, the patient gazes at the doctor and she finalises her utterance. The doctor holds on to the phone and as the nurse anticipates that the doctor probably is going to answer the call, she reaches out for it (see picture C). From the moment the nurse reaches for the phone and the patient has finalised her utterance in line 10 (00:17.80) and until the nurse almost has the phone in her hand and the patient resumes her narrative (00:19:10), 1.3 seconds elapse (see Figure 6.4). The phone-switching event is defined as the primary event pivot. It only causes a minimum of disturbance, which entails that the interaction is briefly put on standby. Most likely the nurse anticipates that the doctor's actions are going to interrupt the current undertaking. Thus, at a critical moment, she both offers and demands that she is going to handle the phone call. The doctor hesitates as he briefly gazes at the phone display to check who is calling before he accepts the nurse's demand (see picture C). Thus, as the patient continues her narrative in line 13, the phone rings for the second time. At the same time, the nurse gets the phone from the doctor who regains eye contact with the patient and resumes the history taking (see picture D). At 00:21:50 the nurse answers the call and walks away while the doctor and patient continue their dialogue in the same manner as before the interruption occurred. Hence, the cognitive system remains intact and its boundaries are recalibrated (see Figure 6.4).

While the nurse handles the phone call, she executes a nested task, which the medical team needs to respond to, but she does it in a way that reduces the chances for cognitive overload, interpersonal breakdowns and task switching. The therapeutic alliance between doctor and patient remains intact. The patient's behaviour indicates that the disturbance or 'noise' in the cognitive system goes almost unnoticed by her, and the doctor and patient continue without any problematic breaks or disturbances.

The team performance is highly coordinated, and it enables values realisation in a constrained situation with a minimum of dysfunctional outcome. As the doctor cannot do two things simultaneously, the nurse enables him to continue with his initial task as she performs the second task for him. This coordination succeeds as the nurse anticipates the flow of actions and the doctor relies on and trusts the nurse's prioritisation. Their coordinated behaviour enables them to embrace complex and diverging expectations and realise multiple constraining values. As the team organises the values in a heterarchy, decisions can be made as a result of emergent properties of the environment combined with expectations for goal orientation. Specifically, it is due to the distributed properties of the cognitive system that multiple values are realised simultaneously without ordering the activities in a predefined hierarchy.

From the emergence of the first event pivot until the system has calibrated its dynamical interaction mode, 5.60 seconds pass. A few moments later, the nurse re-enters and closes the phone conversation while the patient is simultaneously plagued by a bad cough. The whole situation prompts the doctor to pay attention to the nurse to define which issue requires his attention the most (the patient or the interruption). From that moment a small nested activity is embedded in the history taking task (see Figure 6.5).

Figure 6.5 underlines the minimal disturbances the interruption entails after the nurse has responded to the call, and finally it illustrates how the situation has affected the cognitive task of history taking overall.

As the nurse closes the phone conversation *super* (line 22) the doctor orients himself to her (see picture F) and he asks whether it was an important call (line 24). Briefly, the nurse updates the doctor about the particularities, which do not require the doctor's further involvement as she has solved the problem already (see picture G). The doctor acknowledges this update, puts his phone back in his pocket and reorients himself to the patient (see picture H).

To sum up, the doctor and nurse complete this nested task within 7.8 seconds. The interruption proved to be just a trifle and as a result the doctor was exempted

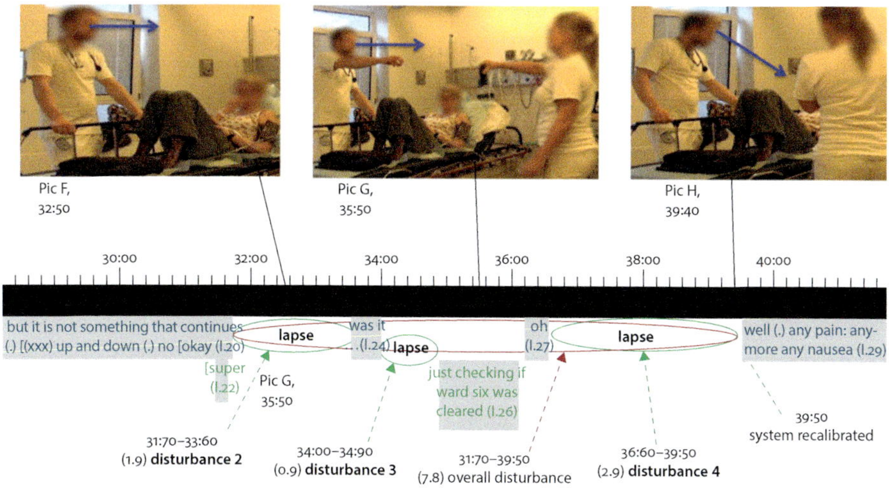

Figure 6.5 Interruptions as non-interruptive

from engaging further in the intentions behind the interruption. If the interruption had required the doctor's attention, this would presumably have been prioritised. Only in this case, it was not needed.

The way the team manages the phone interruption is an exception in my dataset. The interactivity trajectory deviates from standard situations involving interruptions. In the ward, the doctors answer their phones themselves without fail. Experienced doctors tend to answer immediately without taking time to judge from where the call is coming; in a few situations they ignore the calls if the local situation is acute and critical. Novices on the contrary tend to hesitate before they respond as the situated demands for presence and attendance often collide with non local expectations for responding to an authority. However, the delayed response only adds further frustration and cognitive overload as shown in the first case.

Sharing responsibility for dialogical work practice and making use of the team's capabilities as interruptions occur are barely noticed in the coding. A phone call is always an interruption, but the nurse anticipates a line of actions that affords her to manage the interruption, so it never becomes problematically interruptive. As the team members co-act, their actions serve as negative feedback mechanisms, which reduce the risk for task switching regularly leading to human error or harming the interaction unnecessarily. The nurse actively recalibrates the boundaries of the cognitive system. In the beginning she is cognitively loosely associated to the system. Nevertheless, she observes what is happening. Rather than allowing the patient-doctor relation to break down, she enables the doctor to maintain ongoing dialogue and history taking. As she turns around and walks into a corner of the room as she handles the call, she disintegrates with the doctor-patient system. Hence, her task performance does not disturb or interfere with the doctor's task performance to be a consequence for the functionality of the cognitive system.

In the ward, interruptions appear to be imposed on individuals, for instance when a caller seeks to reach a specific practitioner. However, there are alternatives to individual problem-solving. As the latter case showed, relying on the distributed qualities of team constellations enables caring for the patient by prioritising differently in the same situation. The team's coaction enables it to complete a shared project and to meet the broader organisational needs constituted as procedure following as well as local needs in interaction. By acting individually together, they multitask. The overall multitask tolerance is high even when challenged by interruptions, and the team deals with the competing requests in a way that replaces a traditional task hierarchy with a shared task heterarchy. This performance minimises dilemmas and favours several groups of people simultaneously: the organisational system, the medical team and the patient.

4. Wayfinding in emergency medicine

The first case presents a general interruption-driven practice involving a novice doctor operating in a stressful environment. Interruptions lead to cognitive overload as multiple demands constrain local dialogue and task performance. The second case unveils how successful interruption management is achieved through team coordination. The nurse's anticipatory behaviour and the way the team balances multiple expectations simultaneously, enable a dialogical and fluent diagnostic process where the risk for human error is remarkably lower due to the high multitask tolerance of the team. Attention, sensitivity and a caring attitude towards both patient and the general needs of the organisation are the beneficial and functional result of the team's behaviour. Most importantly, the distribution of task performance enables an efficient performance without reducing or losing power and responsibility. As the nurse is not allowed to make decisions within the doctor's domain, she can offload the doctor and facilitate the information processes so that information is given at the right time. As the interruption was just about information passing, no decisions were made, and no responsibility domains were challenged. In other words, the nurse could perform this task just as well and unproblematically as the doctor. Paraphrasing Hodges (2007a) their dialogical behaviour is a form of wayfinding, from which the cognitive system as a whole, benefits both functionally and interpersonally.

As the cases illustrate, patients tend to have a high tolerance to interruptions coming from non-human sources. However, in cases, when healthcare practitioners left the room, the patients often uttered a frustration because of the practitioners' interruptive behaviour: The patients would say to me (I remained in the ward with the patients and their relatives) that it was not because they were interrupted as such, but because the practitioners were gone for an unknown amount of time, and the waiting time was almost intolerable for the patients, who were seeking clarification and expressed a need to being taken seriously. Frustrated and irritated patients do not seem to be the intended outcome of the healthcare practitioners' responses to interruptions; rather, they are unaware of how patients make sense of the situation when they leave the room. On the other hand, the healthcare practitioners appear to be affected by interruptions in the history taking task, and there is a tendency for the novices to attempt to balance multiple expectations in a way that leads to more stressful situations. The novices with less automatised diagnostic skills display a low multitask tolerance as they are cognitively limited, and they spend more time on navigating through the complexity of an interruption-driven situation. Eventually, when a maximum stress level is reached, the novice employs a strategy, which allows for one thing at a time, and they tend to prioritise expectations from non-local systems.

The experienced healthcare practitioners prioritise and handle dilemmas by doing one thing at a time carefully and contain local frustration. In the previous Chapter 5 the doctor simply avoids responding to the interruption and refuses to switch task and eventually, the nurse, a less busy team member at the time, handles the interruption. Thus, the doctor prioritises the current undertaking and contains the stressful situation caused by an increasing noise coming from the interrupting source. Other experienced doctors I have observed, ignore incoming calls as they know the call is diverted to another colleague, and that in 'true' emergencies they will be interrupted by alarm systems etc. However, such deviant and 'disobedient' behaviour is related to culture and expertise, and for a novice it can be difficult to know when not following protocol is useful and acceptable.

CHAPTER 7

Cultural dynamics

Emotions, role hierarchies and touch in emergency medicine

1. The biomedical model in emergency medicine: Cultural challenges and values[1]

Medical practitioners are constrained by cultural dynamics shaped by non-local timescales (Pedersen 2010; Pedersen, 2012; Pedersen and Steffensen 2014, Steffensen and Cowley 2010, Cowley 2011). In real time interactivity, cultural dynamics, such as normative embodied procedures, mesh with situational dynamics that become local affordances for action. When these dynamics diverge and provide different action possibilities they are managed through (dys)functional coordination in the local. As demonstrated in the previous chapter, values are important for understanding the enabling conditions for such coordination as values underlie a self-organising constitution of boundaries in an ecosystem (Hodges and Baron 1992; Hodges 2007a, 2007b). With the theory of values realisation, this chapter investigates how much power cultural dynamics have on situated interactivity, and at the same time how culture is dynamically shaped by embodied behaviour, and eventually how this process relates to the emergence of error cycles. Initially, two main cultural challenges that appeared in the coding are elaborated and related to general cultural challenges in the medical sector. The challenges concern the emotional consequences of a biomedical model in diagnostic processes in emergency medicine and the function of role hierarchies in emergency medical decision-making.

First, the biomedical model in Western medicine favours a logic, which prioritises objective facts over emotional and subjective experiences. This model implies a predefined understanding of proper clinical behaviour. The model thus shapes a specific kind of actions and frames decision-making in situated interaction

1. An earlier version of Sections 7.1–7.2.1 appeared as "Affect and affordances– The role of action and emotion in social interaction" in *Cognitive Semiotics*, 9, 2016. It is reused here with permission from De Gruyter: https://www.degruyter.com/view/j/cogsem and co-author, Thomas Wiben Jensen.

in a fixed fashion, which constrains flexible adaptive behaviour. Put simply, the biomedical model dominates and contributes to a fixed view on healthcare: "The biomedical model has become a cultural imperative, its limitations easily overlooked. In brief, it has now acquired the status of a dogma … Biomedical dogma requires that all disease be conceptualized in terms of derangement of underlying physical mechanisms" (Engel 1977: 130). The biomedical model entails a disparity between patients' experiences of *illness* and the biomedical categorisation and focus on physical symptoms, the *disease* (Putsch and Joyce 1990). With a Cartesian rationalism, the practitioner focuses on the bodily disease as it reveals itself to the observer, and what the patient thinks and utters about his medical situation is secondary: "It has been proposed that the inability to deal with illness is a major failing of biomedicine" (Putsch and Joyce 1990: 1050).

Moreover, the biomedical model argues against emotion-laden interactivity. Especially in the emergency ward, due to the high level of uncertainty and the possible extreme outcome of the medical situation, emotional experiences are ubiquitous amongst both practitioners and patients (Angoff 2002). Anxiety, stress, anger, withdrawal or even hostility are emotional circumstances the patient and healthcare team enact. "Yet physicians are taught to remain detached from participating in these emotions in order to maintain the objectivity thought to be crucial to accurate clinical decision-making" (Halpern 2001: 188). In educational settings, medical students are taught to achieve the "detached concern" and the student learns to objectify and intellectualise emotion-laden experiences as a means to distance himself from his own anxiety and fear and maintain a rational focus on the task (Halpern 2001). In my dataset, this distance is not just symbolic and mental. It is expressed in a physical moving away strategy and a fear of being physically close to or *with* the patient.

From an ecological perspective, emotions are not individual mental representations; they are dialogically tied to interactivity (Jensen 2014a). In a general social context, Goodwin and Cekaite (2018) have made visible how touch is important for the establishment, negotiation and maintenance of valuable relationships. In a similar vein, Dewey argues that emotions are not distinguished in internal biological states and external expressions; instead he defines *situations* as saturated with emotionality (Dewey 1929). Such an approach allows for analysing emotions "as processes of organism-environment interactions" (Colombetti 2010: 157). In contrast to this view, the biomedical model prompts healthcare practitioners to act less dialogically and increase the relational distance between themselves and the patients. In the analyses it is shown how the fear of emotions manifests itself in the way the healthcare practitioners avoid physical contact and attendance with the patient, for instance by relying more on medical verbal explanation than interbodily dynamics. The chances for misunderstanding, frustration and human error increase as practitioners avoid physical rapport with the patient (Putsch and Joyce 1990). Particularly, Dr. Verghese, a physician, professor *and senior associate chair for the Theory and Practice of Medicine at Stanford University School of Medicine in California*, has studied the absence of 'social touch' in contemporary medicine. He continuously underlines how the frequency of, and the time spent on bedside examination are decreasing and how this tendency entails an increasing distance between the patient and the healthcare practitioner. Paradoxically, he argues, in our technological age the most important innovation in medicine is the power of the human hand, which is not acknowledged within the field: "we touch our patients less and less: the physical exam, the skilled bedside examination of the patient, has diminished to where it is pure farce" (Verghese 2009: 1178). Other practitioners within the field of medical education underline how important social touch is and how it is rarely, if ever, a focus area of education: "Learning to effectively use procedural and social touch together is important in limiting risk and, when done well, can enhance the power of the clinical moment" (Searles).[2] Further, Goodwin et al. (2012) argue that "touch constitutes one of the modalities that has distinct temporal qualities; in contrast to speech, touch […] has the potential to endure. […] verbal requests do not need to be repeated; rather, their interactional relevance can be effectively extended through the use of the tactile modality" (Goodwin et al. 2012: 8). That means that laying a hand on a patient's shoulder during history taking, for instance, can be a way of realising multiple values simultaneously as the enduring touch calms the patient (caring) when the healthcare practitioner at the same time is able to maintain a bio-medical focus on the task. Hence when he touches the patient, he can ask relevant questions, and the emotionality of the situation is more likely to be contained in a functional and caring manner.

Unfortunately, within the literature referred to above, the opposite (a bodily less engaged attitude in the medical encounter) seems to be prioritised. This development within the field of medicine is a consequence of the technological advances within the field that prompt practitioners to orient themselves to a representation of the real patient, a patient that is clothed in binary garments, also referred to as the *iPatient* (Verghese 2009). The technological development provides affordances (technological artefacts e.g.), which underwrite the scope of the biomedical model. While the development enlarges the distance to the real patient (see also Chapter 4 and 5), it feeds positively back on the biomedical culture. This is the focus of the first case in this chapter.

Another cultural and general issue of debate concerns the function and consequences of professional role hierarchies in medical decision-making. Role

2. http://www.mbc.ca.gov/Licensees/Sexual_Misconduct/Touch.aspx, May, 18th, 2015.

hierarchies contribute to fixed understandings of who is in charge and responsible for various decision-making processes. Potentially, such hierarchies scaffold efficient subdivision of tasks and responsibility, but they also become a pitfall for individual and monological behaviour when dilemmas emerge, problems arise and the unknown surfaces (Pedersen 2010). This will be investigated in the second case.

While the medical culture is characterised by strong expectations of the different roles in the medical team, practitioners easily please those same expectations. The healthcare sector places medical roles in a hierarchy that is characterised by differences in responsibility, control, authority, knowledge etc. This is not just implicit. Differences appear in artefacts such as salaries, clothes, equipment and even factors such as how practitioners interact and behave. The artefacts function as affordances for acting in hierarchies of fixed roles. Working in healthcare, however, is also working in a learning practice where team members learn from each other. Given this way of thinking, members of a team must accept and also approach knowledge sharing and dialogue. A large part of the problem with role hierarchies lies with a social system that consists in culturally and historically defined norms and procedures, which, in effect, come into conflict with a need for more flexible and collective procedures.

It is hypothesised that cultural dynamics are more powerful than situated affordances in local decision-making processes. The chapter uses two cases in which cultural dynamics clash with local interactivity to investigate to what extent healthcare practitioners draw on non-local cultural affordances (Pedersen 2010) for action and how flexibly they adapt to the changes within the environment respectively.

This chapter pays particular attention to how cognitive events are constrained by cultural dynamics. It uses CEA as a method for identifying the relevant event pivots that connect with non-local understandings of how problems are managed. Therefore, it also draws on longer timescales to show how situation-transcendent dynamics affect local organisation in interaction. Specifically, dialogical theories and values-realisation theory are applied in the analyses. Thus, by applying an ecological values realisation perspective, healthcare practitioners' attempt to navigate and manage such challenges can be investigated as sense-saturated, coordinated self-organising processes, which guide action and lead to results (Hodges and Baron 1992; Hodges 2009). To balance and realise multiple values without violating the boundaries of a cognitive system requires an overview of the situation and an understanding of how experience and cultural norms scaffold and inhibit local decision-making.

2. Case I: The social touch

The first case presents two excerpts, which involve a patient who literally reaches out for the doctor. It investigates what happens when the biomedical model dominates in diagnostic situations and fixates healthcare professionals in a strict problem-solving mode of interaction. It further investigates how and why emotional dynamics of interactivity are suppressed, and it outlines the consequences of this absence of dialogical task achievement. The aim is to demonstrate the challenges a bio-medical perspective entails for dialogical diagnostic situations and how touch appears to be crucial in interactions where the unexpected permeates the situation.

In this situation, the doctor, a young, female novice struggles to get hold of the patient's unstable and critical medical condition. The patient is an elderly woman, who just arrived with 911, and her condition is critical, unresolved and unstable. Her husband sits next to the patient and he plays a key role in the history taking process, as the patient's speech is impaired due to respiratory problems. Below is an illustration of the layout.

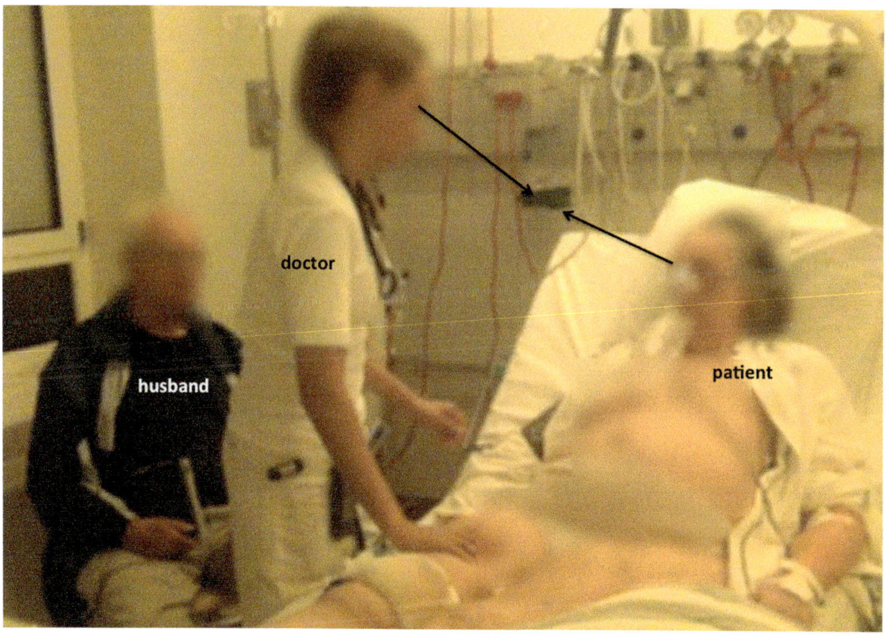

Figure 7.1 Overview of the layout: Touch

2.1 The soothing effect of touch and emotional alignment: Patient-initiated touch

As we enter the interaction, the doctor is faced with the indication of the patient's dangerously unstable oxygen saturation, which is documented by measurements appearing on the screen above the patient. The doctor fixates on medical measurements and the patient and the patient's husband have not been informed about the procedures or general agenda. Rather, they observe the doctor's actions as a step-by-step procedure, without knowing where they are heading in advance. While the doctor keeps observing, they wait. The patient, who is scared as she presumably just had a blood clot in her lung, initiates an emotion-laden interaction mode, which indicates a need for contact. As her speech is impaired due to her respiratory problems, she relies primarily on non-verbal interaction. When the doctor has observed the measurements for 8.7 seconds, the patient reaches for the doctor's hand. This patient-initiated touch seems to surprise and make the doctor uncomfortable to such a degree that she awkwardly withdraws from the interaction. This event is visualised in the following Figure 7.2, which indicates the exact timing of the multiple dynamics in the interactivity and the inter-bodily dynamics that lead to system disintegration.

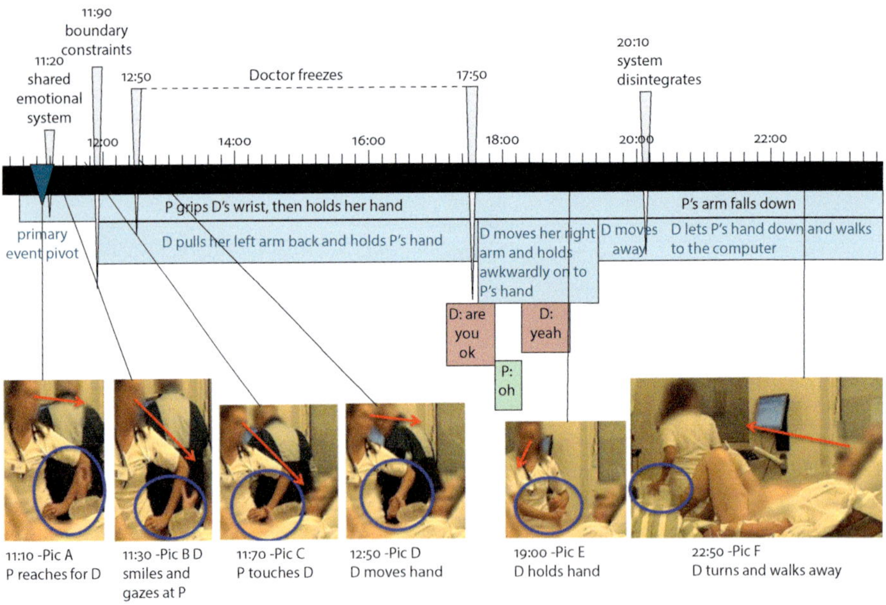

Figure 7.2 Shared emotional system: Touch and task performance

The figure emphasises the behavioural dynamics that affect both the emotional alliance between the doctor and the patient and prompt the doctor to switch task.

Before the patient-initiated touch, the patient and the doctor were not engaged in joint coordination. However, throughout the whole excerpt the patient gazes at the doctor. At 00:10:70 the patient initiates a dialogical movement; she reaches for the doctor's hand (see picture A). This action is characterised as an event pivot, which prompts the doctor to reorient herself to the patient. Thus, 0.6 seconds after the patient initiates the movement, the doctor perceives the behavioural change and gazes in the direction of the patient (see picture B). At that moment, 00:11:30, the patient and doctor align, and a shared emotional system emerges (see Figure 7.2). 0.4 seconds after they have gained eye contact (00:11:70), the patient touches the doctor and holds on to her wrist (see picture C).

According to Hodges (2007a), caring is what makes social coordination and coaction possible. Before this moment, coordination was absent, and the doctor engaged in individual problem-solving. Far from being ignorant, the doctor's individual-oriented behaviour is likely to be caused by stress and overload as her attempt to solve the medical problem reduces her sensitivity to other elements in the situation. However, no matter the cause, the function of the doctor's behaviour results in a need for coordination from the patient's perspective. The patient literally turns the doctor's attention away from the screen towards her, which changes the flow of interactivity. As this happens, the emotional state of the patient is no longer an individual private feeling; it is part of a shared experience, which invokes emotions in the doctor as well, and she smiles at the patient. By so doing, the doctor acknowledges that the patient wants something from her that is different from what a medical, individual-oriented approach provides. The reciprocal relationship between the doctor and patient necessarily makes both parties emotionally accountable for the interaction and to maintain this relationship requires that they coordinate their behaviours. As shown in Figure 7.2, coordination ceases and the shared emotional alliance lasts only a short while. The reason for this termination is analysed after the description of what happens.

Immediately after the patient touches the doctor (0.2 seconds), the doctor reorients herself to the observation task and gazes at the screen as she smiles. She moves her arm further away from her own body and holds the patient's hand in an awkward position (see picture D). This movement and her change in gaze direction, together serve as a boundary condition that threatens the newly established emotional system (see Figure 7.2). If maintained, the emotional and vulnerable relationship between the two needs to be nourished through dialogue. However, the doctor continues to hold on to the patient's hand but her body freezes for 5 seconds as she primarily stares at the electronic display above the patient's head (see Figure 7.2). Thus, 5 seconds later, 00:17:50, the doctor initiates a closure; without looking at the patient, she uses her right arm to remove the patient's hand as she gazes at the patient's medical paper record, which is located next to the patient (see picture E). During this activity she asks whether the patient is all right as she removes her hand (see Figure 7.2). The patient who has difficulty in speaking hardly reacts and as the doctor lets go of the patient's hand, she utters *yeah*, then turns around and walks to the electronic computer with the paper record in her hand (see picture F). The doctor-patient system disintegrates both emotionally and cognitively, and caring dialogue is replaced with monological behaviour. As the doctor fails to care for the patient and as she prioritises the medical task over the interpersonal relation with the patient, the system dissolves (Hodges 2009; Hodges and Baron 1992). Physically, the doctor walks away without scrutinising the intentionality behind the patient's request. There are several explanations as to why the doctor withdraws, which will be elaborated next.

Patient-initiated touch is rare, and it seems to have an interruptive function on the doctor's individual agenda. In this case, the doctor's reaction to the patient's emotional behaviour is minimal and brief. From her body language she appears uncomfortable with the patient's direct contact and she awkwardly removes the patient's hand and puts it down (see picture D-F). Interestingly, the doctor is not uncomfortable with physical touch when she establishes the contact. Several times during the diagnostic event she strokes the patient's arm or thigh and calms her. Yet, when the touch is patient-initiated, she appears uncomfortable and unable to engage emotionally in a dialogical sense. Problems arise when changes in the affordance layout are unpredicted, unusual or afford the doctor to re-prioritise her orientation, in this case from the biochemical patient represented by the screen to the emotional, living patient. Further, the complexity arises when the patient asks for something during a task performance. When Verghese (2008) underlines the importance of the social touch and bedside examination, he also explicates the dilemma that practitioners face in practice:

> When I stroked a patient's palm and caused a twitch of the mentalis muscle under the chin – the palmomental reflex – it was as if I were performing magic. Still, the demands of charting in the electronic medical record (EMR), moving patients through the system, and respecting work-hour limits led residents to spend an astonishing amount of time in front of the monitor; the EMR was their portal to consultative teams, the pharmacy, the laboratory, and radiology. It was meant to serve them, but at times the opposite seemed true. (Verghese 2008: 2749)

Verghese describes the complex field that practitioners navigate in. To realise values that enable caring and efficient work practices depends on the practitioner's ability to adapt to the situation: in this case orient themselves to the patient's needs. The situation is characterised by time pressure, complexity, rapidly evolving and changing information load with high levels of ambiguity, risks and a high workload. In situations like this, it can feel more comfortable to draw on familiar patterns rather than caring. Moreover, flexible adaptation requires situation awareness rather than a predefined hierarchy of task performances. According to the biomedical model, medical problem-solving and emotional alliance with the patient are two interdependent tasks with a clear priority. However, ignoring the emotional patient can have fatal consequences. It can lead to frustration, anxiety and withdrawal, which eventually show on the biochemical scale, for instance when fear causes high blood pressure or when anxiety and confusion inhibit patients in answering correctly to vital questions. Further, such hierarchy is not necessary. Goodwin et al. (2012) show how touch has a long-lasting effect, which can do something very different than verbal utterances. Thus, the doctor could hold the patient's hand as she continued the medical hypothesis generation alongside. The doctor faces a dilemma related to sociocultural issues and beliefs. Time is an explicit local challenge, which complicates decision-making as she meets local demands from the patient and non-local expectations of medical problem-solving. Emotional interaction does not correspond with the "detached concern", subjective and caring dialogue complicates objective medical hypothesis generating and the doctor sees no opportunity to complete both tasks on time.

Part of the dilemma can be solved if the doctor asks for help. While the medical condition is difficult and requires all her attention and possibly even specialised expertise, the dilemma is not only related to the cultural hierarchy of the biomedical model over emotional concerns but is also related to one of formal roles. In the ward there are implicit rules for when it is appropriate to call for assistance. The interviews with the practitioners show that a healthcare practitioner must make sure that he or she has done everything in her power to avert the situation by herself due to lack of resources. Thus, double-checking protocols is common procedure before one asks for help. However, as the patient's condition continues to worsen, the doctor confers with her primary doctor, and they agree to call for further assistance and get a doctor of internal medicine to examine the patient.

The doctor of internal medicine examines the patient. The doctor follows the medical examination intensively and momentarily she observes the medical values on the electronic display. During the course of events, the patient once again reaches for the doctor's hand.

This is visualised in the following figure, which indicates the exact timing of the multiple dynamics in the interactivity prompted by the patient's wish for an emotional alliance.

The situation from before is repeated. As the doctor approaches the patient, she becomes an affordance for dialogue. The patient perceives that the doctor heads towards the end of the ward where she lies, and where the computer and the electronic display are located, and she co-constructs her itinerary by requesting her attention. The doctor walks determinedly towards the patient and responds

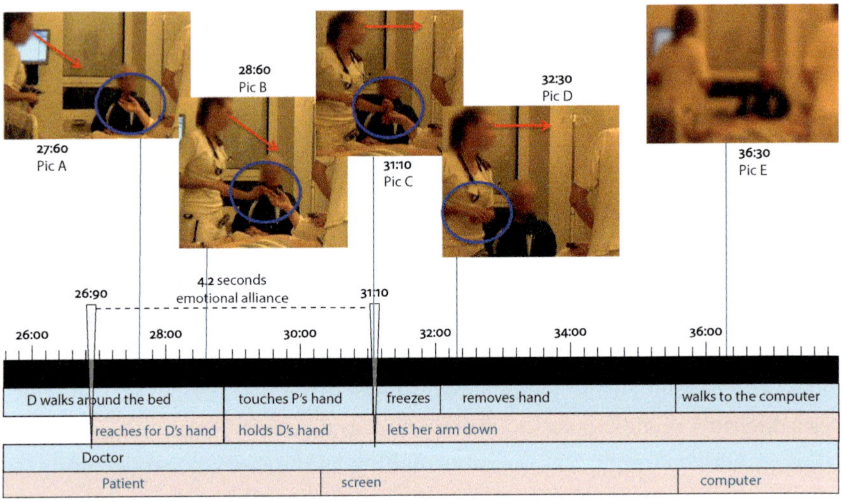

Figure 7.3 Emotional alliances through touch
The blue top layer indicates the doctor's movements. The second pink layer indicates the patient's gestures. The third blue layer indicates the patient's gaze, whereas the final pink layer indicates the doctor's gaze.

by putting her hand out. At 00:28:60 the doctor is just about to hold the patient's hand (see picture B) and she smiles at the patient. The doctor gazes at the patient and for a short moment they are aligned. However, the doctor briefly reorients herself to the screen located above the patient's head. It underlines how the doctor is alert and needs to deal with medical problems as she also needs to contain the emotional alliance with the patient. From the moment the doctor gazes at the electronic screen, only 0.8 seconds pass until the patient lets her hand down again (see picture C). As this happens, the emotional alliance between the two ceases. Due to the breakdown, the patient withdraws and the doctor freezes for a moment before she places her hands on her hips and continues to observe the measurements provided on the screen (see picture D). Finally, the doctor turns around and walks to the computer (see picture E) exactly as she did in the previous excerpt.

During this episode no one speaks. As the doctor and patient align, a special kind of emotional inter-bodily dynamics emerges. As Jensen (2014a) argues, language is inherently affective and emotions are an integral part of language and, thus, interactivity. When socio-physiological constraints are experienced in interaction, their effects shape the interactivity trajectory. In this situation, when looking at the interactivity trajectory, the patient's reaching out for the doctor manifests itself as deviant dynamics in the trajectory. The default dynamic flow is characterised as relatively stable and with few changes. The patient primarily focuses on breathing and neither says nor does anything else while the doctors are occupied with individual medical tasks: examination and observation. Conversely, as the patient interferes with that practice, the dynamical flow changes and the emotional commitment changes concurrently.

For 4.2 seconds the patient and doctor are emotionally aligned, even though the doctor does not gaze at the patient for the last 0.8 seconds of the alignment, see Figure 7.3. Touch and eye contact appear to be important elements for facilitating emotional alignment and commitment. From a biomedical perspective, this situation is not a desirable position for a doctor to be embedded in, and the 'detached concern' does not incorporate such incidents. Hence, an individual-based approach fits the biomedical model, and this could be one reason why the doctor hesitates in the patient-initiated requests for intimacy and closeness. The patient obviously wants something from the authoritative doctor. However, from her embodied behaviour, it appears that the patient primarily seeks contact and a dialogical relationship rather than attempts to *communicate* a specific content. Even though she is inhibited from speaking, she could point, or otherwise indicate a communicative need. Instead she seeks a professional, dialogical relationship by holding the doctor's hand. Holding hands is a dialogical, intimate act that connects individuals and entails moral obligation for caring behaviour (Linell 2009; Hodges 2009). Thus, language is more than a means of communication:

> Roughly put, Saussurian linguistics regarded language primarily as a means of communication. In order to transmit meanings, language employs a more or less fixed code, the features and structures of which can be studied independently. For various strands of literary scholarship and criticism, especially those fostered by hermeneutics, such a perspective on language seemed dangerously one-dimensional. Language was not just or not even primarily a means of communication, but first and foremost the epistemological condition of our existence – the "house of being" (Heidegger). (Benne 2017: 78)

If language is an epistemological condition of our existence, then it cannot be reduced to a code distinct from our bodily experiences. *The house of being* involves complex dimensions of human life and experience: engaging in activities with others, touching things etc. are crucial aspects of language. Moreover, the soothing effect of the touch has been demonstrated in other studies. For instance, a neuroscientific study investigated the relationship between stress relief and holding the hand of another person and concluded that "results indicated a pervasive attenuation of activation in the neural systems supporting emotional and behavioral threat responses when the women held their husband's hand" (Coan et al. 2006: 1032). Even though the attenuation of activation in these systems was limited when the test persons held a stranger's hand compared to their husband's, the effect was still present. In this case, there is a further incitement for the patient to specifically seek the doctor's attention rather than her husband's: The doctor is the key person in the diagnostic and treatment activity. Whether the patient wants to be calmed down, needs specific information or something else remains uncertain as the doctor fails to co-act and align with the patient for more than a few seconds. What is certain is that the patient seeks a close rapport with the doctor. At no time is the patient being included in the medical hypothesis generation, and when the doctors have finished the examination, they continue with hypothesis generation in front of the computer. As the doctors are located around the screen, their backs are towards the patient. The patient then suddenly moves and attempts to sit up in the bed. However, as she raises her upper body the oxygen mask falls off and the doctor of internal medicine immediately reacts by putting the mask back on (see picture F).

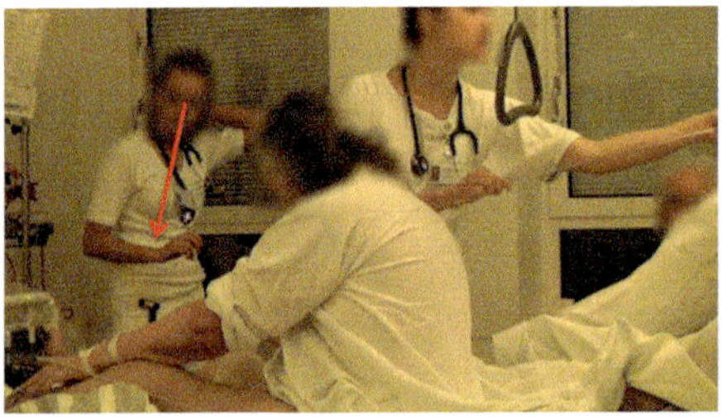

Picture F, 12:38:20

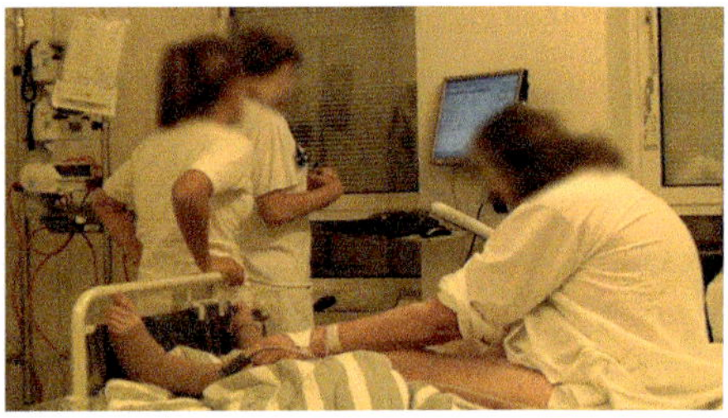

Picture G, 12:53:80

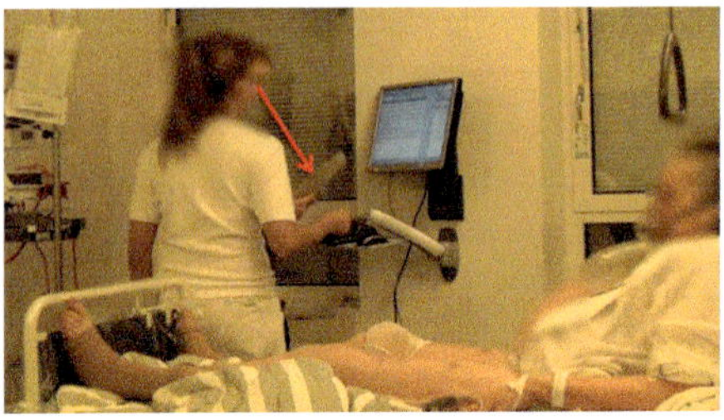

Picture H, 13:05:50

The doctors do not interact with the patient but they move the bed, so the tube attached to the mask is long enough to allow the patient to sit. The patient sits, but she does not look well, her breathing is troubled, and she has a crumpled posture. The doctors leave the patient alone and resume the medical hypothesis generating around the computer (see picture G). After a couple of seconds, the patient falls back in the bed, exhausted and unwilling or unable to say anything (see picture H).

From an observer's perspective, the patient's physical reorganisation does not seem to be related to wishing to sit up instead of lying down. Rather, it appears to be a wish for integration or communication more generally. Her multiple embodied actions are intentionally directed toward the professionals, but they are not perceived as such by the medical team. As they are fixated on medical problem-solving, they do not treat the patient's attempts at dialogue as such.

According to Jensen (2014a: 3) emotions are not individual inner states, but "processes of organism-environment interactions, and given that languaging is seen, not as an abstract semiotic system, but as dynamic adaptive behavior, emotion is to be seen as an intrinsic part of languaging itself." And he continues: "emotions *are* in fact movements; not just within us however, but also movements that connect experiences with situational affordances" (Jensen 2014a: 2ff). The patient's emotional behaviour is identified as a movement of reaching out and an attempt to establish shared coordination that affords dialogue. In the last excerpts, the doctors suppress the emotional dynamics, and the patient's movements remain movements. Finally, the patient falls back in the bed and silence or lack of movement is another emotional interactivity trajectory, which changes the flow of interactivity from dynamic to static, and as mentioned above it harms the patient in the situated interaction: She appears scared and she is excluded from the cognitive system. From a biomedical perspective no errors are detected; however, from an overall viewpoint the situation seems to harm the patient unnecessarily.

In three interrelated excerpts the patient initiates an emotional relationship with the doctor. The relationship is established through touch in the first two examples, but it lasts shortly, and the doctor withdraws and initiates other activities. In the final excerpt the medical team hardly recognises the patient's emotional wish, and after having solved the physical constraints for sitting, they resume their original task. The medical team is acting to realise only one value: caring for the patient through biomedical problem-solving. As they focus on the medical aspect of treatment, the emotional side is undermined. In the long run, such a prioritisation could turn out to be a good prioritisation as the patient's life depends on identifying the underlying causes for the disease. However, as the patient (a) perceives the medical team's professional and serious approach, (b) has difficulty breathing and (c) repeatedly seeks contact, it is likely that she fears for the outcome of her medical condition. Such feelings call for alleviation and can be managed if the doctor relies on the team's capabilities for multitasking. For instance, in other cases, nurses are called in to comfort the patient and therefore caring for the patient in local interaction could be managed if the team distributed responsibility for treatment.

2.2 Emotions in a biomedical perspective

This case reflects the tendency that the medical culture builds on a biomedical model that downplays emotional dynamics and prioritises objective medical problem-solving over interpersonal relations when dilemmas arise. Even when, in the second excerpt, the responsibility of task performance is distributed within the medical team, the doctor fails to interact successfully and continues to prioritise the biomedical model. Because the physician of internal medicine functions as the main cogniser (Galosia et al. 2010) during the physical examination task, the doctor has time to follow up on other issues regarding the patient's general situation, but she does not. As a medical team they are able to realise multiple important values simultaneously: caring for the patient and reaching a diagnosis. As they pursue the latter, they overlook the former. The doctor observes the work of the specialist, which inhibits her in adapting to local demands in the patient-doctor relationship, which again increases the possibility for human error. The doctor's evasive gaze, her reduced sensitivity to what the patient seeks from her, her fixated attention to the biomedical values on the screen and the evolving critical situation all afford the doctor to continue as she has done thus far. The doctor's continuous focus on the medical measurements engages her in abstract cognitive activity, which serves as positive feedback mechanisms as her awareness of the situation becomes reduced. In the end, the behaviour results in a negative outcome: The patient becomes excluded from the cognitive and dialogical system.

Furthermore, the analysis demonstrates how the biomedical model contributes to the doctor's prioritisation. Even though the situation escalates, the doctor waits (too) long to call for assistance. As the doctor of internal medicine arrives, the doctor does not rely on the cognitive ability of the cognitive system and the system remains unable to realise multiple values. As the biomedical model is prioritised, the trajectory is characterised by individual and monological behaviours and it leads to unnecessary consequences: The patient suffers from the lack of coordination.

3. Case II: Re-enacting role hierarchies[3]

I now turn to a case, which focuses on the dynamics that constitutes meaning. Special interest falls on how two healthcare professionals shift from a state of being a coordinated medical team to a state of negotiating what to do next. I zoom in on a situation in which a 92-year-old woman has been hospitalised with a proximal femur fracture (a hip fracture). At the hospital she is received by a medical team consisting of an experienced nurse and a novice doctor, who has worked at the

3. Sections 7.3–7.3.7 were originally published as "Meaning emergence in the ecology of dialogical systems" in *Psychology of Language and Communication*, 20, 2016. It is used here with permission of Sciendo: https://content.sciendo.com/view/journals/plc/plc-overview.xml and the co-author, Sune Vork Steffensen.

ward for only a couple of days when the recordings took place. The asymmetry between the two practitioners leaves them in a precarious position: On the one hand, the role of the "doctor" entails certain legal and cultural obligations to take the lead, and on the other hand, newcomers in teams tend to take a position of "legitimate peripheral participation" (Lave and Wenger 1991).[4] One would expect that the tension between two sets of expectations on a cultural timescale plays out in the interpersonal dynamics on an interactional timescale (Steffensen and Pedersen 2014). An overview of the setting is given in Figure 7.4.

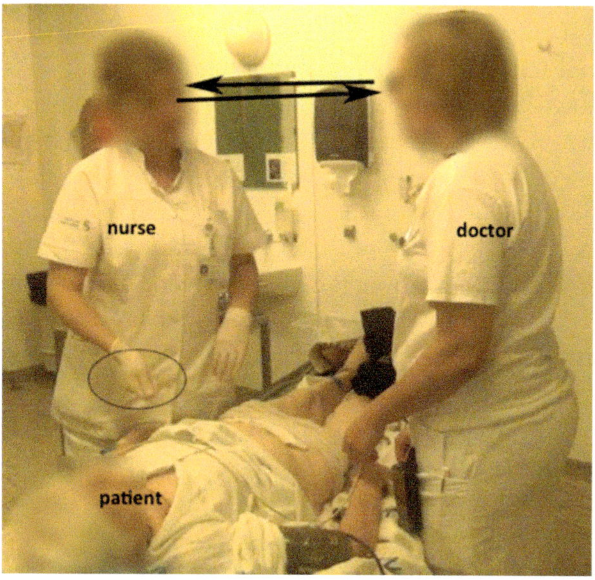

Figure 7.4 Overview of the layout

As the patient has been diagnosed with a hip fracture, the treatment of the patient will include orthopaedic surgery. However, before the patient is ready for that, the medical team must go through a number of pre-treatment procedures, including pain alleviation and stabilisation of the patient's other bodily functions. Our focus is on a single procedure in the pre-treatment phase that relate to the latter, namely the patient's ability to urinate and defecate. In our case, the medical team – in accordance with standard procedures – performs a urinary catheterisation. The urinary catheterisation is a rather trivial procedure, but the *decision* to perform it depends, not on rules, but on a judgment based on the mobility of the patient. In our case, the decision becomes an interesting *cognitive event* because the team

4. In a Danish context, these cultural expectations are sometimes referred to as doctors having a "Tarzan syndrome": They are expected to deal with everything themselves, and asking for help is a sign of weakness.

decides *not* to perform the procedure despite a high number of indications that catheterisation is indeed necessary. The event illustrates how meaning in the dialogical system emerges in the interplay between sociocultural regularities, individual expectations, knowledge about medical procedures, perceptual pick-up of information about the patient and situated decision-making.

From a procedural point of view, the decision to perform a urinary catheterisation has three phases, which are all saturated with meaning-making: First, the team must identify a need (i.e., the team must come to see it as a meaningful procedure to consider); second, they must examine a number of informed arguments pro and con the procedure; and third, the team, or one of the participants in it, must conclude (either through wordings or through action) that the arguments in favour of catheterisation outweigh those against. In the vast majority of our ethnographic material, these phases are collapsed into a single action: Practitioners "just know" that catheterisation will be needed sooner or later, and the arguments in favour of the procedure are so well-established that it is hardly even seen as an argumentation. Accordingly, the procedure is "just carried out". However, in this case the medical team diverts from the three procedural phases; they go through the second phase two times: The first time they do *not* reach the conclusion that they need to insert a catheter while they do the second time (at a later stage in the pre-treatment procedure). As the decision not to perform a urinary catheterisation significantly diverts from the standard medical procedures at the department, the question from a cognitive point of view obviously becomes: *What happened when they decided not to catheterise the patient?*

In what follows I analyse this event in fine-grained detail. Below follow the approximately 60 seconds in which the relevance of catheterisation and the decision not to catheterise are played out.

Transcript 7.1
Danish original

```
1.  34:01:10, P:   jeg har s jeg har sådan en (.) ble p[å
2.  34:03:50, D:                                       [ja:: det har du
3.  34:04:60, P:   ja
4.  34:05:00, ps.  (0.8)
5.  34:05:80, D:   øhm
6.  34:06:40, ps.  (0.7)
7.  34:07:10, N:   vi skulle jo nok lægge et kateter
8.  34:08:60, ps.  (0.9)
9.  34:09:50, D:   ska vi det? (.)
10. 34:10:20, N:   eller (.) det er ikke nødvendigt måske
11. 34:12:30, P:   (xxx) [det det det næ det plejer jeg [ikke
12. 34:12:60, D:         [na:rj det er da ikke nødvendigt hvis ikke du plejer at bruge
                   kateter
```

13. 34:15:30, N: [nej jeg tænker nogen gange med mobilisering til bækken og sådan noget men det kan vi jo nok godt↓
14. 34:19:20, ps. (0.7)
15. 34:19:90, N: få et bækken ind under når du skal tisse og sådan↑
16. 34:22:80, P: ja [det ved jeg-
17. 34:23:10, N: [men det virker som du er rimelig god alligevel til og lige at få
18. 34:26:40, ps: (0.8)
19. 34:27:20, P: ja bortset fra at øh den der den gør ondt
20. 34:30:30, N: ja:=
21. 34:30:70, D: =men nu lægger jeg jo FIC-blokken
22. 34:31:80, N: ja
23. 34:32:40, D: tror du tror du ikke vi klarer [°°uden°°
24. 34:33:80, N: [vi gør det jo tit men men men lad os bare prøve at se
25. 34:36:60, D: ja <u>det</u> ved jeg ik så [det det er jo det kan da godt være vi [ska det er dig øh
26. 34:37:40, N: [ja
27. 34:38:40, N: [ja men det er jo folk der [ik øh ka:: ka bevæge sig så godt og jeg synes egentlig hun er rigtig god
28. 34:40:20, P: [altså jeg har jeg har jeg har den der på gulvet med min mave
29. 34:45:20, D: med maven [der driller den er [lidt tynd (.) ja
30. 34:45:80, P: [ja [ja ja
31. 34:48:20, N: lad os bare lige øh (.) nu prøver vi bare li:ge at lægge det her så
32. 34:50:80, D: e ellers det [jeg tror det er dig de::r er me::st øh
33. 34:51:30, N: [ja jeg tror nemlig (0.1) ja (0.1) vi ser det lige an (0.3) fordi jeg synes egentlig også at øh det er realistisk og
34. 34:57:90, D: det er jo begrænset hvor mange bækkener jeg lægger
35. 35:00:10, P: ja
36. 35:00:70, D: eller hvad hedder det
37. 35:01:30, N: ja (smiling)
38. 35:01:70, D: så (laughs)

English translation

1. 34:01:10, P: I have a I have such a (.) diaper o[n
2. 34:03:50, D: [ye::s you have
3. 34:04:60, P: yes
4. 34:05:00, ps. (0.8)
5. 34:05:80, D: ehm
6. 34:06:40, ps. (0.7)

7. 34:07:10, N: we should probably insert a catheter
8. 34:08:60, ps. (0.9)
9. 34:09:50, D: we should? (.)
10. 34:10:20, N: or (.) that is not necessary perhaps
11. 34:12:30, P: (xxx) [that that that no: I do [not
12. 34:12:60, D: [no:: that should not be necessary if you do not usually use a catheter
13. 34:15:30, N: [no I think sometimes with regards to the mobilisation to the bedpan and such but I guess we can manage that↓
14. 34:19:20, ps. (0.7)
15. 34:19:90, N: place a bedpan under when you need to go to the toilet and such↑
16. 34:22:80, P: yes [I don't know
17. 34:23:10, N: [but it seems like you are pretty good anyway to just get
18. 34:26:40, ps: (0.8)
19. 34:27:20, P: yes except from ehm that this one it hurts
20. 34:30:30, N: ye:s=
21. 34:30:70, D: =but now I am going to perform the FIC block right
22. 34:31:80, N: yes
23. 34:32:40, D: don't you don't you think we manage [°°without°°
24. 34:33:80, N: [we often do it but let us just try and see
25. 34:36:60, D: yes <u>that</u> I do not know so [it it is well it might be that we [should that is you eh
26. 34:37:40, N: [yes
27. 34:38:40, N: [yes but that is people who are [unable eh to move so easily and I actually think she is rather mobile
28. 34:40:20, P: [well I have I have I have this one on the floor
29. 34:45:20, D: with the stomach [that is a bit tricky it is [a bit diarrhoea like (.) <u>yes</u>
30. 34:45:80, P: [yes [yes yes
31. 34:48:20, N: let us just eh (.) now we are ju:st trying to give this so
32. 34:50:80, D: o or this [I think it is you who a::re the mo::st eh
33. 34:51:30, N: [yes because I believe (0.1) yes (0.1) we will just wait and see (0.3) because I actually also think that eh it is realistic and
34. 34:57:90, D: after all I only place a limited number of bedpans
35. 35:00:10, P: yes
36. 35:00:70, D: or what is it called
37. 35:01:30, N: yes (smiling)
38. 35:01:70, D: so (laughs)

By matching the procedural description of the decision process with the transcript the following key transition points in the cognitive trajectory are identified: (a) the relevance of dealing with the patient's urinary function emerges in line 1 (P: *I have such a (.) diaper on*); (b) the initial suggestion to catheterise is expressed by the nurse in line 7: *we should probably insert a catheter*; and (c) the decision to rely on using a bedpan for her urination is taken in line 33 when the nurse says: *we will just wait and see (0.3) because I actually also think that eh it is realistic*. In the terminology of CEA, these three transition points are *event pivots*: They indicate when the problem becomes relevant, when the argumentation begins and when a decision is reached and confirmed.

What makes this particular event so interesting is that the nurse's initial judgment will be carried out much later in the pre-treatment process, but it is overruled in this sequence as they reach the conclusion not to catheterise and instead rely on a bedpan. As this outcome is a direct result of the meaning processes in the dialogical system, the emergence of meaning is best investigated by zooming in on the relevant event pivots and transition points that indicate changes in the specific *meaning configuration* of the dialogical system, and hence the focus on these transition points gives insight into the overall meaning-making trajectory.

Investigating the trajectory thus gives us the opportunity to investigate how the two agents create different meanings (understood as organism-environment relations) and how they reach a decision through meaning coordination. Thus, based on changes in the agents' meaning-making in relation to the task, this sequence is segmented into seven phases (see Table 7.1).

Table 7.1 Seven phases in the meaning configuration in the dialogical system

Phase	Line	Meaning configuration
I	7–12	The nurse suggests catheterisation The doctor does not concur with catheterisation
II	13–18	The nurse repeats her suggestion to catheterise the patient The doctor is silent
III	19–23	The catheterisation suggestion is related to the patient's pain
IV	24	The catheterisation suggestion is related to the department's procedures
V	25–27	The doctor reconsiders catheterisation The nurse argues against catheterisation
VI	31–32	The doctor reconsiders catheterisation The nurse argues against catheterisation
VII	33	The nurse concludes that catheterisation is not necessary

The seven phases are visualised in Figure 7.5 below. In what follows, the trajectory described in Table 1 and Figure 7.5 will be elaborated on in detail by zooming in on each of the seven phases.

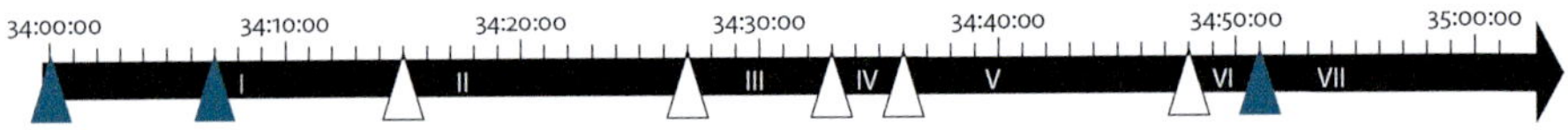

Figure 7.5 The emergence of meaning in decision-making. The arrow indicates the cognitive trajectory, the blue triangles indicate event pivots, the white triangles indicate phase transitions. The phase transition points and event pivots segment the trajectory into the seven phases listed in Table 7.1

3.1 Phase I: Making medical procedures meaningful

The first phase concerns the nurse's proposal to consider urinary catheterisation. Her proposal is prompted by the patient mentioning that she is wearing a diaper (line 1). This utterance is identified as an event pivot because it prompts the nurse to interrupt the procedural flow in the medical team by suggesting catheterisation as the proper solution to an anticipated problem of urination.

In theoretical terms, the coordinated multi-agent system is perturbed, and the two practitioners reorient themselves to each other as relevant affordances for their meaning-making activities. This reorientation is observable from the nurse's gaze behaviour. Thus, when the nurse begins on her proposal (in line 7), she gazes at the patient's body, but at the end of her utterance, she re-directs her gaze to the doctor. Hence, the dialogical system undergoes a centrifugal movement where they move from a coordinated state with joint attention to a less-coordinated state where they need to achieve a shared interpretation of the situation. This process of coordination depends on a centripetal movement that gives rise to meaning dynamics in the situation, and from an observer's point of view, this meaning is observable in their bodily orientation. Thus, the nurse makes the hip area of the patient's body relevant through her gaze, and both doctor and nurse pay attention to that part of their environment, which hence becomes a shared affordance for meaning and subsequent action. The nurse's combination of verbal prompting and gaze becomes an affordance for restoring the multi-agent system: The nurse makes it clear what action must be initiated, and by pointing to relevant features in the environment, she prompts the doctor to perceive the same meaning. But the doctor does not follow the nurse's lead. After a pause of 0.9 seconds (line 8), the doctor questions the nurse's suggestion explicitly: *We should?* (line 9). Thus, the patient's initial utterance becomes an affordance for very different action possibilities. In this way several meanings emerge: The nurse argues for catheterisation; the doctor does not concur.

Since the decision on whether to catheterise or not is based on how mobile the patient is, the doctor's utterance *we should?* (line 9) indicates that catheterisation was not part of the doctor's pre-treatment plan, either because she does not share the nurse's judgment or because she never even thought of it as a relevant procedure to consider. Accordingly, the doctor's hesitation creates a relational ambiguity: On the one hand, if the doctor rejects the nurse's judgment, the role hierarchy and cultural expectations dictate that the doctor has the right and obligation to make the final decision; on the other hand, if the doctor's reaction is caused by her surprise because she did not take a relevant procedure into consideration, priority is normally given to the one in the best position to overview the situation, and in this case that is the most experienced participant: the nurse. Evidently, the ambiguity cannot be easily resolved, and hence two meanings co-exist in an interpersonal negotiation that needs to balance both a clinical aspect and a cultural role aspect.

From the nurse's subsequent utterance – *or (.) that is not necessary perhaps* (line 10) – it is clear that she picks up on the first of these two aspects: She modulates her proposal into a question so while she initially proposed a procedure, she now asks the doctor whether this is a good idea. While the doctor's contribution to the reasoning has been minimal, the sequence has created a conclusion (catheterisation is not necessary) and a line of argumentation (a rejection of the nurse's judgment) that the doctor is prompted to adopt. It is not based on an elaborate argumentation, however, but such an argument is quickly reconstructed. To come up with an argument, the doctor uses the patient as a cognitive resource (line 10 and 11). The patient is made relevant by the nurse: When she utters that catheterisation is perhaps dispensable (line 10), her gaze moves from the doctor to the patient. In this way, the patient becomes involved in the negotiation, and she states that she does not usually need a catheter. The doctor uses this statement and frames it as a warrant for her own opinion (line 12): *no:: that should not be necessary if you do not usually use a catheter*. As the doctor addresses the patient with the deictic 'you', she changes her orientation (in gaze, body position and in verbal utterance) from the nurse to the patient, leaving the nurse as a less significant component in the system as she becomes a temporary observer of what is going on.

The information provided by the patient has a significant impact on the meaning processes in the interaction. It confirms the doctor's line of argumentation, and because the multi-agent dialogical system so crucial in medical teamwork is dissolved, the role hierarchy means that the doctor is positioned as the main cogniser, i.e., as the one who is going to make the decision. However, from a medical point of view, the patient's information is utterly useless. Whether the patient needs a catheter or not, is *not* a question of whether the patient normally uses one, but only a question of her present condition. The only relevant question is whether her broken hip complicates or even prevents her from going to the toilet or using a bedpan or not?

In conclusion, including the patient as a relevant source of information in the decision-making process does not contribute any valuable information regarding the clinical problem that needs to be solved. However, integrating the patient has a direct impact on the dynamics in the system as it enables the doctor to dissolve the initial meaning ambiguity by reaching a conclusion in a way that is consistent with the provided, though irrelevant, information. She avoids rejecting the nurse's proposal, but the price is high: She relies on irrelevant information and her conclusion is invalid.

3.2 Phase II: Embodiment as an affordance for meaning

In the cultural context of a medical department in Denmark, the doctor is the main responsible for patient treatment, and in the end, she has the authority and the obligation to decide what to do. Instinctively, it seems as if a decision has already been reached in the previous phase: the nurse proposed a pre-treatment procedure, but the doctor rejected it. In the ethnographic material it is extremely rare that such decisions are questioned, and if one reads the transcript of the second phase, which runs from line 13–18, it visualises that the nurse on two instances concurs with the doctor's decision: *but I guess we can manage that↓ [and] place a bedpan under when you need to go to the toilet and such↑* (line 13–15) and *it seems like you are pretty good anyway to just get* (line 17). But she also expresses her disagreement with the emerged conclusion: First, only once during this sequence does the nurse interrupt another interlocutor, namely the patient. Not only does she interrupt the patient, she does so while the patient is sharing her experiences with using a catheter (line 11), which, as we saw, is the utterance that implicitly, and logically fallaciously, supported the doctor's hesitation. Second, the nurse expresses an outright disagreement: *no*, she says in line 13 in response to the emerged conclusion in the first phase. Third, she expresses a vague concern with the implications of the conclusion: *I think sometimes with regards to the mobilisation to the bedpan and such* (line 13).

Her concerns are vaguely phrased, but they are accentuated and amplified by her embodied behaviour. Thus, the phase transition marks a change from verbal argumentation in Phase I to embodied performance and visualisation in Phase II. This change in the trajectory comes to the fore when she anticipates the line of actions in case the patient needs to urinate. This anticipation is articulated in a whole-bodied narrative of how the bedpan is difficult to place under an impaired patient. She refers to her experiences from previous situations with the words *sometimes with regards to the mobilisation* (line 13), and at the same time she engages in an embodied visualisation of the physical constraints in placing a bedpan under the patient. In the following the nurse's visualisation is scrutinised (cf. picture A-D in Figure 7.6 below).

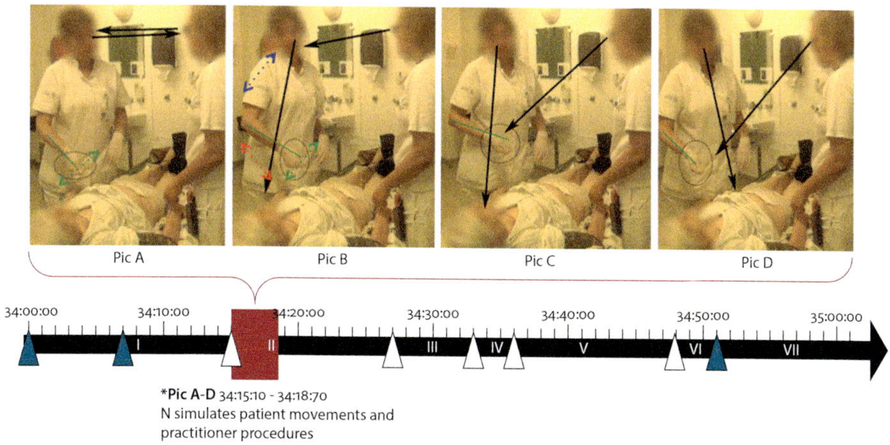

Figure 7.6 Decision-making in Phase II. In picture A-D, the nurse wiggles her hips and torso from side to side as she moves her right hand back and forth. These body movements visualise the physical constraint when arranging a bedpan. Simultaneously, the nurse utters: No i think sometimes with the mobilisation to the bedpan and such *(line 13)*

The nurse performs the situation for both the doctor, whom she needs to convince in order to make the "right" decision, and the patient, who will feel the consequences of the decision. As the nurse verbally refers to the process of placing the bedpan (line 13), she performs a series of embodied movements: She wiggles her hips and upper body from side to side while she moves her right arm back and forth. The arm movements simulate the actual bodily movements required in placing a bedpan under the patient (see Figure 7.6), and the simultaneous wiggling of hips illustrates the movements of the patient during the process of placing the bedpan. In other words, in this small scenario the nurse performs the actions of two agents: the nurse placing the bedpan and the patient moving her (fractured) hip. The nurse simultaneously communicates the bodily consequences to the patient and the constrained working condition to the doctor. Using her own body as a display, she creates affordances for perceiving the future consequences of a particular procedure. By so doing, she prompts the dialogical system to restore a joint meaning and a joint interpretation. This centripetal movement is seen in Figure 7.6, where the doctor first gazes at the nurse's head (picture A-B) but soon after turns her attention to the movements of the nurse (picture C-D). Such a reconfiguration in the dialogical system, in which the participants attend to each other's embodied behaviour, gives rise to new patterns of meaning-making: They temporarily suspend their orientation to the task and the patient in order to calibrate how they perceive the problem of urination and the potential solution of catheterisation. In the overall treatment procedure, verbal symbols have functioned as nudges that impacted on their joint orientation to the patient (Rączaszek-Leonardi 2011), but now meaning-making emerges from the embodied behaviour as they orient themselves to each other. During the narrative the doctor carefully observes how the nurse plays out the scenario through embodied movements. When the nurse has demonstrated the problem, she stops moving her body. Interestingly, in immediate continuation of this dramatised intermezzo, the nurse contradicts her own concern by estimating that they probably *can* mobilise the patient in order to place the bedpan: *but I guess we can manage it*↓ (line 13) as she nods 'yes' and gazes at the doctor. So, while she creates the bodily affordances for the doctor to make the centripetal movement towards the nurse's perspective, she engages in an opposite movement towards the perspective that the doctor entertained in Phase I. This double movement leaves the doctor in a tense position: If she picks up the embodied information and is convinced by the nurse's scenario, she has to ignore the subsequent estimation – and *vice versa*. Placed in this tension, the doctor hesitates (cf. the pause of 0.7 seconds in line 14) as she makes a noticeably facial expression, which resembles a kind of lip-pursing grimace response (see Figure 7.7). The doctor does not respond verbally, but she wrinkles her nose and pouts her lips in a remarkable way.

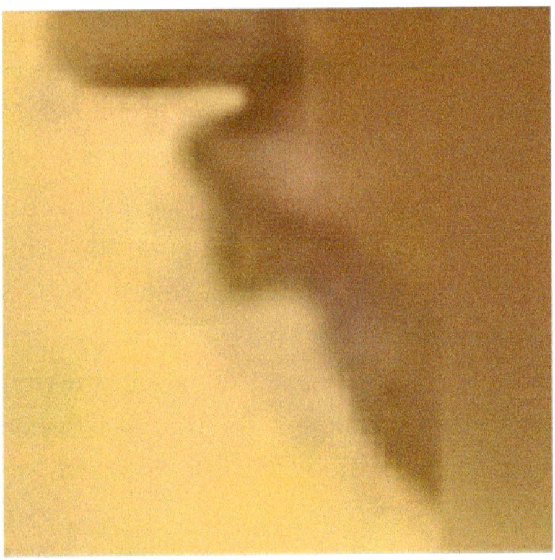

Figure 7.7 The doctor's lip-pursing grimace in line 14

While the meaning embedded in this grimacing cannot be determined, it can be extrapolated from her subsequent behaviour, in particular the fact that later in the sequence she attempts to align with the nurse's position, arguing that the nurse is the most experienced of the two (line 32). If the doctor's meaning trajectory changes through the seven phases, this particular moment is a viable candidate for the first occurrence of some sort of concern pertaining to her initial position. If so, the embodied knowledge of the nurse turns out to be an important affordance for the doctor to change her mind. The nurse's expertise is observed in the way she manipulates the affordances in the environment of the dialogical system: She indicates what is relevant through embodied behaviour (gaze, movements, and wordings), and the meaning that emerges is a direct result of this embodied expertise. When encountering the nurse's affordances for meaning-making, the doctor freezes as she is prompted to reconsider the consequences of her initial decision. Since the doctor does not respond directly to her utterance in line 13, the nurse continues her turn by elaborating the *that* in line 13 by explicating that *that* refers to *plac[ing] a bedpan under when you need to go to the toilet and such* (line 15). As she now directs her turn to the patient, she shifts from the doctor-nurse *we* (line 13), to the patient *you* (line 15).

The patient also picks up on the nurse's visualisation. While she does not have the medical expertise to decide whether it is possible to place the bedpan or not, the nurse's bodily visualisation has a strong illustrative power that enables her to imagine the situation in a tangible way beyond verbal explanations. Obviously, to wiggle one's hips and torso is not a preferable activity with a hip fracture, and the nurse's whole-bodied meaning-making prompts the patient to utter her doubt about whether this is doable or not (line 16). However, for the second time the nurse counters her own objections. This time she compares general cases with the patient in question: *but it seems like you are pretty good anyway to just get* (line 16).

As we reach the end of Phase II, we see that both the doctor and the nurse have moved from their initial position to a position characterised by doubt and meaning equivocality. Both agents have formulated immediate interpretations of the situation, and both agents have undergone changes in their perspective, which results in confusion because in the end only one decision can be made. Ideally, a necessary step is to align and calibrate the system so that it is able to act based on a shared meaning. In this case, however, the attempt to do so has created even more confusion and insecurity in the dialogical system.

3.3 Phase III: Emergent changes in perspectives

The dialogue so far has led to a point where the nurse doubts her own suggestion, the doctor doubts her rejection of the nurse's suggestion and the patient is expressing uncertainty and insecurity. In Phase III, which covers a small excerpt in the transcript (line 19–23), the doctor voices her last attempt to legitimise her rejection of the nurse's suggestion. She is prompted to do so by a short exchange between the doctor and the patient: The patient informs the medical team that her hip hurts (*this one it hurts*, line 19), and the doctor responds that the FIC block will remove the pain. Her conclusion from this exchange is expressed as a hesitant request for confirmation: *don't you don't you think we manage °°without°°* (line 23). That they can manage the situation without catheterisation is thus linked to the FIC block, but that is another fallacious conclusion: The fact that the patient does not normally use a catheter does not warrant the conclusion that she should not be catheterised, but at the same time the conclusion that catheterisation is not needed is not warranted by the patient needing to be anaesthetised. Given that the doctor in fact expresses a concern with her own pre-treatment administration less than three seconds later, her hesitancy may indicate that she is in a process of realising that her argument is flawed: The relevant clinical question is whether the patient will be sufficiently medicated to permit the bedpan placement without hurting the patient.

An experienced emergency medical practitioner such as the nurse knows that already. But insisting on bringing these considerations to the fore in the medical team's meaning-making would conflict with the doctor's reliance on patient-provided information. It would also disturb the delicate balance between being the experienced practitioner and being the inferior in the role hierarchy. As a consequence, the nurse has been silenced, and she abstains from expressing her opinion any further. Instead, she replies with two minimally responsive *yes* (line 20 and 22) to both the patient's and the doctor's utterances. This dialogical behaviour where her meaning is withdrawn from the systemic reasoning altogether changes the interactional dynamics further. Thus, while the doctor's request for confirmation in line 23 functions as a conclusion, it also calls for the nurse to take a more active role in the meaning-making process.

At this point in the cognitive trajectory, the coordination in the dialogical system is constrained and this constraint inhibits the system from moving on. In order to get back on track, the system needs to recalibrate and dampen its meaning dynamics: They must agree on what to do next. Such a decision requires either a powerful autonomy, through which a single agent overrules the other and simply decides what to do, or a shared meaning-making process through which the dialogical system as a whole decides what to do.

3.4 Phase IV: Cultural dynamics in situated meaning-making

In Phase IV (line 24) the two states of individual autonomy and system autonomy co-exist as a tension in the dialogical system. The phase consists of only one utterance, and it is defined as a distinct phase because the line of argumentation changes: For the first time in the exchange, the general procedures in the department become part of the meaning-making. This happens as the nurse refers to catheterisation as a standard procedure at the department: *we often do it* (line 24). She draws on non-local resources (Steffensen 2015) in the meaning-making of the dialogical system as the pronoun *we* evokes a general team of professionals (Linell 2009) who often choose to catheterise. This strategy scaffolds her situated meaning-making by drawing on experience and general practice. Hollan et al. (2000: 178) elaborate:

> *Culture is a process that accumulates partial solutions to frequently encountered problems.* Without this residue of previous activity, we would all have to find solutions from scratch. We could not build on the success of others. [...] This is tremendously enabling. But it is not without cost. For culture may also blind us to other ways of thinking, leading us to believe that certain things are impossible when in fact they are possible when viewed differently.

The power of culture is re-enacted as the nurse appropriates sociocultural voices, and thus she presents a powerful perspective on the joint meaning-making of the dialogical system. After all, the widespread use of catheterisation is an important perspective for a novice doctor who has no experience with this part of pre-treatment. Hence, the nurse makes non-local aspects of general practices highly relevant.

Essentially, the nurse seems to attempt to dissolve the impasse of the dialogical system by empowering the system by providing useful information. But the nurse's reply is ambiguous: Immediately after the prioritisation of systemic autonomy, she undermines the joint meaning-making of the system by downplaying the importance of the department's general procedures. She does so by scaffolding the novice doctor's individual autonomy in an explicit support for the doctor's plan: *but let us just try and see* (line 24). The ambiguity is striking: On the one hand, the nurse speaks with an authority grounded in her knowledge and expertise, which calls for catheterisation, and on the other hand, she argues against this decision.

3.5 Phase V: The doctor and the nurse swop position

How does a sensitive dialogical partner react to such ambiguity? The doctor has the nurse's support for a pre-treatment plan, which does not include catheterisation, but at the same time the doctor is aware that this plan goes against departmental procedures. The result is striking: In Phase V (line 25–27) the doctor and the nurse swop positions! The nurse complies with the non-catheterisation plan, arguing from the perspective of the relative mobility of the patient, and the doctor shelves her initial conviction, explicitly picking up on the nurse's reference to departmental procedures: *it it is well it might be that we should that is you eh* (line 25). Precisely when the doctor accepts the nurse's suggestion, the nurse withdraws her suggestion on the pretext of identifying the patient as relatively mobile, even though the 92-year-old patient is in a great deal of pain and complains about her physical condition several times (line 19 and 28). As a result, both the doctor and the nurse have made a *meaning U-turn* based on their information pick-up *and* on the dynamics in the dialogical system.

The nurse has drawn the doctor's attention to social affordances in the environment, and the doctor has enacted her lack of expertise. While this change could have led to a systemic reconfiguration where they decide on a new and better pretreatment plan, the outcome is different. In the next two phases, the doctor's confession of her inexperience thus becomes an affordance for the nurse to maintain the doctor's systemic position – and her face (Goffman 1959).

3.6 Phase VI-VII: Functionality and dysfunctionality in the dialogical system

During the overall event, multiple suggestions have been evaluated in the team, and both their meaning-making and their positioning in the dialogical system have undergone significant changes. The result of these oscillations in the dialogical system is the emergence of a decision: In Phase VI (line 31–32) the nurse concludes: *let us just eh (.) now we are ju:st trying to give this so* (line 31) and shortly after the doctor explicitly refers to the nurse as the expert: *o- or this- I think it is you who a::re the mo::st eh* (line 32). In Phase VII (line 33) the meaning-making trajectory reads a temporary end point in the shape of a publicly stated decision: *we will just wait and see (0.3) because I actually think that eh it is realistic and.* This decision is the cognitive result of 42.2 seconds of reasoning. It functions as the primary event pivot in the sequence, as this decision defines the overall sequence as one of meaning-making and reasoning.

From these two phases, the self-organising nature of the decision-making process is evident: The decision is not the result of any pre-conceived pre-treatment

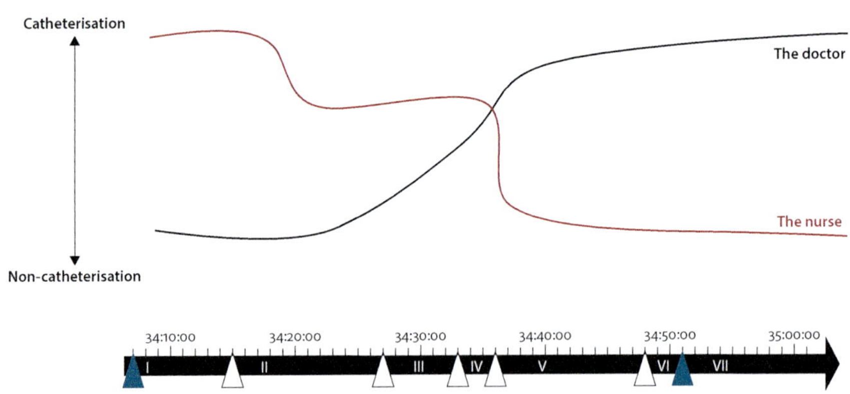

Figure 7.8 The figure illustrates how the two agents move through a logical space between the decision terms: Catheterisation and non-catheterisation. The figure is not intended as a quasi-mathematical model, but rather as a heuristic illustration of movements between the two decision terms, catheterisation and non-catheterisation

plans, which the practitioners try to realise. Indeed, both agents in the system abandon their initial arguments and come to sponsor the intuitions of the other agent (cf. Figure 7.8).

This oscillation indicates that the decision is less the result of medically informed reasoning, and more a result of how the role hierarchy and the protection of professional face take the lead. From a strictly functional point of view – as favoured in the tradition of Distributed Cognition (Hutchins 1995a; Perry 2010) – the system becomes dysfunctional because it allows task irrelevant considerations to constrain the reasoning process. The two practitioners mesh their inter-bodily dynamics with experience and medical expertise, and this process gives rise to meaning and decisions, as well as to insecurity, confusion and frustration. The dialogical system thus has to balance medical decision-making and interpersonal emotional processes. As can be seen from Figure 7.8, these dynamics lead to a decision that is predominantly determined by the position the nurse takes at the end of the sequence. In the dynamics of the dialogical system, the nurse takes the lead and secures that a decision is made. But the price is high for at the same time she puts herself in a non-expert position by withdrawing her experience-based proposal and deciding to do what the doctor initially argued for.

From a purely medical point of view the decision is not based on best practice and expertise but on interpersonal caring and an orientation to hierarchies and practices for decision-making. The case demonstrates that in real-life situations, decisions are not made in a vacuum but embedded in meaningful interpersonal relations shaped through the processes of maintaining each other's face (Goffman 1959) and orienting themselves to role hierarchies that exist between different professional groups (Pedersen 2010).

3.7 Epilogue: On the poverty of phenomenal reports

A few hours after the recordings, both the doctor and the nurse were interviewed as part of the ethnographic work at the ward. During her interview, the doctor told the researcher that "*the nurse was right*". It turned out that it was not possible to locate the bedpan under the patient, and they had to insert the catheter at a later and more complicated stage in the pre-treatment process. This caused a delay in the treatment plan, and it harmed the patient unnecessarily. According to the doctor, she was wrong, and the nurse was right: "*as the nurse also said*", she explained, catheterisation did indeed turn out to be necessary.

Evidently, the doctor did not experience the situation as shared decision-making with equally shared responsibility for the decision they reached: She identified herself as the main responsible for the decision. Such an approach to decision-making is widespread in the medical world: "Errors are regarded as someone's fault, caused by a lack of sufficient attention or, worse, lack of caring enough to make sure you are correct. [...]. While the proximal error leading to an accident is, in fact, usually a "human error," the causes of that error are often well beyond the individual's control" (Leape 1994: 1852).

The nurse reached a similar conclusion in her posttreatment interview: The collaboration went well, but as it is often the case, the doctor had not listened carefully to what she, as a nurse, had to say. Thus, in the post hoc interviews, both the doctor and the nurse reach the same conclusion about responsibility: The nurse was right about the work procedure, but she was overruled by the doctor. However, their experience of their team performance does not match the actual coordination shown in the data. Initially, the doctor rejected the nurse's proposal, but that changed as the nurse informed the doctor about possible future complications and departmental procedures. Thus, from the data a gradual change of perspective in the doctor's meaning-making was identified, even to the degree that she realises that the nurse, as the more experienced of the two, should take the lead: *I think it is you who a::re the mo::st eh* (line 32). The fact that they both report a sequence of events, which do not match their behaviour *in situ*, is a powerful testimony to the fragility of phenomenal reports: The widespread cultural narrative of dominant doctors and inferior nurses frames their interpretation of the events they went through a few hours earlier.

What is so striking about the catheterisation case is, first, that it exemplifies decision-making without a singular agent making the decision and, second, that it points to the importance of non-local processes in local decision-making. As regards the first point, if rationality was unbounded (cf. Secchi 2011), a decision-making process could in principle be completely computational and logical. But since that is not the case, decision-making relies on meaning-making processes. The scrutiny of the example has shown that even though the two main cognisers are two meaning-making individuals, it is the dynamics within the overall dialogical system that leads to the decision not to catheterise. Thus, the cognitive outcome of the process is a result of how the two practitioners shift between being a multi-agent-system with a shared, tightly coordinated agency and a loosely coupled dialogical system through which the individual brings forth an understanding based on each their professional backgrounds and each their expertise. Joint meaning-making thus emerges as the agents shift between centripetal and centrifugal dynamics in the system, e.g., by (a) pointing to relevant affordances in the environment so that new meaning emerges as new information is picked up and made relevant for the whole system, (b) by enacting and embodying their medical-cultural knowledge in the situation, which allows for evidence-based meaning-making and decision-making in the dialogical system and (c) by evaluating the meaning that emerges in the dialogical system.

Secondly, taking an ecological perspective on the meaning-making processes, the example reveals how cultural dynamics affect local decision-making. Culture transcends individual reasoning, and it is constantly re-enacted as an emergent phenomenon. Decision-making processes are shaped by previous episodes so that the practitioners' actions reflect embodied understandings of multiple cultural phenomena, for instance role hierarchies, systemic norms, physical and procedural limitations, personal experience and caring for human beings in complex situations.

When one studies cognitive dynamics in dialogical systems, one has to take into consideration how the system is saturated by (a) the agents' non-local experiences of sociocultural and institutional procedures, (b) the team's compliance with non-local expectations about how decision-making is managed (role hierarchies etc.) and (c) situated affordances for specific actions. Crucial to a team's general success is the ability to balance procedures and interpersonal dynamics by caring for both the persons in the dialogical system (in our case, patients, colleagues and oneself) and the task to be solved by the system (in this case, diagnosis, examination and treatment).

4. Breaking down traditions

In the first case, the doctor is fixated on medical measurements on the screen as she struggles with diagnostic hypothesis generation and this behaviour leads to a constrained situational sensitivity to local changes within the patient domain. With Martina et al. (2014) this lack of situational awareness and ability to build good rapport with the patient is partly due to an incomprehensive teaching practice:

> Although nonverbal communication is addressed in many medical school curricula, the focus tends to be on body language and use of gestures rather than the intimacy of touch. Yet physical examination is a dynamic process of engagement. For example, as we examine a patient, we perceive on multiple levels – not just the presence or absence of physical signs, but also the patient's comfort and emotional state. In turn, the patient responds to us – reading our facial expressions, interpreting the pressure of our fingertips, and responding to the gentleness (or lack thereof) to inform how he or she will proceed within the consultation.
>
> (Martina et al. 2014: 1314)

Verghese (2008) argues that medical students must learn how to use clinical skills at the bedside with real patients and by observing master clinicians. Moreover, he claims such a dialogical approach will bring about cultural change and nourish one's sensitivity and perceptual system to identify local relevant dynamics (Verghese 2008). Hence, the relationship between healthcare practitioner and patient becomes more bodily, more caring and more situated, and it can be balanced with the biomedical model and demands for providing clear diagnoses. The doctor is further constrained by sociocultural norms and procedures – originating from the biomedical model – to separate and prioritise medical calculation over emotional and interpersonal relationships. In this case, the doctor is rather confident in using self-initiated touch to calm the patient in the examination process. However, when the patient touches the doctor, she withdraws and leaves the patient in an emotionally distressed state.

The second case investigated the complexity and constraints of cultural dynamics in local interaction. Specifically, the analyses show how culture with a constant focus on local errors and individual blame pervades local treatment activities without anyone being fully aware of it. It leads to the hypothesis that many failures and errors are never identified for what they really are if self-reports or complaints are the mechanisms used to detect such processes. This is why observations of real-life situations are vital if learning is to be achieved.

By emphasising the value of an ecological approach, decision-making is not an individual, mental task but a shared process with shared responsibility maintained through coaction. This viewpoint is far from how practitioners experience what they do and how decisions are made in real-time.

To establish an interpersonal relationship based on co-presence and attention, participants need to coordinate priorities. Collective and effective coordinated problem-solving thus depends on sharing and caring. When these values are not present, felt or shown, distributed cognition is to some extent dysfunctional. In the first case, the doctor does not share her concerns explicitly, which results in lack of coordination. In the second case, the nurse is a moral being, who fails to balance different tasks and values in the system because she relies too much on one value (caring for the doctor's face). The team coordination entails the establishment of a frozen role hierarchy, which serves as a constraint and hindrance for adaptive flexible behaviour. *When medical teams believe in role hierarchies, they become real in their consequences*,[5] which means that when cultural dynamics are automatically re-enacted in local interaction, they serve as feedback mechanisms in that particular situation. Positive feedback mechanisms emerge in interactivity imbued with latent conditions for human error. In this case, experiences of how role hierarchies shape action patterns become a positive feedback mechanism nourishing that specific expectation and inhibiting a flexible orientation to local situational dynamics.

5. This is a paraphrasing of the Thomas theorem: "when men define situations as real, they become real in their consequences" (Thomas and Thomas 1928: 571–572).

To conclude, this chapter points to the importance of investigating what is beyond the micro-sociological scale of conversation. The way healthcare practitioners generate cognitive results is characterised by enacting embodied experience, sociocultural norms and situational dynamics.

CHAPTER 8

Medical teams of experts and novices

An educational perspective

1. Why study teams?[1]

This chapter investigates how teams make sense. It pays attention to the benefits of thinking of a team as a cognitive system with sense-making qualities different from those of individuals. As mentioned in Chapter 1, human errors are frequently related to a perceived lack of communication and coordination. This problem has given rise to an interest in studying this phenomenon further; thus over the last decades, there has been an increasing interest in conversational issues in healthcare. Communication skills such as team performance (e.g. Grumbach and Bodenheimer 2004; Manser et al. 2009; Manser 2009; Husebø et al. 2011) have been implemented in healthcare practices in order to train practitioners in safe and efficient patient care. There is an overwhelming literature on teamwork and communication skills (e.g. Senge 2006; DuBrin 2004; Glaser 1994), but it primarily pays attention to individuals within the team. Much is left out when the objective of analysis is solely individual action rather than the cognitive system, no matter its size (Hollan et al. 2000). Furthermore, Paradis et al. (2014) argue in a recent review that "the fundamental insight that interprofessional interactions in intensive care do not happen in a historical, social, and technological vacuum must be brought to bear on future research in intensive care if patient safety and quality of care are to be improved" (Paradis 2014: 230). And Hindmarsh and Pilnick argue that:

> despite the wealth of studies of health-care teams and medical practice, we are left with little understanding of the skills that enable medical staff to come together for a duration of an operation and coordinate their work such that they are seen as professionals: competent in the practices that form the foundation to this community. (Hindmarsh and Pilnick 2002: 141)

---

1. Sections 8.1–8.3.3 were originally published as "Insights and their Emergence in Everyday Practices: The Interplay between Problems and Solutions in emergency medicine" in *Pragmatics & Cognition*, 24, 2017. It is reused here with permission of John Benjamins: https://www.benjamins.com/catalog/pc and co-author, Per Linell.

The literature focuses on organisationally prescribed team constellations in order to scaffold individual patient care programs etc. (Hindmarsh and Pilnick 2002). However, ad hoc constellations rather than stable assemblages are employed in emergency wards teams. In such cases, the focus is not "to decide on patient care removed from the presence of the patient, but to coordinate their contributions to actual care work in situ, in the moment and with the patient" (Hindmarsh and Pilnick 2002: 140). When ad hoc teams emerge, multiple issues are at stake. For instance, the level of expertise, the knowledge about medical equipment, the interpersonal relationships amongst some team members and the presence of bystanders (for instance medical students) are all constraints within which "the team has to build enough rapport to be able to manage the health and safety of the patients under their care. Indeed, their ability to collaborate successfully is critical and can significantly affect the quality of patient care" (Hindmarsh and Pilnick 2002: 141).

Managing cognitive events in emergency medical teams is difficult, both due to how such teams are constituted and because of the problems they face. Emergency medical teams are led by medical practitioners who have to deal with presentations of sometimes highly ambiguous symptoms, incomplete information and a high degree of specialisation of the team's members. In terms of organisational literature, emergency medical teams are "fluid teams" (Edmondson 2012) whose "teaming" depends on gathering experts into temporary groups "to solve problems they're encountering for the first and perhaps only time" (Edmondson 2012: 74). Edmondson (2012: 74) elaborates: "Think of clinicians in an emergency room, who convene quickly to solve a specific patient problem and then move on to address other cases with different colleagues, compared with a surgical team that performs the same procedure under highly controlled conditions day after day".

Given these conditions, the educational challenge for a department of emergency medicine is daunting. Faced with patient narratives and symptoms that differ from textbook diagnoses and descriptions of diseases, medical novices have to become experts capable of making critical decisions while managing fluid teams in an unpredictable clinical context. Furthermore, the fact that different areas of responsibility are tied to specific formal roles entails expectations for certain role hierarchies. However, as is often the case in emergency departments, the majority of doctors are novices, who work with experienced nurses, a constellation that might lead to frictions and tensions within the team, see Chapter 9. Thus, medical practitioners also need knowledge of *how* medical teams function, *how* practitioners interact, and *how* to develop the skills required. Rather than emphasise medical knowledge, this chapter therefore examines the management of real-time cognitive events in the emergency medical team. The team's expertise depends on subtle modes of coordination that may be particularly important in emergency settings where medical teams face unpredictable cases, unpredictable resources, time pressure and the pressure to make critical decisions quickly and determinedly.

This chapter investigates two cases with ephemeral and unique teamwork constellations. The first case investigates how such a team constellation is an opportunity to engage in ongoing interactivity and test common procedures in the ward in a way that scaffolds learning. By showing how cognitive insights depend on the ability to embed and link the slow, non-local narratives in fast real-time dynamics, the term "expertise" extends to involve more than individual mental activity and embodied skills: Expertise depends on historical agents that draw on interactivity.

The second case demonstrates the benefits and efficiency of organising work procedures within a team. Specifically, it demonstrates how recalibrating the boundaries of the cognitive system, coordinates teamwork *with* and *without* the patient, and how different members within the team perceive changes in the layout of affordances differently. It pivots on how habit and expertise are required by linking a team's perceptual capabilities with an individual's own experience. Showing how negative feedback mechanisms contribute to a team's functional coordinative behaviour and joint sense-making, gives us an understanding of the possible benefits such a composition imparts on practical cognition. If an emergency ward works with an anticipatory approach to human errors, it can arrange work practices in accord with such insights to stimulate teamwork and increase chances for effective and dialogical outcomes.

1.1 Problems and solutions in an ecological perspective

On the ward, medical teams repeatedly solve problems. Some are highly complex and unique whereas others seem to be recurring and simple as the solutions emerge naturally because expertise is enacted almost automatically in the situation. It is suggested that successfully managing cognitive events (whether complex or simple), depends on the individuals' ability to coordinate and integrate situated real-time demands with cultural routines, rules, conceptualisations and power relations. In terms of theory, such cultural conditions can be understood as situation-transcending (Linell 2009), distributed (Hutchins 1995a) and ecological (Gibson 1979/86; Hodges 2009; Steffensen 2013; Jensen 2014a; Pedersen 2015). Such processes are characterised by a complex interplay between local and non-local enabling conditions.

The underlying assumptions of an ecological approach to problem-solving are hardly compatible with the classical models of cognitive practices. A recent review of the cognitive literature on clinical problem-solving and diagnostic decision-making (Elstein and Schwarz 2002), reaches the overall conclusion that in this context reasoning should be described as a process of hypothesis-testing. In experimental settings, this comes about through artificial set-ups with a 'game-like' function. The game-like function comes about in the experimental design based on tricking the participants into cognitive traps when they try to move forward to solve the task, i.e., when they try out moves to win the game. Hence, the participants are sometimes even misguided or misled into a constructed problematic situation (Vallée–Tourangeau 2013; Cowley 2014a; Steffensen et al. 2016), which may enhance frustration and make them search for a bedrock in the core aspects of "pure" reasoning. The logic seems to be that when they come across an *impasse*, individuals will retreat to reasoning logically and systematically. While this approach may generate important insights into a limited domain of constructed problems, it is not obvious that the dynamics and the results will be applicable to broader contexts of natural task performances in which problem-solving is nested.

Ecological problem-solving contexts are constituted by heterogeneous sets of dynamics and logics. As demonstrated in the analysis, problem-solving is less about pure mental reasoning than about trusting each other, working together and picking up information in a rich and dynamic environment. Furthermore, problems are rarely isolated and subject to binary choices as they appear to be in many experimental settings. In real life, they are rather messy, unclear and nested in a broader context of multiple actions. Consequently, this classical scientific approach to problem-solving has been adopted by organisations and it has led to a practice whereby attention is paid to individuals and their personal, mental thinking processes, their verbal accounts and how they follow written instructions or share information, etc. (Reason 2005, 2008; Pedersen 2015). Such mentalistic approaches assume that problems can or must be known before solutions. For example, it is often believed that problem-solving consists of an investigation of solutions found by medical hypothesis generation used to guide the data collection and to develop a diagnostic plan. Elstein and Schwarz (2002) point to the problematic aspects of dealing with real-life cognitive problem-solving in such a simplistic way. According to them, the hypothetico-deductive approach does not really apply to situations in which experts engage in familiar situations, as "their speed, efficiency, and accuracy suggest that they may not even use the same reasoning processes as novices" (Elstein and Schwarz 2002: 730). Thus, different types of methods are applied in different reasoning contexts based on the observation of physicians' flexible approach to problem-solving. In the view of Elstein and Schwarz, simple problems are solved by pattern recognition whereas complex problems require a more thorough and systematic reflection based on hypothesis generation and testing.

In this example it is argued that an ecological alternative to that of Elstein and Schwarz (2002) is needed if the aim is to account for the variety of problem-solving activities that appear in real life. Recent cognitive ethnographic research indicates that many problems are not solved by individuals. Many problems are not isolated processes, but instead constitute an interconnected problem heterarchy, and they are often unspecified and emerge ad hoc. Yet again, many problems are not solved by logical deduction as they relate to, e.g., emotional dynamics in the interaction (Pedersen 2015; Klein 2015; Jensen and Pedersen 2016). From an ecological perspective, problem-solving should not be viewed as an example of how an individual or a team deals with a simple or complex problem based on hypothesis-testing, pattern-matching or categorisation. Rather, it is recommended that the focus be on results emerging from a cognitive system (Hutchins 1995a, 2014; Pedersen 2015; Steffensen et al. 2016). The emergence of results often reveals a pathway inconsistent with a fixed structure of problem identification, reasoning and action, which the first example illustrates.

2. Case I: The emergence of insight: Linking local perceptions with experience

In case I, interest falls on how a nurse is able to identify and link a solution in the here-and-now to a non-present challenge or alleged problem on the ward by using her experience as a particular way of picking up relevant information.

While insights are identified as local changes in interactivity trajectories, they often impact the individual's non-local memories of previous situations too. Observing a solution enables you to identify the nature of previous situations in a new perspective as being flawed or problematic, for instance. In this case it is thus underlined how such an insight emerges as a nurse observes and makes sense of a successful procedural performance and relates this information to performances in the past. The insight enables a problem analysis, which in this context, enables her to problematise standard procedures on the ward. Generally, such standard procedures have been characterised by tacit ignorance and are being problematised in the situated interaction due to the emergence of local insights. While the insight relates to local and non-local operations of professional procedural performance, it further enables anticipatory problem-solving as the nurse is able to take precautions against problematic task performances in the future.

In case I the medical team consists of an experienced nurse and a novice doctor, who had worked on the ward for only a couple of days when the recordings took place. The medical team has just decided which procedures should be initiated: the performance of a femoral nerve block (*FIC-block*). This specific standard procedure becomes the basis for learning. After the patient has been informed about the pre-treatment process and the procedure has been explained to her, a few procedural steps are required. First, the doctor needs to identify (via palpation) and mark (usually by pen) the needle insertion site. Second, the skin area must be disinfected before the doctor can insert the needle. Third, the *doctor* must perform the FIC-block itself. Under normal circumstances, the third step is impeded by the fact that the marking (first procedural step) is made by pen, and the ink often disappears when it is cleaned with alcohol (second procedural step). In standard situations, a consequence of this challenge would be that the doctor needs to allot a lot of cognitive effort to memorise exactly where the mark was in the first place when the third procedural step is to be executed. Figure 8.1 is an overview of the setting.

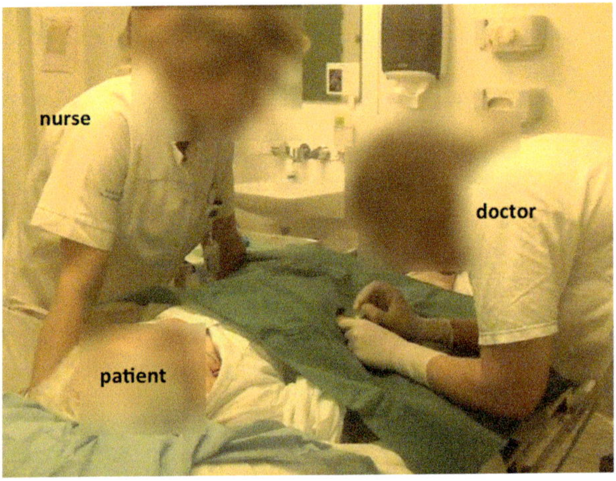

Figure 8.1 Overview of the layout

2.1 Defining the event and its phases: Reverse problem-solving and learning

Within the overall situation of preparing and performing the FIC-block, there are nested events. One event is an emergent problem-solving activity, which is a result of serendipity, as performing the FIC-block offers perceptual affordances to the experienced nurse, which can lead to safer and more efficient work practices in the future. Following CEA, we categorise this event as a *learning event* as the observation of the task performance leads to an insight that allows information to be incorporated into existing procedures in new ways.

As we enter the interaction, the doctor has completed the first two steps and she is about to insert the needle. The nurse stands by and is ready to assist if any complications occur. In other words, we enter the conversation *in medias res* when the focus is narrowed down to the learning event that can be identified when the nurse perceives an unfamiliar procedure and expresses an interest in the alternative method which the novice doctor uses.

Transcript 8.1
Danish original

1. 43:52:00, N: har du lavet sådan en afmærkning i huden
2. 43:54:10, ps. (0.5)
3. 43:54:60, D: ja: kan du se det
4. 43:55:50, N: ja (.) hvordan har du gjort det

[. . .] (25.5) (The patient complains about pains in her hip)

5. 44:22:40, N: men øh hvad har du lavet den der afmærkning med
6. 44:25:10, D: jeg har taget en øh prop fra ø:h de der saltvandssprøjter
7. 44:27:80, ps. (1.2)
8. 44:29:00, N: okay
9. 44:29:20, ps. (1.5)
10. 44:30:70, N: det var ret smart
11. 44:31:20, ps. (0.8)
12. 44:32:00, D: ja men fordi [ellers så forsvind (.) narj men det er fordi eller så forsvinder det jo når man tegner det med kuglepen ik
13. 44:32:40, N: [det tror jeg aldrig jeg har set før
14. 44:36:50, ps. (0.8)
15. 44:37:30, N: ja når du vasker a[f
16. 44:38:10, D: [når jeg vasker af ik
17. 44:38:90, N: ja
18. 44:39:30, D: så øh (.) nu skal du se så er det denne her jeg kommer ned så
19. 44:40:60, N: det har jeg nemlig os (.) tit tænkt på

English translation

1. 43:52:00, N: did you make such a mark in the skin
2. 43:54:10, ps. (0.5)
3. 43:54:60, D: ye:s do you see that
4. 43:55:50, N: yes (.) how did you make it

[. . .] (25.5) (The patient complains about pains in her hip)

5. 44:22:40, N: but eh what did you make the mark with there
6. 44:25:10, D: I took a eh a plug from e:h those saline needles
7. 44:27:80, ps. (1.2)
8. 44:29:00, N: okay
9. 44:29:20, ps. (1.5)
10. 44:30:70, N: that was pretty clever
11. 44:31:20, ps. (0.8)
12. 44:32:00, D: yes but because [otherwise they disap (.) no: but it is because otherwise it disappears you see when you draw with a pen right
13. 44:32:40, N: [I do not think I have ever seen that before
14. 44:36:50, ps. (0.8)
15. 44:37:30, N: yes when you wash it o[f
16. 44:38:10, D: [when I wash it off right
17. 44:38:90, N: yes

18. 44:39:30, D: so eh (.) now you will see then it is this one I put down so
19. 44:40:60, N: I have actually (.) often thought about that too

The analysis will identify four phases: (1) cognitive puzzlement, (2) explanation, (3) observation as insight and (4) contextualisation of learning. Thus, the analysis is structured into four phases that will be investigated in relation to one another. The phases reflect different dynamics and functions that all lead up to an understanding of how each phase contributes to the cognitive insight which is later perceived as such. As mentioned earlier CEA directs the focus towards how phase transitions are enabled and on the enabling conditions for the transitions categorised as event pivots (Steffensen 2013: 201), i.e., as conditions pivotal for the emerging route of the event. Thus, from a CEA point of view, the event pivots are identified as important events in the trajectory, which lead to noticeable changes. The event pivots and their connected phase transitions are visualised in Figure 8.2.

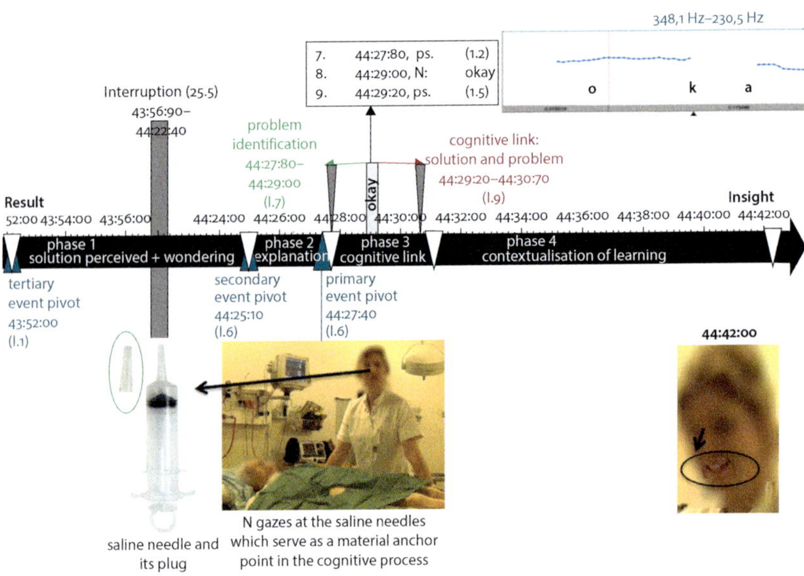

Figure 8.2 The interactivity trajectory visualises how local observations are linked to phase transitions and the generation of insight

As mentioned above, the needle insertion site is usually marked with ink, which disappears instantly when it is cleaned with alcohol. However, this novice doctor marks the insertion site with the plug from a saline needle (see Figure 8.2), which leaves a temporary depression in the patient's skin. This action deviates from how expert doctors on the ward perform the procedure. Because the novice doctor has only worked on the ward for two days, she has learnt the procedure elsewhere and brings a new perspective to the ward. Alternatively, she simply chooses what seems obvious as she has not yet learnt routinised work procedure of the ward. Within the overall interaction, something noticeable happens when the nurse observes the procedure: the interaction dynamics change. The marking serves as an event pivot as it indicates a break from the original procedural workflow to a phase saturated with cognitive puzzlement (see Figure 8.2). The beginning of the event is thus identified in the nurse's question in line 1 – during which the doctor marks the patient's skin with the plug – because it is at this point that the doctor's performance triggers the nurse's interest, which leads to surprise and a conversation about medical procedures and general work procedures. In this first phase, cognitive puzzlement (lines 1–5), we observe the nurse's sense-making as a mere concern for the operation of marking (how it is done) rather than non-local awareness (that the marking procedure is better than marking with ink that disappears). Until now the dynamics reveal puzzlement and an interest in obtaining more information. Intrigued by the appearance of the mark, the nurse asks how the doctor has learned to mark the skin in this particular way (lines 1 and 5).[2] Such an exchange is not standard practice on the ward. First, from a medical perspective, the procedural steps are of no relevance to the nurse since only doctors perform these procedures. Second, time constraints often inhibit practitioners in conversational debates during diagnosis or treatment activities, and third, the perfectionist culture often prevents practitioners from exposing their inexperience, especially when the patient is listening. Accordingly, the nurse's question in many ways indicates a deviation from standard practice. Here, it develops as a clinical detour where the cognitive system is able to recalibrate its function flexibly throughout the interaction.

2.2 Explanation and procedural observation as insight: The materiality of thinking and professional vision

The second and third phase, the two intermediate phases, are explained as a logical transition prompted by the nurse's question in line 1. But as shown below, they reveal unexpected results. The second phase is constituted around the doctor's answer (line 6). However, the most salient aspect is not merely that the doctor replies to the nurse's question (as one would expect from a micro-sociological perspective), but more the embeddedness of the answer in the material-medical

2. The nurse receives no answer to her question in line 1 as the interaction between the two is interrupted by the patient's complaints of pains during the insertion process as well as a beeping coming from the electronic screen. However, after these disturbances have been managed by the medical team (25.5 seconds later), the nurse rephrases her question (line 5) and gazes at the doctor.

environment. The doctor's wordings and the integration of the material environment into the interaction add value to the nurse's cognitive sense-making. The doctor points and gazes towards the saline needles as she verbally answers the nurse's question: *I took a eh a plug from e:h those saline needles* (line 6). The material embeddedness of the answer affects the trajectory and the nurse's thinking. Therefore, it is shown in detail what affords the initial interest and sudden change in the trajectory that leads to a phase transition.

As the doctor utters *those saline needles*, she guides the nurse's visual attention to the actual location of the saline needles because she gazes and points in their direction. This utterance, accompanied by the doctor's gazing and pointing, is marked as the event pivot that changes the phase of questioning into a phase of *explanation* (see Figure 8.2). As the nurse perceives the answer (line 6), it changes her subsequent strategy for exploring the affordances constituted by the doctor's procedure. The nurse has listened and is turning the information into a coherent hypothesis or explanation. She hears and sees that the mark is made with the help of saline needles available on the ward, but this explanation is insufficient to the nurse. The nurse thus engages with the affordances in a way that, once again, changes the interactivity trajectory considerably. Silence and fixation become the functional criterion for defining a new phase in the event. The third phase transition is identified as *observation as insight* because the nurse now sees the marking procedure as something more than just a marking procedure. It emerges in the moment the nurse gazes at the needle in the middle of line 6 when the doctor is in the process of explaining and pointing. The visual discovery of the needles thus serves as a crucial event pivot. As the nurse visually perceives the needles, the doctor has finished her explanation; the nurse fixates her gaze and she freezes for a moment (see Figure 8.2). Again, the materiality of the needles plays an important role in the nurse's cognitive sense-making. A lapse of 1.2 seconds (line 7) emerges as she gazes at the needles. This is the only time in the event trajectory when the nurse is not in motion, which indicates that she starts connecting the local interactional dynamics (emotions, perceptions, sounds, objects, wordings) to non-local cognitive memories, i.e., situation-transcending sense-making. In other words, the actual materiality of the saline needles becomes closely coupled with the nurse as the cognitive system reconfigures the nurse's cognitive processes. They serve as a material anchor point (Hutchins 2005) for reflection, and 1.2 seconds later she bursts out into *okay* (line 8). Another lapse of 1.5 seconds follows (line 9) before she concludes: *that was pretty clever* (line 10). During those 2.9 seconds, *something* suddenly made sense to the nurse. To sum up, multiple dynamics in the cognitive event trajectory indicate that she links the anchors (the needles, the wordings etc.) to the creative procedure (the marking). Finally, the nurse links the anchors to the procedural challenge of the practice of the department in general (the disappearing ink). It is relevant to treat the nurse's perception of the mark and the needle as phenomena with rich information beyond their physical contours. She sees the mark as something more than a mark, something with value to her professional agency.

Gibson contrasts his ecological approach to visual perception to those communicated in general textbooks and handbooks (Gibson 1979/86: 1), which ground their explanations of perception in physiological models of the retinal image.[3] He defines them as shallow because they separate sensations from knowledge: "our reasons for supposing that seeing something is quite unlike knowing something come from the old doctrine that seeing is having temporary sensations one after another at the passing moment of present time, whereas knowing is having permanent concepts stored in memory" (Gibson 1979/86: 258). Gibson's alternative, his theory of information pickup, closes the gap between perception and knowledge as individuals become aware of the world by living in it: by feeling, tasting, seeing, smelling it, etc. His approach to visual perception corresponds with our ecological take on insight and problem-solving activity. This notion of perception as an extension of knowing applies to the nurse's action.

In the following, we zoom in on how knowing relates to sense-making and perception. Within the same context, multiple actions contribute to learning. The insight is enabled by multiple local and non-local conditions. The non-local conditions concern the nurse's understanding of general practice and work procedures whereas the local conditions relate to the doctor's explanation, her pointing and her gazing at the needles (the solution). With CEA, such conditions are marked as event pivots, which lead to the insight and consequently to the learning result, which can be used to improve practice. However, other studies have emphasised the function of shifting gaze during insight problem-solving (Lichtfield and Ball 2011). For instance, they have shown how cueing individuals' attention towards relevant visuospatial components increases the likelihood of task success (Lichtfield and Ball 2011). Similarly, in this case we observe a result of cognitive work embodied in the nurse's tone of voice supported by her fixated gaze during the first lapse (line 7) when the doctor has pointed in the direction of the needles, cueing the nurse's attention towards the solution. While the nurse identifies the information just perceived as relevant, she starts wondering, thinking, hesitating,

3. "Direct perception is what one gets from seeing Niagara Falls, say, as distinguished from seeing a picture of it. The latter kind of perception is *mediated*. So when I assert that perception of the environment is direct, I mean that it is not mediated by the *retinal* pictures, *neural* pictures, or *mental* pictures. *Direct perception* is the activity of getting information from the ambient array of light. I call this a process of *information pickup* that involves the exploratory activity of looking around, getting around, and looking at things." (Gibson 1979/86: 147 [italics in original])

and then she comes up with a worthwhile connection. In phase one, the nurse only observes or notices the doctor's acts , but as she links her prior observations with more perceptual cues, she makes direct sense of the information picked up in ways that lead to insights. In other words, the nurse has identified the marking as a solution to a challenge or a problem. However, it is a non-local problem in the sense that it is not grounded in the local context of interaction. Her thinking is *situation-transcendent* (Linell 2009) or *sense-saturated* (Steffensen 2013), which means that she understands her environment in terms of her history as a professional, a process she only later reflects upon (phase four). Finally, it is relevant to point out that the nurse is only able to make sense of the environment in the way she does due to her level of expertise as it provides her with a *professional vision* (Goodwin 1994, 2000a). Goodwin has written extensively about this notion, for example in the work of archaeologists, who learn to see details and nuances in dirt that are invisible to the untrained eye. When iterative actions and interactions sculpt categorical patterns and shapes over time, they provide the interlocutors with a professional vision, an expert view that is often materialised into "objects of knowledge that become the insignia of a profession's craft: the theories, artefacts and bodies of expertise that are its special and distinctive domain of competence" (Goodwin 1994: 606). The nurse's experience and professionalism enable her to see the marking and the saline needles as resources beyond the local situation, namely, for general medical practice. The moment she realises that the mark and the needles are solutions to general procedures she becomes engaged in embodied cognitive work. This engagement is reflected in her fixation behaviour (Figure 8.2), her conversational pattern as well as her vocal pitch. A measurement of the pitch patterns was performed, and a clear change was noticeable: The nurse's *okay* in line 8 stands out; this utterance is visualised in Figure 8.3.

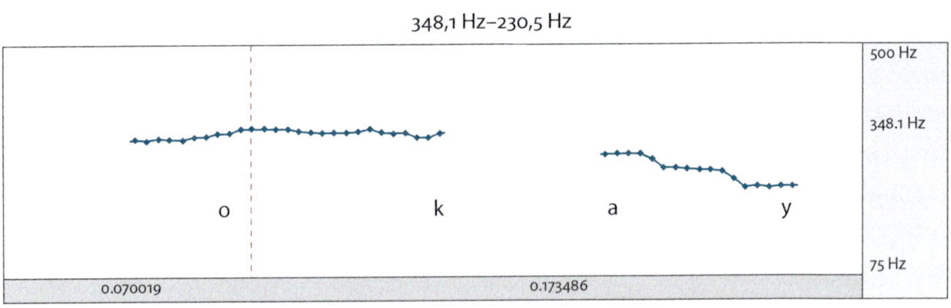

Figure 8.3 Maximal pitch of 'okay': 348.1 Hz. Pitch range for 'okay' in line 8: 118 Hz

First, a lapse followed by a delayed response (acknowledgment or evaluation) is a noticeable event since nothing else requires her attention at that exact moment; she is visibly not attending to any other work procedure or perceptual affordances. Further, at no other point in the conversation does the nurse's vocal pitch get close to the level of 350 Hz. Her average pitch during the whole event is around 250 Hz, and the second highest pitch point is in line 4 at the end of the question where it reaches 300 Hz. Her *okay* thus marks a shift in interactivity, and it is placed between two lapses (1.2 seconds and 1.5 seconds in line 7 and line 9), which surround the 0.2 seconds of the utterance. Until the first lapse, she did not explicitly reflect on the general applicable function this procedural approach could have, and after the second lapse she provides a rather explicit expression of praise (line 10). Later, she relates the doctor's method to a more general procedural level beyond the local situation: *I have actually also (.) often thought about that* (line 19). The lapses and the noticeable change in pitch underscore a deviation from her pitch baseline. Thus, the example underlines how thinking is embodied and doubly dialogical and that interaction theories are alternatives to the individualist *Theory of Mind* (which holds that one's mind is largely hidden from others) (Gallagher and Hutto 2008).

In early CA literature (e.g. Heritage 1984) the acknowledgement *okay* and the assessment *that was clever* have been described as *change-of-state tokens* (Heritage 1984), which– in a sense – are indications of new insights (however minimal). They can also be interpreted as a way of assisting the doctor in maintaining face by acknowledging the new information the nurse has received. But the interaction also provides the nurse with a richer understanding. Consequently, the nurse – as an individual – has learnt something. While the doctor provides the solution, the nurse makes the cognitive link between a local solution and a general challenge on the ward. The *okay* is more than a verbal stance marker accounting for new information. The vocal pitch deviates noticeably from the pitch baseline in the global trajectory in this sequence. The pitch change and gaze fixation are part and parcel of the physiological and sociological dimensions of sense-making processes. They do not just indicate or point to changes in perception or cognitive activity; they are cognitive actions in themselves. Moreover, the change in the nurse's gaze pattern is salient as she suddenly fixates on the *material solution*: the saline needles. The needles become a perceptual anchor, and as such a part of the distributed cognitive system. To make a link between local embodied experience and abstract and general situations takes time and requires cognitive effort. Thus, taking the two isolated lapses, the gaze pattern and the rapid timescales of pitch as evidence, it is shown how cognitive insights are facilitated in a team beyond micro-sociological collaboration and individual mental processing.

2.3 Contextualisation of learning

Only a few moments after the nurse has issued her *okay*, we get he results of the cognitive process as she links the local situation to the general practice on the ward (lines 10, 13 and 19). This final part of the interaction constitutes the fourth phase of the event: the contextualisation of learning (see Figure 8.2). The nurse makes explicit that the perceived solution connects with a general challenge that she often faces: *I do not think I have ever seen that before* (line 13) and *I have actually (.) often thought about that too* (line 19). The *that (too)* at the end of line 19 refers to the problem. In this specific context, she combines her new, locally achieved knowledge (the insight) with the non-local *that* in a way that is recognised as *problem identification*, and as she utters *that*, she smiles in a noticeable way, which she has not done previously during the overall conversation (see Picture B in Figure 8.2). In fact, her actions can be characterised as both problem identification and learning (Figure 8.2). The nurse's behaviour and the cognitive results that emerge add to our understanding of the enabling conditions for insights in interactivity. The nurse benefits from the cognitive system. She does not herself come up with the solution. Rather, she ("dialogically") uses the doctor's actions and products of action (the marking), her verbal utterances (explanations) and the material environment (the saline needles) as a means to solution-finding, problem-identification and anticipatory problem-solving (they anticipate a solution to a long-standing challenge). Thus, the cognitive result is an outcome of trustful coaction between nurse, doctor and the environment, with the doctor as the main agent and the nurse as the main cogniser.

This case is interesting as "the marking challenge" or the problem in a sense is absent, or at least backgrounded. The problem is not in front of the nurse and the doctor; it is a problem that exists beyond this activity, in the past and potentially in the future. The nested cognitive results, which emerge in situ, might lead to anticipatory problem-solving in similar future situations. Further, only the nurse knows the character of this procedural hurdle, which in the light of the new procedure can be phrased as a problem, and although the doctor has known the solution for some time at least, she has not identified it is a solution to a problem. Further, this situation-transcendent activity reflects the dialogicality of cognition; the nurse's sense-making is best explained beyond a representational level of perception. However, what she observes is related to her own experience on the ward, which is why the nurse and the doctor do not see the same challenge. In line with the theory of direct perception, the nurse sees it as something valuable in relation to general work procedures whereas the doctor sees it as a natural procedure that is not in need of any explanation. In other words, the situation-transcendent nature of cognition is what allows the nurse to define and anticipate a procedural challenge, which is non-existing to the doctor. The problem is not to be seen or solved, but to be deduced (found) during information pickup (Gibson 1979/86) based on material anchors, experience and aided by a professional vision (Goodwin 1994).

3. Case II: Team performance, professional evaluation and the patient's roles

In the following case example, the medical team consists of multiple team members, and most of them are from other departments. Similarly, it emphasises how sense-making teams benefit from and construct a shared expertise. The case demonstrates a transient team constellation in which most team members do not know each other beforehand. The atmosphere is calm despite the acute situation. The interpersonal relationships are continuously managed *in situ* in parallel with medical evaluation, hypothesis generation and patient involvement. While this team performs successfully (they reach a conclusion, the patient is satisfied and the dialogical relation is characterised by professionalism and respect), the enabling conditions for the team's ability to collaborate as excellently as it does are not immediately obvious. What appears to be the opposite of patient involvement turns out to be an example of professional caring and clear distribution of work tasks. The medical team is able to work efficiently because the practitioners jointly concert their actions in a flexible cognitive system with both tightly and loosely assembled relationships.

The medical team consists of an experienced primary doctor, who has the overall responsibility, a gastrointestinal surgeon, who has been called in for assistance, a medical student, an experienced nurse and a paramedic. While the doctors and the medical student constitute a relative stable team, the nurse is occupied with individual tasks and the paramedic observes at a distance as part of his further educational progress. The patient is a middle-age male, who arrived

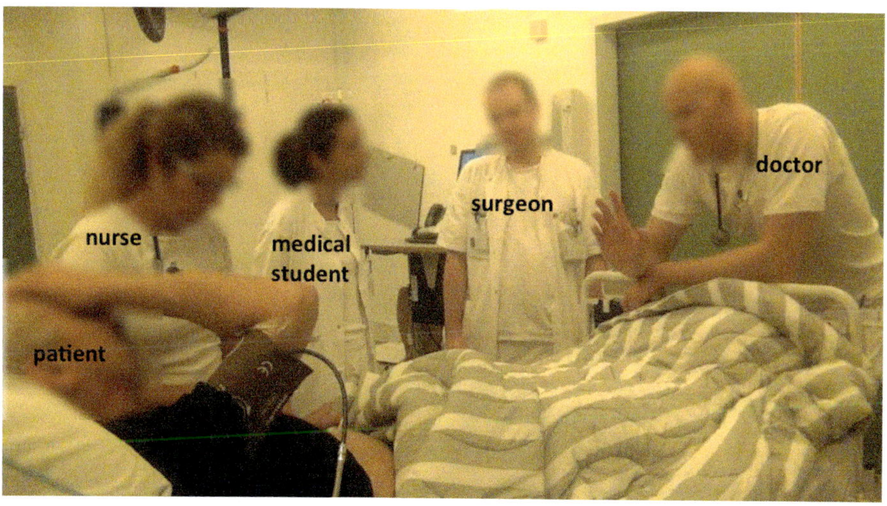

Figure 8.4 Overview of the layout: A sense-making team

with stomach cramps. He was instantly treated with morphine to reduce his pain and is now calmed down, but his condition is still acute.

3.1 A collaborative team: The organising power of gaze

At this point, the doctors summarise and evaluate the patient's narrative to decide how they should come up with a plan for further treatment. Specifically, they need to decide whether they should initiate surgery or gather more information about what causes the tremendous pain, and they need to reach a decision immediately. On the one hand, if they choose not to operate, they waste time, money and resources on providing diagnostic imaging and analysis, and that might have consequences for the well-being of the patient if it ends with surgery anyway. On the other hand, surgery without substantial information may lead to unnecessary action, and in this case, it could be a serious interference that could have been prevented. Based on the medical measurements they have just interpreted (blood tests etc.), the patient's own narrative, information from the medical record and real-time observation of the patient, the two scenarios are discussed. In other words, they do not know the exact problem – what is causing the pain – and based on insufficient information, they need to decide what to do. The sequence presents itself as follows:

Transcript 8.2[4]
Danish original

```
1.  05:37:20, D:    °og så har der været et døgns varende diarré som jeg heller ikke
                    kan forklare°
2.  05:40:50, S:    °°ja°° (.)°nej°
3.  05:41:50, ps.   (0.7)
4.  05:42:20, P:    jeg [havde j
5.  05:42:40, D:        [og der havde han så rigtig ondt i maven da han kom ik
6.  00:44:20, ps.   (0.4)
7.  05:44:60, P:    jeg havde jo regnet med det var s bare sådan noget øhm=
8.  05:46:80, S:    bare det ikke e::r en kronisk smerte syndrom eller noget der er
                    ved at udvikle sig (xxx) plejer ikke at præsentere sig sådan her
                    (.) det plejer at komme snigende ikke os
9.  05:53:60, D:    ja
10. 05:54:00, ps.   (1.0)
11. 05:55:00, S:    spørgsmålet er om vi skulle have noget billede-diagnostik på det
                    (.) elle:r en scan
```

4. In the transcript, S stands for surgeon.

English translation

1. 05:37:20, D: °and then there has been this diarrhoea for about a day which I cannot explain either°
2. 05:40:50, S: °°yes°° (.) °no°
3. 05:41:50, ps. (0.7)
4. 05:42:20, P: I [just I
5. 05:42:40, D: [and at that time he had a real pain in the stomach when he arrived right
6. 00:44:20, ps. (0.4)
7. 05:44:60, P: I just thought it was s a kind of a ehm=
8. 05:46:80, S: as long as it i::s not a chronic pain syndrome or something that is about to develop (xxx) usually not presenting itself like this (.) it usually progresses slowly right
9. 05:53:60, D: yes
10. 05:54:00, ps. (1.0)
11. 05:55:00, S: the question is whether we should have some imaging on this (.) o:r a scan

The two doctors are absorbed in the diagnostic process and, as we enter the conversation, the doctor lists unresolved circumstances in a low voice to the surgeon (line 1). Both doctors are facing the patient, but they gaze at his body and more specifically at his stomach, which is the locus of the medical problem. Momentarily, they briefly gaze at each other but at no time at the patient.

The medical student observes the overall situation, but she has, qua her role as a doctor *in spe*, an interest in the medical problem-solving managed by the

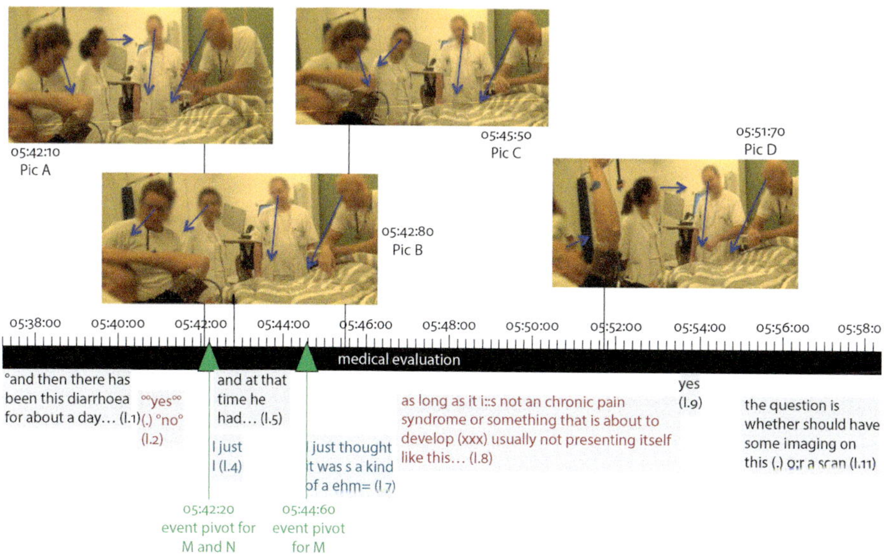

Figure 8.5 The function of team management of changes in the layout of affordances

two doctors, who are also the main cognisers in this event. During this excerpt the medical student and the nurse remain silent. The nurse is occupied with a procedural task.

The figure illustrates how interruptions are managed in accord with how the situation develops. In the figure, event pivots are indicated, but as will be explained, the pivots only become affordances for action for some parties within the team.

All practitioners are occupied with the medical problem-solving and no one gazes at the patient's face (see picture A). The patient covers his eyes with his hand, which narrows down his visual system. However, as a 0.7- second pause is made (line 3), the patient takes advantage of the break to share his concerns, but the doctor immediately interrupts him. Only 0.2 seconds after the patient begins to utter *I [just I* (line 4), the doctor continues the narrative with the surgeon. None of the doctors responds to the patient's remark, either verbally or non-verbally; consequently, the patient stops himself in the middle of his utterance. While the doctors continue as if nothing happened, both the nurse and the medical student gaze immediately at the patient's face. Only 100 milliseconds pass from when the patient starts his utterance until the two practitioners turn their heads. The patient's utterance is identified as an event pivot for the nurse and the medical student, who react to his speech at the exact same time (see Figure 8.5). The nurse temporarily suspends her task and looks up while the medical student ignores the medical interaction and orients to the patient (see picture B). Neither of the doctors changes their visual orientation. After 2.3 seconds the nurse resumes the medical task, and only the medical student continues to gaze at the patient's face, for 8.3 seconds in total.

As soon as the doctor has completed his utterance, a new 0.4-second pause is made, and the patient once again tries to contribute with his own view: *I just thought it was s a kind of a ehm=* (line 7). This time the surgeon cuts off the patient just as the patient was about to explain what he thought was the matter with him. This time only the medical student gazes at the patient's face. The rest of the team, in contrast, 'non-react' to the patient's remark even though he speaks loud and clear (see picture C). After this non-reaction, the patient removes his arm from his forehead and grabs on to the handle in the ceiling. The patient holds on to the handle, which entails a more participatory behaviour as he is able to gain eye contact with the doctors. As this happens the medical student stops gazing at the patient and continues to learn from the medical evaluation (picture D).

From a micro-sociological perspective, it is relevant to dwell on the timing of the patient's interruption and interference. The patient takes the turn at a relevant place. His verbal expression is coordinated in accordance with the doctor's utterances. Thus, as the doctor's turn is complete, the patient takes the next turn. However, the response remains absent. Rather than being an example of insensitive and non-dialogical behaviour, investigations of whole-bodied coordination reveal quite the opposite picture. With the interactivity perspective, a multi-scalar approach includes dynamics beyond the enchronical scale of interaction. By tuning in on how gaze serves as a coordinating resource, which allows for flexible and dynamical organisation within the team, it demonstrates how the team is functionally defined by individual roles and priorities. The doctors continue their professional evaluation of the patient, the medical student stands by and takes note of the overall situation, and the nurse reacts and observes to see if something critical emerges, and then soon resumes her task.

Efficient and coordinated teams are defined as individuals who perform differently but share a common objective and priority (in this case diagnosis and pre-treatment). This excerpt pivots on how the team co-acts via coordination of gaze. Thus, through gaze, the patient's request is responded to, but it is not treated as an affordance for dialogue. Moreover, caring for the patient in the long run requires other situated actions (Pedersen 2010, 2012; Hodges, 2007a, 2007b).

In this case, the changes in the cognitive system do not lead to task switch (interaction with the patient). The apparently non-dialogical behaviour is not a consequence of reduced sensitivity or stress; rather, it is an expression of overview, clear priorities and efficient distribution of responsibility. The organising power of gaze is seen in the team's ability to perceive and act on relevant changes. They adapt smoothly to the situation with a minimum of cognitive effort and disturbance. Even though the situation is acute, the team perform calmly and professionally. The work of the healthcare professionals is highly coordinated. In this moment, it is not the time to bring in the patient's ideas; they will only disturb a focused argumentation amongst the doctors, who are also under time pressure to come up with a plan for further treatment.

Interestingly, the actions of the medical student deviate from the rest of the team members. While the cognitive event trajectory indicates a smooth interactivity trajectory, where potential event pivots remain *potentialities* for the medical team (the patient's utterances do not lead to a change in the cognitive agenda), the medical student freezes and her gaze is fixated at the patient's face for 8.3 seconds. To the nurse, the first utterance of the patient becomes a minimal disturbance, which briefly disrupts her work. For the medical student, both utterances of the patient become event pivots, which make her unable to attend the medical evaluation for 8.3 seconds. The medical student might perceive the patient's expression as an affordance for dialogue, but constraints such as her position as the lowest in the professional role hierarchy, the fact that she is the least experienced in the team and her role as an observer rather than a full member of the medical team, could be explanations as to why she stays focused on him for a long time, yet ends up doing nothing. Another explanation is that as a novice, she relies on the experienced team's sense-making and learns from their behaviour. The nurse immediately identifies the non-critical comment and the doctors continue to complete another important task. The medical student does not have the same expertise as the other team members, who are all highly experienced practitioners. Intuitively, she might not have the same sense for how to prioritise and balance multiple values: caring and moving on in terms of interpersonal communication and medical evaluation. In previous case examples, novices often attempt to realise multiple values simultaneously, which leads to salient changes in the interactivity trajectory and is often enabled by stress, confusion and frustration. In this case, the team maintains a constant interactivity pattern even though changes are enacted. However, they have no consequences for the functionality of the cognitive system: The patient's interruption is not a difference that makes a difference, to paraphrase Bateson (1972).

A verbal expression is a social affordance for integrating behaviour. In this concrete example, however, it is *not* picked up as an opportunity for dialogue. Dialogical expertise is related to the ability to instantly know when and where to pick up on changes in the layout of affordances. The medical cognitive system is able to reconfigure its boundaries as the gazes of the various team members indicate a precise distribution of responsibility and tasks.

Coordinated and efficient team performance is characterised by the team's ability to distribute responsibility and adapt flexibly to changes in the environment rather than by following predefined and fixed procedures about who should do what in predefined scenarios. Learning opportunities are more easily apprehended within teams than in individual-based situations as people inspire and constrain each other. As healthcare professionals, given their reciprocal relationship, co-articulate, co-act and coordinate, they become bound up with each other's distinctive medical histories and ways of performing as professionals (Thibault 2014). As this happens, medical teams co-modify and co-adapt *in situ*, which results in coaction enabled by conditions that relate to multiple timescales and which link endogenous and exogenous conditions for interactivity (Thibault 2014). The medical student perceives the actions of the team and over time her expertise becomes richer and more automatised. Such automatisation is what characterises the team's sense-making processes. Further, when experts make sense in real life, they do not only follow social rules. They balance multiple tasks and values, which, depending on the situation, entail a behaviour, which is unpredictable in advance. The "right thing" to do, both interpersonally and medically, emerges *pari passu* with the act of perceiving what to do with what the environment offers, and with the ability of the cognitive system to adapt to the changes in situ. In this case *conversational ignoring* is necessary if caring for the patient is to be realised in the long run. Emergency medicine is to some degree about routine practice, and there are numerous procedures and protocols that enhance work practice and contribute to safe and standardised outcomes. However, unexpected and sudden changes unpacked in milliseconds give the practitioners limited opportunity to reflect. Generally, while novices allocate a lot of cognitive effort into rule-following processes, experienced practitioners rely on expertise defined as an embodied intuition equipped with experience over time (Merleau-Ponty 2012). In this case the experienced team relies on an embodied historicity, which releases cognitive power to important tasks. This case example emphasises the importance of team performance. Much can happen simultaneously, and joint sense-making emerges as interactivity connects individual behaviours in a shared trajectory.

In the final excerpt the case is turned around. The patient comments on the team's medical evaluation and his comments require immediate response and explicit attention from the medical team. The patient becomes a part of the cognitive system as the doctors manage to re-organise its boundaries through coordination of gaze, body movements, tone of voice and change in vocabulary.

3.2 Managing boundary constraints in a cognitive system

This excerpt investigates the interactional constraints when the two main cognisers (the surgeon and the doctor) evaluate the patient in a precise, medical language while the patient is present. In continuation of the previous excerpt, the two doctors share their thoughts just to ensure that they agree that they have reached a shared and respectable decision. Attention is given to the team's shared coordination of repair and recalibration of the cognitive system as the patient utters a relevant concern.

Transcript 8.3
Danish original

```
1.  06:12:80, D:   næ:: [det synes jeg er en fin ide
2.  06:13:00, S:        [jeg tænker vel bare vi skal have god indsigt i abdomen i
                   hvert fald [ik så så vi: øh kan med sikkerhed sige: ikke (.) er
                   noget galt
3.  06:15:20, D:              [ja
4.  06:19:00, D:   ja
5.  06:19:30, S:   inden vi begynder o:g og lukke op i dig og kigge ind
6.  06:21:60, D:   ja ja men det synes jeg er en ([xxx) er en udmærket approach
7.  06:22:70, P:                                   [nu må I sgu da lige styre jer
8.  06:24:90, ps.  (0.6) (all laughing, except P)
9.  06:25:50, D:   VI STÅR O:G (.) OG SNAKKER OM VI SYNES DET ER EN GOD IDE OG LIGE
                   AT TAGE DEN LIDT MED RO FØRST↓
10. 06:30:00, ps.  (0.4)
11. 06:30:40, D:   O[G LI:GE STARTE MED NOGET (.) pænt ik
```

12. 06:30:50, P: [før I åbner mig op
13. 06:33:60, S: jo=
14. 06:34:00, D: =ja
15. 06:34:50, P: nu havde jeg det lige så godt
16. 06:35:30, S: ja::
17. 06:35:70, ps. (0.8) (student and paramedic laugh)
18. 06:36:50, P: (x[xx)
19. 06:36:80, S: [vi starter med at tage e en sca en CT scanning ik↑
20. 06:39:50, P: jo
21. 06:39:80, ps. (0.9)
22. 06:40:70, S: af maven
23. 06:41:20, ps. (0.6)
24. 06:41:80, P: °ja°=
25. 06:42:20, S: =og så ser vi: på den og får den beskrevet af en røntgenlæge
26. 06:44:50, ps. (0.6)
27. 06:45:10, P: °okay°
28. 06:45:90, D: det var ikke pænt sagt↓
29. 06:46:60, ps. (1.2)
30. 06:47:80, P: nårh (xxx)
31. 06:49:80, D: nå så skriver jeg en journal (.) og så ø:::h bestiller jeg en CT
(.) og så kommer han op til dig og så: øh: °må vi se på det°

English translation

1. 06:12:80, D: no:: [I think that is a good idea
2. 06:13:00, S: [in any case I think we need a good idea about what is going
on inside the abdomen right [well so so we: eh can with certainty
say: nothing (.) is wrong
3. 06:15:20, D: [yes
4. 06:19:00, D: yes
5. 06:19:30, S: before we decide to: open you up
6. 06:21:60, D: yes yes but I that is a ([xxx) a sensible approach
7. 06:22:70, P: [you need to get it together guys
8. 06:24:90, ps. (0.6) (all laughing, except P)
9. 06:25:50, D: WE ARE JU:ST (.) TALKING ABOUT WHETHER WE THINK IT IS A GOOD IDEA TO
JUST
TAKE IT KIND OF EASY TO BEGIN WITH↓
10. 06:30:00, ps. (0.4)
11. 06:30:40, D: A[ND JU:ST START WITH SOMETHING (.) nice right
12. 06:30:50, P: [before you decide to open me up
13. 06:33:60, S: yes=
14. 06:34:00, D: =yes
15. 06:34:50, P: I was just starting to feel well
16. 06:35:30, S: ye::s
17. 06:35:70, ps. (0.8) (student and paramedic laugh)
18. 06:36:50, P: (x[xx)

```
19. 06:36:80, S:    [we will first take a a sca a CT scan right↑
20. 06:39:50, P:   yes
21. 06:39:80, ps.  (0.9)
22. 06:40:70, S:   of the stomach
23. 06:41:20, ps.  (0.6)
24. 06:41:80, P:   °yes°=
25. 06:42:20, S:   =and then we: will go through that and have it described by a
                   radiology doctor
26. 06:44:50, ps.  (0.6)
27. 06:45:10, P:   °okay°
28. 06:45:90, D:   that was not a nice thing to say↓
29. 06:46:60, ps.  (1.2)
30. 06:47:80, P:   well (xxx)
31. 06:49:80, D:   well then I will write a record (.) and e:::h I order a CT (.) and
                   then he will come back to you and the:n eh °we will take it from
                   there°
```

The surgeon emphasises that the next step is to get sufficient insight into the abdomen. As the surgeon utters, *with certainty say:*, both doctors nod in agreement and they have eye contact. Until this moment the two physicians have constituted a relatively stable cognitive system; they have gazed at the patient's stomach and momentarily at each other. They have spoken in a lower voice, which further demarcates the boundary of the cognitive system. This constellation changes as the doctors are about to reach a conclusion and utter this in a way that prompts the patient to participate in the interaction. In contrast to the previous interruptions, the doctors treat this one as an affordance for dialogue. This is visualised in the following Figure 8.6.

Overall, the figure visualises how the medical team is able to manage a potentially critical situation by moving from medical evaluation to dialogue with the patient and back to professional discussion again. The team uses two repair strategies, which enable them to recalibrate the cognitive system in a way that allows for patient inclusion without losing sight of the professional task. What enables the team to manage this challenge efficiently and dialogically, is investigated below.

As the doctors have reached a decision (line 4), the surgeon nods towards the patient's stomach and gazes in the same direction when uttering: *before we decide to: open you up* (line 5). As he utters *to: open*, he gazes at the patient's stomach, but as he continues his verbal utterance *up* (the rest of line 5), he changes his visual orientation and gazes at the doctor (see picture B). Linguistically, the deictic "you" in line 5 refers to the patient and indicates a shift in the interactivity as the conversation now involves the patient. Both the *open you* and the gaze towards the patient serve as a primary event pivot, which leads to patient involvement (see Figure 8.6).

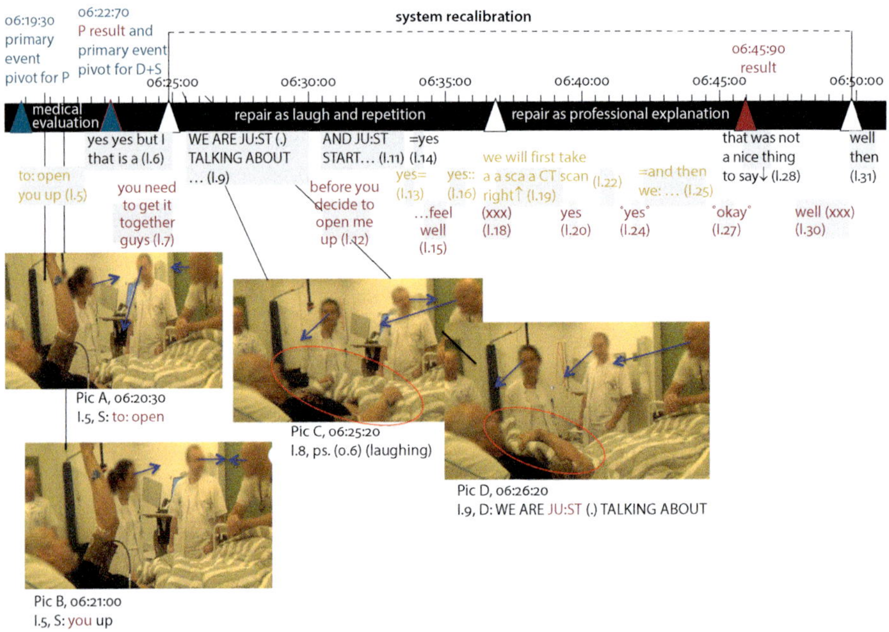

Figure 8.6 System recalibration

Prior to line 5, the patient was a medical object of discussion and the doctors mainly addressed him in third person 'he' (see the previous Transcript 8.2, line 5) or parts of his body (the abdomen) (see Transcript 8.3, line 2). Yet, the deictic "you" reconfigures the relations in the cognitive system, so the patient is now directly addressed. The whole process seems ambiguous, though. On the one hand, the surgeon indicates a transition from the diagnostic process to an informational period when the patient is being informed about what they have discussed and their recommendations for further treatment. But, where the deictic "you" refers to the patient, the nod towards the stomach both points to the patient as a subject and to the stomach as an object.

The surgeon never gains eye contact with the patient. He gazes briefly at the patient's stomach while the doctor remains focused on the surgeon, and the surgeon immediately regains eye contact with the doctor (see picture B). At no time have the doctors gazed at the patient and after this explicating episode, the doctors re-establish a dyadic relation. Thus, the surgeon both attends and disattends to the patient. However, when the doctor utters *yes yes but I that is a ([xxx)* (line 6), the patient grabs the handle and raises his head. Immediately the doctor gazes at the patient's face. As the patient raises himself up in the bed, the patient utters *you need to get it together guys* (line 7), after which the patient falls back into bed and lets his arms down. This action serves as a crucial primary event pivot for the doctors as they immediately react to patient's utterance; they laugh and the patient immediately pulls up the duvet just under his chin and holds on to it in a noticeable way as if he wants to protect the exposed part of his body, the uncovered stomach (see picture C and D). From when the surgeon has completed the utterance *before we decide to o:pen you up*, 06:21:70, line 5, until the patient responds 06:23:00, line 7, 1.3 seconds pass. While it is old news that surgery is a possible action, the patient seems to respond to the *wordings* in the context *to: open you up*. The patient repeats these words in line 9: *[before you decide to open me up*. Goodwin (2013) explains how individuals often reuse resources that are provided previously in the context in order to build new actions. The cooperative act entails a change in the interactivity trajectory as the wordings of the surgeon's professional evaluation is repeated to create a tragicomic atmosphere (they all laugh). Goodwin argues that this process of "systematically modifying that structure to build something new, is a central, distinctive feature of human action, one that makes it possible for human culture and knowledge to accumulate in a systematic fashion" (Goodwin 2013: 9). Thus, for this action to be meaningful and possible, the patient and the medical team must share a cultural understanding of such cooperative action. As competent members of a shared cultural and cognitive system they are able to cooperatively make sense of the linking between the surgeon's and the patient's perspectives respectively, and as a result they laugh. The surgeon's deictic reference (*you*), the patient's verbal interruption and his physical protective embodiments are important event pivots, which serve as affordances for dialogue. Thus, the result is a dialogue in which laughter and professional explanation recalibrate the cognitive system (see Figure 8.6). Prompted by the specific wordings, *open you up*, the patient's dramatic and demonstrative action becomes a way of combining seriousness with drama. After the patient has uttered that they should take it easy and covered his stomach with the duvet, the medical team bursts into laughter (line 8). The laughter within the team and the act by the patient frame the situation as a tragicomic event where the patient seems shocked and at the same time responds to the laughter with an ambiguous act that is both serious and comical. With the duvet as a "safeguard layer", the interpersonal relationship between the patient and the doctors is potentially exposed and constrained. All laugh except the patient. Just as the patient has pulled up the duvet, the surgeon suddenly takes a couple of steps to the side and forward as he moves away from the doctor and closer to the patient (see picture C and D). For several moments and until this moment, the surgeon has not moved as the two physicians have established a relatively stable relationship. This relationship is now changed by the physical reorganisation, the actions of the patient and the laugh that connects all members as a shared team.

The patient's feelings are ambiguous. Nevertheless, several dramatic actions indicate a kind of shock condition, which changes the flow of interactivity noticeably. In other words, unless the interpersonal relationship is further constrained, the doctors will need to handle the situation professionally and dialogically. While the two doctors previously ignored the patient's utterance, they now respond to his concerns immediately, both verbally and in bodily movements. The doctor raises his volume distinctly as he utters that they were indeed agreeing on taking it easy to begin with (line 9), and he gazes at the medical team and at the patient's face. Moreover, they speak louder, the surgeon radically changes his position, so he faces everyone in the ward and the vocabulary is less specialised and serious, and in this way the cognitive system recalibrates and reconfigures its boundaries. For 11.9 seconds the doctor manages the situation by responding to the patient's interruption and the laugh is an important coordinative factor in this interpersonal repair (see Figure 8.6).

As the patient continues the tragicomic form and states *I was just starting to feel better* (line 15), the medical team laughs once again. The paramedic and the medical student continue to laugh. Again, the patient contributes to the dialogue (line 18); only this time the surgeon interrupts and changes the tragicomic genre to a serious and professional one. As the surgeon interrupts, he changes the phase of repair through laughter to one of professional explanation (see Figure 8.6). The surgeon's interruption, his professional explanation and his embodiment enable him to recalibrate the system so that a serious approach can be maintained. The other team members stop laughing and the surgeon explains the factual medical procedures of the situation. As the surgeon addresses the patient and explains and summarises what is going to happen, he uses the category "stomach" rather than "abdomen", which was the preferred term in the interaction with the doctor.

Later on, as the surgeon utters *have it described by an x-ray doctor* (line 25), the doctor covers his mouth with his right hand. He then removes it a bit and scratches his chin as he responds to the earlier reaction by the patient with the comment: *That was not a nice thing to say*↓ (line 28). Exactly 24.0 seconds after the surgeon has uttered the 'critical' comment in line 5, the doctor makes a very late repair (the result prompted by the primary event pivot in line 7). This response makes the doctor appear understanding and empathetic because he puts himself in the position of the patient. When the practitioners move outside their own medical domain and 'observe' their utterance as critical wordings (*open you up*) from the perspective of the patient, they see the critical aspect of their formulation (that was not a nice thing to say). Thus, the major challenge in this case is to balance different professional domains. The doctors need to exchange their medical hypotheses in a professional domain, which sometimes expands to or interferes with the domain of the patient. There are no rules for how the patient should be included in medical dialogues. As I have shown, it depends both on inter-bodily dynamics (laughter, gesture, words, gaze) and the overall situation (e.g. time constraints). A verbal utterance from the patient in itself is not an affordance for dialogue. Sense-making is enabled by far more complex and dynamic features than verbal patterns.

A functional cognitive system produces a coordinated agency. This seems to match the experience of the team. While the doctor excuses himself for being impolite, he was not the one who uttered the critical comment. However, the atmosphere and mood do not seem to be caused by one or two words uttered in isolation, but by the flow of interactivity that has been guided by shared activities. The cognitive system entails shared activity as an ongoing accomplishment, which is not about what single individuals do, but about how a team acts within ongoing processes in interactivity. The medical team's laughter, the surgeon's professional explanation and the doctor's late repair serve as negative feedback-mechanisms, which enable the self-organisation of the cognitive system and recalibration of the interactivity trajectory (see Figure 8.6).

4. The benefits of team performance in an educational perspective

In the first case example, insight emerges as specific non-local and situated work domains are linked. The nurse learns from the collaboration with the doctor and the result of this is one of the major advantages of team performance. In emergency medicine, the team constellations are often ad hoc, and teamwork is challenged by the vulnerability of exposing one's expertise and knowledge in new situations and in new interpersonal relations in which level of expertise and knowledge are explicit in tasks, procedures, and formal and informal roles. Within such constraints, team members need to be open, vulnerable and able to share and change strategies as the situation changes and plans prove unsuccessful. Thus, safe and dialogical team performance relies on trust and confidence with the tasks, roles and work practices. If the culture works against such criteria, functional team performance is inhibited (Pedersen 2010). However, ad hoc team constellations also scaffold unique possibilities for learning. When teams are fixed, standard procedures are automatised and become tacit, which is a valuable quality in highly structured and known environments. However, in the emergency wards much relies on the team's ability to respond to the unknown. In the first case example, insights emerge as the nurse perceives a new approach to a standard procedure. If the team constellations become fixed, such learning opportunities decrease, as new correlations are unlikely to emerge to the same extent as in new constellations.

In the final cases, it is exemplified how error cycles are more likely to be managed efficiently in teams than in situations that are handled individually. The team members are perceptual detectors who jointly enlarge the visual system, and in this way pico-scale changes are more likely to be identified and encountered in a team as multiple goals can be accomplished at the same time. Thus, effective coordination and distribution of tasks, roles, and responsibilities release cognitive power to maintain the overview of the overall interactivity.

Finally, expertise is a crucial factor in successful and efficient problem-solving in stressful environments, and by combining novice and experienced practitioners in teams, learning is much more likely to emerge as a result of meaningful interactivity than from intuition when practitioners operate individually. The experienced practitioner is able to point to changes in the layout of affordances and thus the feedback-mechanisms become explicit for the less skilled practitioner. Merleau-Ponty underlines the importance of bodily experience when acquiring new habits:

> Acquiring a habit as the reworking and renewal of the body schema presents significant difficulties for classical philosophers, which are always inclined to conceive of synthesis as intellectual synthesis [...] the subject does not weld individual movement to individual stimuli, but rather acquires the power of responding with a certain type of solution to a certain form of situation.
>
> (Merlaeu-Ponty 2012: 143)

In this sense, habits and expertise are neither reduced to abstract knowledge nor automatic reflex, but rather "knowledge in our hands, which is only given through a bodily effort and cannot be translated by an objective designation" (Merlaeu-Ponty 2012: 145). Further, when Merleau-Ponty exemplifies how a blind man's stick ceases to be an object for the man (or merges into our body schema causing an extended peri-personal function (Kirsh 2013)), the same explanation applies to the function of individuals within a team. From a cognitive perspective, when coordinated, the individual team members cease to be distinct properties in the system as they perform as one functional system. Thus, the medical student learns from being part of the team's sense-making activities. Most likely she is not explicitly aware of the particular sense-making values the team realises, but by engaging in interactivity, her body schema is saturated and changed by the local interaction. By extending Merleau-Ponty's idea of how the individual habituates oneself to an environment of objects, to include interactivity, the qualities of working in teams become clear. By emphasising the value of interactivity, the effect of language is unavoidable. In a team we do not just absorb each other as objects; we trust and rely on second-hand perception (Steffensen 2013; Gibson 1966). Thus, if trust is missing, coordinated sense-making is less likely to happen. In relation to this case, the medical student would not accept the team's decision of non-dialogue, for instance.

When the novice works individually, learning takes place – as Merleau-Ponty emphasises – through bodily effort to respond to the environment in a certain way. Thus, when the novice works in a team, she relies not only on individual perceptions, but also on second-hand perceptions, and in this case, it enables the student to skip a level compared to individual learning settings. As the team non-reacts to the patient's utterance, the novice continues to gaze at the patient. Even though she does not know why the team acts as it does in the situation, she comes to experience the functional output. Indeed, by working in a team, the team members share the responsibility for dialogue and, as they concert movement, talk and action, the team jointly recalibrates its boundaries, for instance in cases of unfortunate utterances.

Finally, both cases reveal the learning potential of teamwork. Working in teams increases the chances for negative feedback mechanisms in the system as each team member can recalibrate the system in different ways depending on expertise and situational affordances for action. Thus, in relation to human errors, much can be learned from understanding the underlying dynamics of successful team coordination. The overall analysis encourages an anticipatory approach to human errors where work practice is arranged in accord with its insights. Knowledge about human errors does not need not to be extrapolated from observing human errors in themselves; rather, by observing successful coordination, latent conditions for errors can to some extent be minimised in advance.

CHAPTER 9

Documentation in the electronic medical record

The function of gesture, voice dynamics and gaze

1. Integrating typing and verbal interaction

One of the main obligatory tasks in the ward is documentation in the electronic medical record. This main task is time-consuming and takes a lot of effort during the overall diagnostic task. Previously, documentation was completed outside the emergency room with pen and paper. Today, technological artefacts and software programmes have modernised the task. Moreover, the process is managed next to the patient to enhance dialogue during the process and to detect potential misunderstandings *in situ*. All doctors complete this task, but the way they do it differs hugely. Coding brings forth two overall interactivity trajectories in relation to task performance. First, it brings forth a dialogical trajectory rich on embodiment, which enables the inclusion of the patient during documentation. Second, it brings forth a monological and sequential trajectory in which embodied behaviour is constrained by the practitioner's fixation on the computer, which excludes the patient from being part of the cognitive system. Performing this task dialogically requires that the doctor is able to mesh both artefact and patient interaction: in other words, integrating typing and verbal interaction during documentation.

Writing and typing have been viewed as a code with a one-to-one correspondence to language in interaction (Kravchenko 2011: 33). However, a radical view within linguistics distinguishes writing and speech as ontologically different cognitive activities (Kravchenko 2007, 2011; Love, 2004, 2007; Linell 2005). If the intention of the ward is to achieve dialogical task performance, it is required that the healthcare practitioner is able to mesh and navigate smoothly in and out of the distinctive cognitive processes of typing and patient-interaction. This challenge entails a focus on how dialogical documentation processes are achieved. As this chapter will show, such smooth navigation requires the implementation of creative, embodied strategies. Thus, the chapter investigates healthcare professionals' different use of embodied resources, especially gesture, gaze and voice dynamics as they perform the obligatory task in front of the computer. It further identifies general constraints for a rich, embodied behaviour in the task, such as meshing typing activities and verbal interaction or using artefacts and being sensitive to inter-bodily dynamics, for instance.

> Clearly, a good deal of expertise in the system is in the artifacts (both the external implements and the internal strategies)–not in the sense that the artifacts are themselves intelligent or expert agents, or because the act of getting into coordination with the artifacts constitutes an expert performance by the person; rather, the system of person-in-interaction-with-technology exhibits expertise.
>
> (Hutchins 1995a: 155)

As Hutchins emphasises, the expertise, which a person-in-interaction-with-technology gains, is unique. Documentation in the electronic medical record reduces the chances for human error as the information is standardised, the output is readable, and the process is fast compared to handwritten medical record-keeping. Moreover, the chronological step-by-step commands on screen structure the task and hence the interaction with the patient. While the electronic procedures secure a uniform and comparable documentation outcome, they likewise dictate, as in other task performances, a hierarchy of relevance, which does not necessarily correspond to the relevance of the specific patient.

Generally, the number of electronic artefacts in the medical ward is increasing drastically and the risk of such technological advancements is that the patient becomes secondary in parts of the diagnostic task. Often the implementation of such artefacts is based on the assumption that electronic equipment unambiguously scaffolds cognitive processes in a way that increases efficiency and standardises output. It is hypothesised that such artefact optimism is grounded in an economical cost-benefit metaphor that does not consider contextual issues and emotional dynamics as potential constraints for efficient and logical task performance. As analyses in Chapter 4 and 5 have shown, the way that artefacts are handled is crucial to outcome.

It is hypothesised that the more profound use of embodied resources such as gesture, voice dynamics, gaze and movement during task performance, the more fluidly the two different activities will be managed and the more aligned the patient and the practitioner will be. Attention is thus given to how rich embodiment prompts understandings, affords participatory behaviour, scaffolds precise pain localisation, enhances memory of specific non-local and local experiences and enables the achievement of nested activities. In particular, focus is on how the use of gesture, gaze and voice dynamics contribute to the achievement of a cognitive task. With the interactivity perspective, the function of such embodied resources is intertwined with the articulation of verbal utterances and the material environment (Streeck et al. 2011; Goodwin 2000a, 2013). In that sense, embodiment is a biosocial resource, which enables coordination and mutual attunement (Cowley 2011).

In the following, it is investigated how three doctors perform the documentation task very differently and depending on the function of embodied dynamics, contribute to a monological or dialogical interactivity trajectory. The first part focuses on how a doctor follows protocol and document required information in the electronic medical record in accordance with guidelines from medical textbooks. While no dysfunctional output is identified in this case, it becomes clear how performance based on fixed rule-following diverges from best practice when it is compared to performances based on a flexible and creative approach. The second and third cases focus on how two doctors mesh procedures with situational affordances in a way that enhances efficiency and dialogical relationships. Specifically, they use embodied resources as a means for identifying pain areas, description of symptoms, enaction of memory related to the medical narrative and, finally, to achieve multiple goals simultaneously.

The analyses use the interactivity-based framework to investigate how doctors rely on multiple timescales and material dynamics in the cognitive system. With CEA the cognitive event trajectories unveil how, from a medical point of view, relevant event pivots go unnoticed amongst the doctors. Furthermore, distributed language including ecological theory of gesture (Streeck 2010, Goodwin 2013) is applied to show the valuable significance gestures have for dialogical cognitive outcomes.

2. Case I: The iPatient is only a model of the patient

The following case presents two paradoxes in the documentation activity. First, it pivots on the paradox that while the doctor follows protocol, she becomes inhibited in performing the task efficiently and dialogically in a way that serves the patient's understanding of what is going on. The second paradox relates to the fact that while the members in interaction do not perceive the situation as constrained, an observer's perspective provides an adverse and critical evaluation. This will be discussed on the basis of a comparative analysis of the case and the two consecutive examples of best practice.

The situation of case I is characterised by a doctor's step-by-step procedure following. She has just completed obligatory steps in the diagnostic process (history-taking and physical examination) and as we enter the conversation, she is performing the documentation task. The patient is an old man with a light degree of dementia. Lately, he has been falling, and during the history taking the doctor has difficulties uncovering exactly what causes the patient most problems in his everyday life. He has been complaining about pain in his one leg and foot, but his GP, who has referred him to the ward, indicated other medical issues as primary; see Figure 9.1 for an overview of the layout.

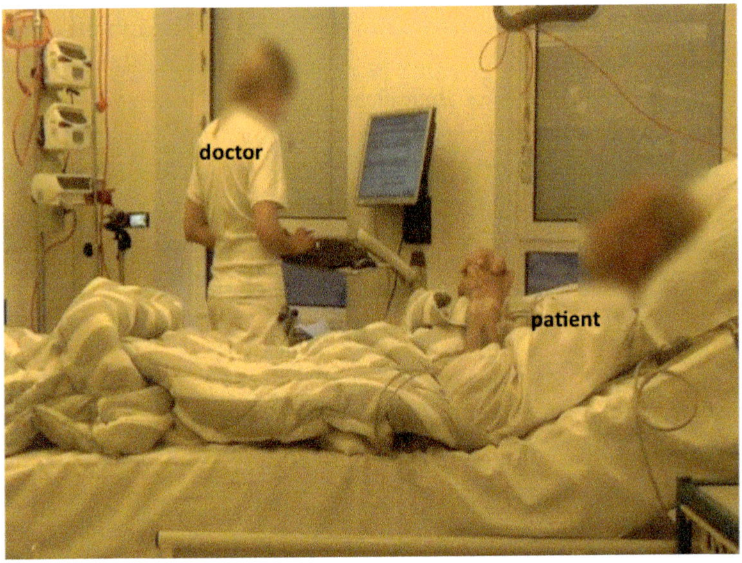

Figure 9.1 Overview of the setting: Individual task performance

Irrespective of the GP's concern or whether the patient is right, the doctor needs to document the patient's concern in the record and thus engage in dialogue to represent his narrative as accurately as possible. The doctor chooses to achieve this goal by relying on memory of previous history taking as she types on the keyboard. This strategy is commonly used and does not conflict with procedures in the ward. While this documentation task requires her attention, she focuses exclusively on the writing-reading activity and turns her back to the patient. Her orientation to the binary patient on the screen fits the analysis in 4.3.1 in which another novice doctor prioritises the distributed patient over the real patient.

Further, when the Polish philosopher Alfred Korzybski stated that "the map is not the territory", he referred to how scientists often mistake models of reality for reality itself (Korzybski 1931). In this case, the doctor similarly mistakes or treats the distributed patient – represented by medical measurements and written narratives in the electronic medical record – for the real patient who lies in bed next to the doctor.[1] This problem is not new. Thus a current dilemma relates to how healthcare practitioners prioritise between interaction with the real biological patient and the iPatient (Verghese 2008) or distributed patient (see Chapter 4, Section 3.1):

> iPatients are handily discussed (or "card-flipped") in the bunker, while the real patients keep the beds warm and ensure that the folders bearing their names stay

1. There are multiple cases identical with this one that show how the doctors are constrained by the electronic computer during the documentation task.

> alive on the computer. [...] If one eschews the skilled and repeated examination of the real patient, then simple diagnoses and new developments are overlooked, while tests, consultations, and procedures that might not be needed are ordered. (Verghese 2008: 2749)

Thus, as the doctor completes the documentation task, her interaction with the patient dissolves. For 3 minutes and 31 seconds only silence appears on the sound track of the recordings. Thus, she reads silently in the medical paper record, gazes at the screen or types information into the system, just as the procedures order her to do (see Figure 9.2).

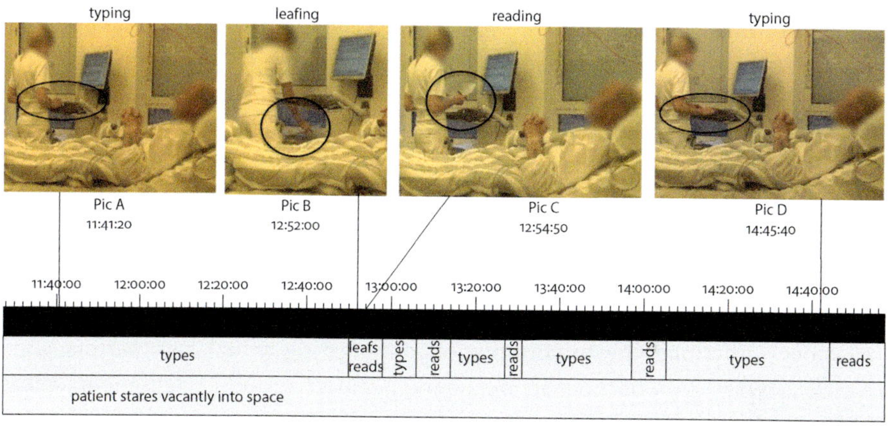

Figure 9.2 Monological behavioural trajectory

The figure represents the patient's "silent" trajectory. As she switches between reading in the papers and typing, the doctor completes the documentation task individually. The trajectory is representative for the overall task performance. Momentarily, she asks a question of clarification, and then continues to operate individually. Clarification happens on the basis of what the doctor needs to clarify. The patient then answers but does not know what the result of their interaction is as the conclusions in the record remain unspecified to him.

In this excerpt, the silence becomes tangible. The doctor stands with her side to the patient. The patient lies in bed and he is not part of the process; nor is he informed about what is going on. From Figure 9.2 no issues, problems or disruptions seem to emerge. No changes in the interactivity trajectory (for instance frustration, confusion, hesitation or the like) are detected. In other words, the involved participants do not seem to experience dysfunctionality. The patient lies in bed with his hands clasped and stares vacantly into space. The four pictures (A–D) visualise the process from the beginning to the end of the excerpt. During the whole scenario, the patient does not change his position at all. The interaction is characterised as non-dialogical and can potentially create emotional tension between the doctor and the patient.

The material organisation of the cognitive system narrows down the doctor's visual system and inhibits her ability to perceive dynamics that are played out beyond the system's boundaries. As she does not interact with the patient, she rarely uses gestures. This approach is error-prone. For instance, it is mandatory that the healthcare wards document the anamnesis in a precise, standardised and scientific, medical terminology. Thus, the doctor needs to translate the patient's explanations into a shared and established medical vocabulary. Hence it can be valuable to engage the patient in this process. When the doctor bases documentation on information generated by electronic artefacts and on memory of previous interactions, the patient is excluded from the part of the conclusion process. He is likely to lose the overview of what is being documented, and potential misunderstandings are not validated in the local situation. The doctor neither meshes tasks, nor does she use gestures. *How* to perform this task in an embodied manner has never been taught. Only the technical and procedural level of documentation, for instance how the software works and what should be documented etc., has been scrutinised in practice. However, as no changes appear (no issues emerge), nothing in the environment prompts the doctor to do so. This ”problem free” trajectory underlines the importance of investigating actual task performance as well as what goes on beyond members' perspectives and phenomenological accounts of problems.

The doctor completes her job in accordance with general procedures, but she reduces her scope of attention and separates the cognitive system from the patient, and this collides with the general principles for dialogical task performance. Seen in isolation, however, nothing critical is identified in relation to her task performance. However, it is argued that latent error cycles are more prevalent when the event trajectory reveals individual and monological documentation processes. By comparing silent and monological interactivity trajectories with dialogical modes of task completion, the quality of dialogical strategies becomes obvious. Thus, in the following, two cases of dialogical task performance are presented. Together they show why dialogical performance is important and effective for all parties involved.

3. Case II: Voice and body dynamics as event markers

This case involves a young man, who has just entered his thirties. He suffers from diabetes and he has lost both legs due to diabetes related complications. He is a known patient with a complicated medical history. During the last couple of months, he has been in and out of the hospital and this time he arrived via 911 due to severe chest pains. The doctor is an experienced primary doctor and after she has briefly examined the patient, she begins the documentation process. During the documentation process, the doctor also takes the patient's history and she meshes these two tasks. Compared to the first case, in which the doctor relied on memory of the previous history taking process, this doctor performs all tasks simultaneously. The excerpt specifically pivots on how she, using her tone of voice to explicate and demarcate different cognitive events, enables the patient to keep track and gain knowledge about where in the process they are and how important the distinct processes are. The setting is illustrated below.

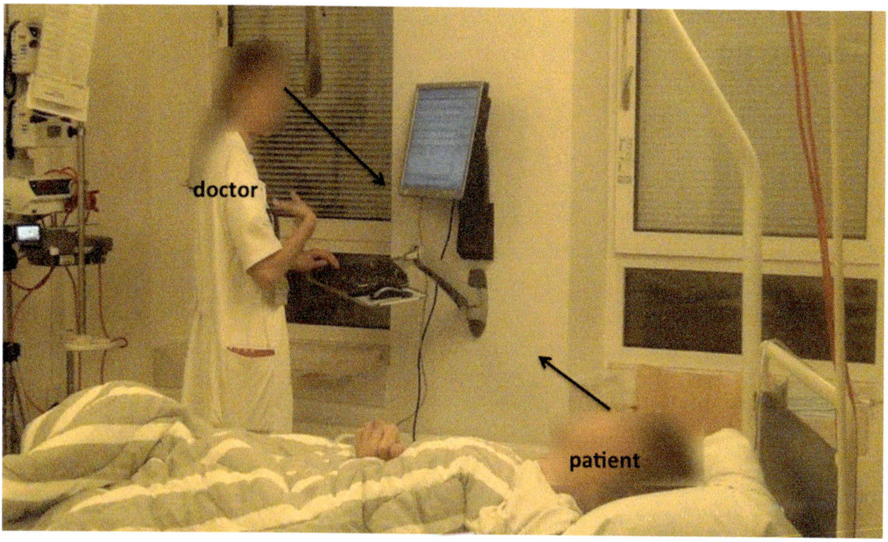

Figure 9.3 Overview of the layout: Voice dynamics

The doctor is obliged to document information about the patient's broader life situation as well as particular illness specific circumstances. These circumstances are explored through standard and general questions as well as more sensitive and context-specific questions. Generally, the doctors rarely make interactional distinctions between these types of questions (see Chapter 5, Section 3.1). This doctor, however, uses her tone of voice differently to indicate changes in types of questions, their relevance and the level of expected engagement. This vocal-based distinction is important since standard questions often seem either irrelevant, embarrassing or even silly from the patient's perspective (do you smoke?, are you pregnant?, do you drink alcohol on a daily basis?, do you suffer from headaches? etc.), contrary to more particular and contextualised questions (where did the pain arise?, what did you do when the pain arose, how do you feel, are you frightened etc.). In particular, this doctor uses three different voice dynamics to demarcate the different status and function of her questions. Cowley (2011) emphasises how prosodic realisation in general intertwines with bodily coordination and leads to an overall utterance-activity: "At all times, however, *digital signalling* (Ross 2004) is coordinated with bodily expression and prosody. In the resulting utterance-activity, vocal and non-verbal expression are integrated by bodies that adjust to an event in a cultural world" (Cowley 2011: 3). The three variations performed by the doctor are termed (a) truncated voice dynamics, (b) fluid voice dynamics and (c) staccato voice dynamics. They are exemplified and discussed in the following.

Transcript 9.1
Danish original

Excerpt 1 truncated voice dynamics

```
1.  D:  synsforstyrrelser svimmelhed hovedpine
```

Excerpt 2 fluid voice dynamics

```
2.  09:10:60, D:    du kommer med 112 på baggrund af brystsmerter
3.  09:13:20, ps.   (4.5) (P nods 'yes')
4.  09:17:70, D:    °°godt↓°°(.) fortæl mig hvad du lavede da du fik
                    ondt i brystet
```

Excerpt 3 staccato voice dynamics

```
5.  D:    okay↓ (0.7) ø:h (0.5) så lignede (4.1) smerten
          i brystet (1.1) fra sidste (0.8) indlæggelse
          (0.5) men værre
```

English translation

Excerpt 1 truncated voice dynamics

```
1.  D:    visual disturbances dizziness headache
```

Excerpt 2 fluid voice dynamics

```
2.  09:10:60, D:    you arrived via 911 because of chest pains
3.  09:13:20, ps.   (4.5) (P nods 'yes')
4.  09:17:70, D:    °°okay↓°°(.) tell me what you did as the chest
                    pains came
```

Excerpt 3 staccato voice dynamics

```
3.  D:    okay↓ (0.7) e:h (0.5) so similar (4.1) to the
          pain in the chest (1.1) from the last (0.8)
          hospitalisation (0.5) but worse
```

The three different voice dynamics relate to different interaction strategies that facilitate task achievement in a dialogically efficient way. These strategies enable the doctor (a) to get brief and summarised information, (b) to allow the patient to elaborate on specific elements in the narrative and (c) to explicate conclusions as final outputs in the record. Further, these vocal dynamics relate to variations of syntax, linguistic content and contextualisation. All the voice dynamics mark an event type with a specific function. With truncated voice dynamics, the doctor is able to cut off unnecessary information around the keywords she needs the patient to respond to. Due to the context, the doctor is able to comprise three questions into one verbal utterance, and thus she avoids constructing complete sentences such as: *did you suffer from visual disturbances*? By uttering single nouns, her utterance is succinct and articulated in a monotone voice rhythm. Using elliptic sentences – or basically single words – allows her to mark the activity as distinct from the rest of the interactivity. In this case, she demarcates the function of standard questions from more emotional and personal questions that are not situationally relevant. Indeed, these questions are needed, but she briefly goes through them with a minimum of elaboration. Because the patient treats the sequenced questions as affordances for short answers as 'yes' or 'no', the doctor and the patient perform in an efficient and coordinated fashion. The doctor implicitly hints at the "obligatory bureaucracy" as she utters these words rapidly and with a monotone voice. Moreover, her tone of voice, her economical use of relevant words, her body position towards the screen and her strict invitation to answer briefly make her appear efficient, authoritative and concise. Consequently, the doctor saves time and completes this nested task efficiently together with the patient as she elegantly prioritises her time and the patient's needs in relation to the overall goal: coming up with a diagnosis.

While the doctor appeared straightforward and concise in the case of truncated articulations, she appears differently engaged and dialogical when it comes to other types of questions. For instance, when the doctor needs elaborated and particular information that requires the patient to contextualise information, she uses a narrative strategy that prompts the patient to engage in dialogue: *you arrived via 911 because of chest pains (4.5) °°okayy↓°°(.) tell me what you did as the chest pains came* (excerpt 2, line 2+4). The doctor's dialogical structure affords a contextualised and detailed answer. Further, the tempo is slowed down and the voice dynamic is more melodious, fluid and soothing compared to the previous example. In this way the doctor indicates that this part of the interaction has another status, function and priority. Compared to other situations, doctors often initiate history taking with the broad question: *tell me what happened?* In this situation, the doctor creates the beginning herself: *you arrived via 911* (excerpt 2, line 2). This strategy saves time and contextualises her state of thought as well as marks the specific part of the patient's narrative she wants him to elaborate: *tell me what you did as the chest pains came* (excerpt 2, line 4). The doctor keeps focus on the screen until the end of her utterance, and as she then gazes at the patient, she further marks a transition relevance place (Sacks et al. 1974) in the dialogue where the patient is expected to contribute. This approach entails an efficient information elicitation, which is characterised by confident prioritising, making it easy for the patient to follow the flow throughout the event.

Finally, the doctor enacts a third voice dynamics pattern, which makes the patient aware of how her interpretation of the patient's narrative is documented in the record. As she types in the information, she utters in a staccato-like tone of voice what she writes. There is, however, a delay between the moment she utters something and the text appearing on the screen, which momentarily causes her to pause at syntactically unusual places: *so similar (4.1) to the pain in the chest (1.1) from the last (0.8) hospitalisation (0.5) but worse* (excerpt 3). This strategy of read-aloud keeps the patient as part of the interactivity, and by explicating the cognitive task, the patient becomes aware of each step in the process. Furthermore, as the doctor marks the shift in the process, especially through her prosody, the patient performs his role as patient differently by shifting between contributing to the process and fading into the background. The doctor thus relies on her embodied resources in a way that enables completion of different tasks. Notably, she utters *what* she writes and thus she is able to maintain the interpersonal relationship with the patient. The patient, in turn, is able to sanction or reject the doctor's conclusions, as he knows exactly how the doctor interprets their dialogue. Thus, writing and documentation is meshed with summarising for the patient so that they at no time break down the joint cognitive system.

All three voice dynamics (truncated, fluid and staccato) are unique forms of embodied behaviour that mark shifts between distinct events with different functions during history taking and documentation. The dynamics enable the patient to distinguish between different purposes and elements during these nested tasks. This doctor, who has a long record as a professional in the ward, has developed an expertise, which enables her to prioritise easily *in situ* and deal with multiple issues simultaneously. The doctor's capability to enact various vocal dynamics is related to her skilled expertise: "Utterance-activity arises as we make and track phonetic gestures (Fowler 2010) that prompt us to hear utterance types. Using different time-scales, rich linguistic memory evokes experience (Port 2010) that gives wording a particular sense" (Cowley 2011: 4ff). The doctor enacts different vocal and non-verbal behaviours as she knows how the different forms of behaviour, each in their own way, enable and constrain task performance. As she knows what is relevant to do, her whole-bodied actions can be interpreted as a way of integrating slow sociocultural processes with fast real-time coordination. Based on her general non-situated understanding of best practice, she performs and adjusts her voice dynamics in relation to the patient's actions. Thus, with an ecological perspective on language (Cowley 2011; Hodges 2007a; Fowler 2010; Thibault 2011; Steffensen 2011), the functional outcome of language is a result of the doctor's history of embodied coordination (her skilled behaviour) meshed with the patient's capabilities for local interaction. The functional result emerges as the non-local experience is coordinated locally.

4. Case III: Gestures as cognitive resources

Case III involves an elderly female patient with a complicated medical history, and during her hospitalisation she is particularly troubled with abdominal issues, and among other serious complications she has suffered from rectal bleeding. Her husband sits at the end of the bed. The doctor is a novice, but in contrast to most other novices, he does not use pen and paper during history taking. In this excerpt he uses his body to facilitate sense-making for both patient and himself.

Transcript 9.2
Danish original

```
1.  06:00:00, P:   jo ja: det gør ondt nu går det jo ned og så går det op her
2.  06:58:40, ps.  (0.6)
3.  06:59:00, D:   op der
4.  06:59:60, P:   ja
5.  07:00:10, D:   okay=
6.  07:00:60, P:   =jeg er lidt øm
7.  07:01:80, D:   der er du lidt øm (.)
(xxx)
8.  07:51:60, D:   godt↓ (.) så hvis vi nu tager det hele engang her [altså igennem 14
                   dage har du haft opkastninger [(.) i forbindelse med at du sådan
                   har rejst dig (.) og det kommer en gang imellem nogen gange er det
                   der [nogen gange er det der [ikke (.) ja↓ så har du været utilpas
                   (.)
9.  07:00:00, P:                                                      [ja
                                                   [ja
                      [ja                          [ja
10. 08:01:40, P:   ja (.)
11. 08:02:10, D:   og så har du haft sådan tiltagende af maveomfang [(.) dels så var
                   du lidt stø[rre (.) og dine ben er også [hævet op
12. 08:04:50, P:                                                    [ja
                              [ja
                                                        [ja
13. 08:07:10, D:   og så samtidig så er det blevet lidt værre med din åndenød som du
                   [ellers har haft igennem mange år
14. 08:09:50, P:   [ja
15. 08:11:00, P:   ja (.) det er altså at så skal jeg ligge mig ned [al
16. 08:13:40, D:                                                    [ja (.) og du har
                   ikke haft feber (.) og du fik så fat i vagtlægen i dag som valgte
                   at indlægge dig
17. 08:17:80, P:   ja
18. 08:18:60, D:   o::g hvad hedder det du har ikke sådan decideret mavesmerter men
                   der sidder sådan lidt noget der sådan kravler lidt i benene [og lidt
                   op mod læ[nden herop
```

```
19. 08:23:20, P:                                                [ja
                          [ja herop
```

English translation

```
1.  06:00:00, P:   yes ye:s it hurts now it runs down and then it moves up here
2.  06:58:40, ps.  (0.6)
3.  06:59:00, D:   up there
4.  06:59:60, P:   yes
5.  07:00:10, D:   okay=
6.  07:00:60, P:   =I am a bit sore
7.  07:01:80, D:   there you are a bit sore (.)
(xxx)
8.  07:51:60, D:   okay↓ (.) so if we qo through it all now [well over the last 14 days
                   you have vomited [(.) when you kind of got up on your feet (.)
                   and it emerges now and then [sometimes it is there sometimes it is
                   [not yes↓ then you have been unwell (.)
9.  07:53:70, P:                                             [yes
                             [yes
                                        [yes
                   [yes
10. 08:01:40, P:   yes (.)
11. 08:02:10, D:   and then your stomach began to distend [(.) partly you were a bit
                   big[ger (.) and your legs are [swollen up too
12. 08:04:50, P:                                           [yes
                      [yes                     [yes
13. 08:07:10, D:   and then at the same time it has become a bit worse with your
                   breathing difficulty which you [actually have had for many years
14. 08:09:50, P:                                  [yes
15. 08:11:00, P:   yes (.) well it is that then I need to lay down [al
16. 08:13:40, D:                                                   [yes (.) and you
                   did not have any fever (.) and then today you got hold of the doctor
                   from the emergency services who chose to hospitalise you
17. 08:17:80, P:   yes
18. 08:18:60, D:   a::nd well you do not have stomach pain per se but you feel as if
                   something is kind of crawling around in your legs [and a bit towards
                   the small of your [back around here
19. 08:23:20, P:                                                     [yes
                                     [yes around here
```

The doctor switches constantly between history taking and documentation, rather than completing one task at a time as in case I. The interactivity is iterative and characterised by loops of asking for information, typing into the system, asking for information, typing into the system, seeking clarification etc. During this process, the patient is not left alone for longer periods of time and when the doctor interacts with the patient, he steps away from the computer and faces the patient. This physical orientation allows him to engage in dialogue without being constrained by the materiality of the computer. This is different from the previous case in which the doctor meshed the two tasks but. For instance, as she places her hands on the keyboard when she asks questions, she is ready to document the answer immediately.

In this medical encounter the novice doctor has initiated his history taking and he asks the patient to locate and describe her pains. The patient uses her left hand to indicate the exact extension of the pain on the right side of her body (see picture A).

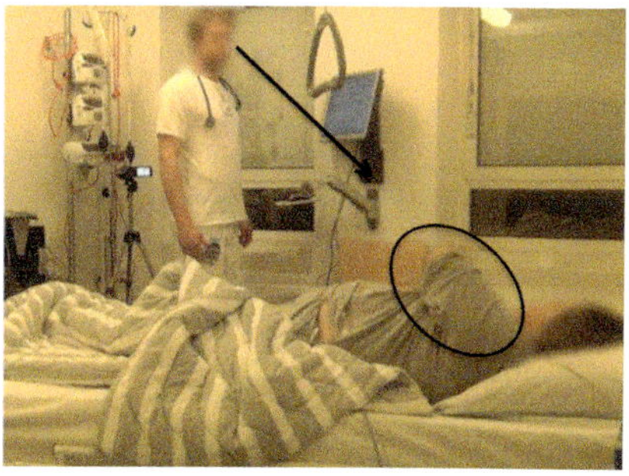

Pic A: 06:58:00
I.1, P: it moves up here

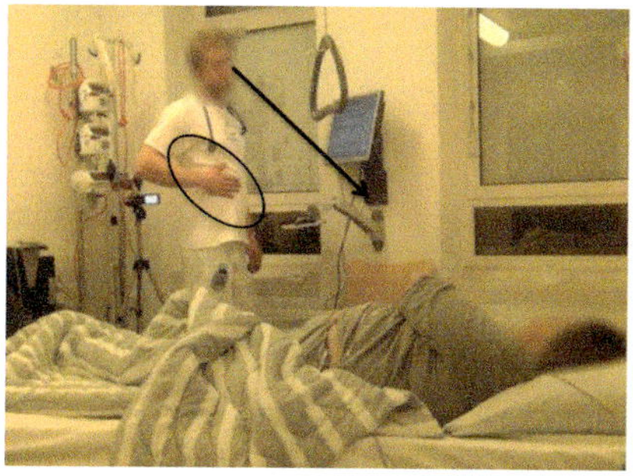

Pic B: 07:03:00
I.7, D: a bit sore (.)

The doctor gazes, not at the patient's face but at her gestures. The doctor then seems surprised by the patient's vocal and gestural location of her pains and he repeats the utterance as he emphasises <u>*there*</u> (line 3). Four seconds after the patient has pointed out the area of pain, the doctor replies to her utterance and a brief pause emerges as he touches his own body similar to the place where the patient has indicated the area of her pain in line 1 (see picture B).

The doctor and the patient engage in joint sense-making as they come up with a shared understanding of pain location while coordinating inter-bodily dynamics *in situ*. The doctor appears intrigued by the perceived pain area, and he starts to simulate the patient's embodied movements to localise the pain area through (physical) self-touch. Rather than relying on verbal questions or observations alone, the doctor inhabits and learns about the patient's world (Streeck 2010). This means that what he gains from observing the patient's localisation of pain and the value he gains from asking her to describe the pain area, is different from what he gains from self-touch. Further, as the patient touches her right side, the doctor touches his right side and as they observe each other's interdependent self-touching gestures, they jointly adjust their movements and make sense of where the pain is located. Thus, they do not use gestures as a means of information processing or expression; rather, as they coordinate their gestures, meaning emerges from the coordinating behaviour:

> Rather than perceiving gestures as part of language, an ecological perspective is proposed [...] This broader account of gesture requires a different conception of the human body than is commonly presupposed by researchers of "non-verbal communication": a model of the body not as an instrument of expression, but as a skilled (knowing) inhabitant of worlds. (Streeck 2010: 223)

In Streeck's view, an ecological account of gestures treats gestures as "symbolic body action evolved from the body's practical engagement with the world" (Streeck, 2010: 237). While he emphasises the importance of the cognitive and embodied aspect of gestures, he remains focused on how the gesturer contributes to the organisation of interaction by anticipating the *next moment* (Streeck 2010: 225). As his ecological perspective is a valuable contribution to conventional multimodal studies, his heuristic of ecologically different modes of gesturing (Streeck 2010: 226) could be expanded with a focus on how whole-bodied interactivity contributes to joint sense-making (Linell 2009, 2015). With the interactivity-based framework, the ecology of gestures requires an analytical focus on coaction beyond sequences of gesturing. As shown above, the doctor and the patient come closer to a shared understanding of pain location as a result of their embodied co-articulation (Thibault 2014).

After the doctor has asked extensive clarifying questions, he summarises the patient's narrative in a rather extraordinary fashion. By relying just as much on his non-verbal resources as medical categories during the process, he explicitly shows and tells the patient how he interprets their joint construction of the patient's narrative. By so doing, he integrates two domains: the objective medical domain and the subjective patient domain. Further, as he wraps up the patient's narrative, his gestures prompt the patient to keep focused on the narrative and recall memory in relation to body parts and pain areas in a way that verbal utterances alone cannot do.

The doctor's embodied actions constitute a cognitive activity, which the patient is part of. The patient replies to how the doctor *enacts* the movement of pain within a given body area, for instance the stomach (see picture H), the lumbar area (see picture G) etc. The gestures enable a shared understanding and validation of the medical symptoms and their locations. The doctor refers to specific physical places that become visible in a here-and-now context. For instance, as the doctor utters *towards the small of your [back around here* (line 18), he determines the exact boundary between the lower ribs, the hip bones and the lumbar area, which the average patient may find difficult. Thus, in this case, the doctor's gestures function

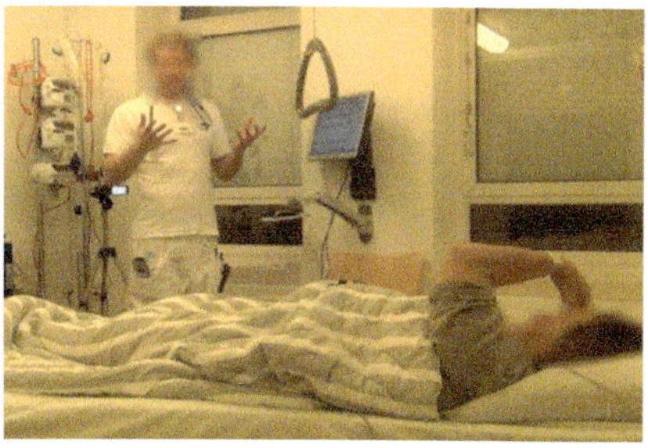

Pic C: 07:56:70
I.8, D: got up on your feet

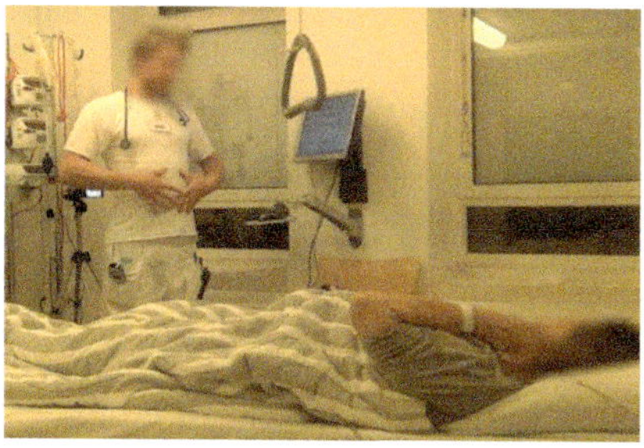

Pic D: 08:03:50
I.11, D: your stomach began to distend

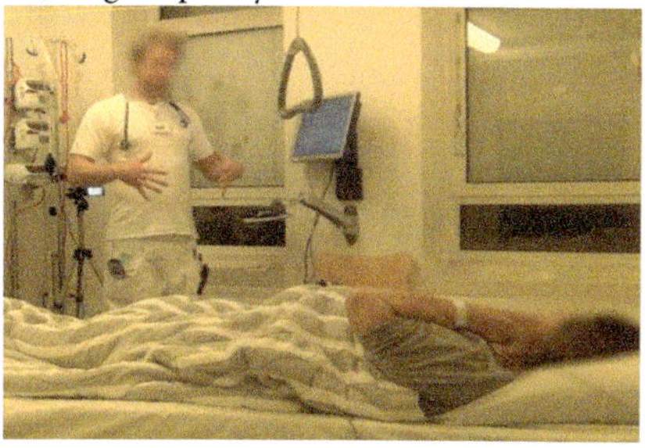

Pic E: 08:04:00
I.11, D: your stomach began to distend

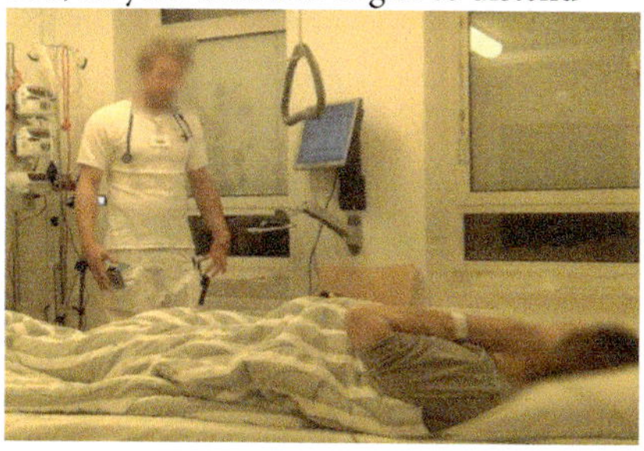

Pic F: 08:06:50
I.11, D: your legs are [swollen up too

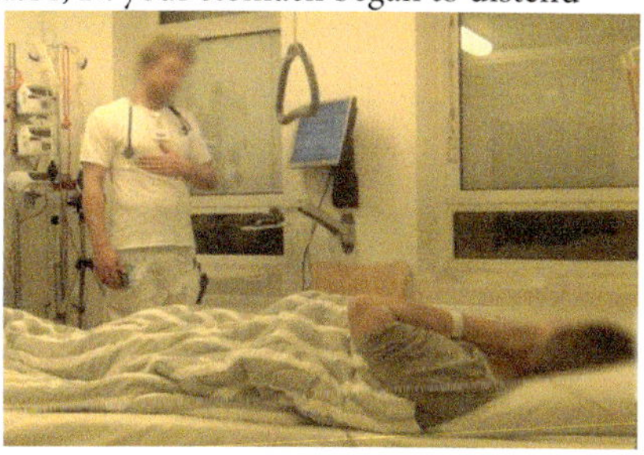

Pic G: 08:08:90
I.13, D: a bit worse with your breathing difficulty

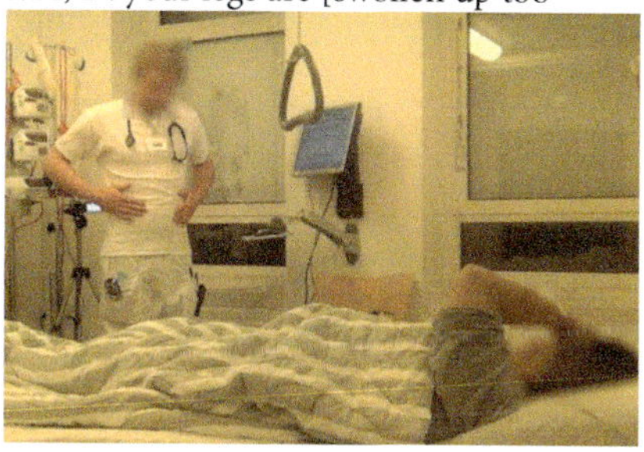

Pic H: 08:20:20
I.18, D: you do not have stomach pains per se

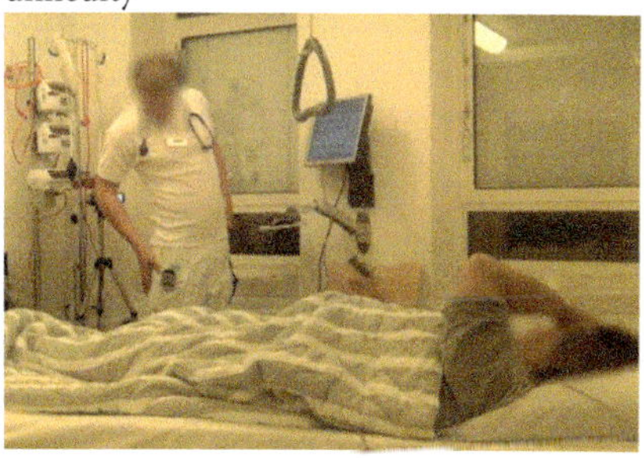

Pic I: 08:21:70
I.18, D: something is kind of crawling around in your legs

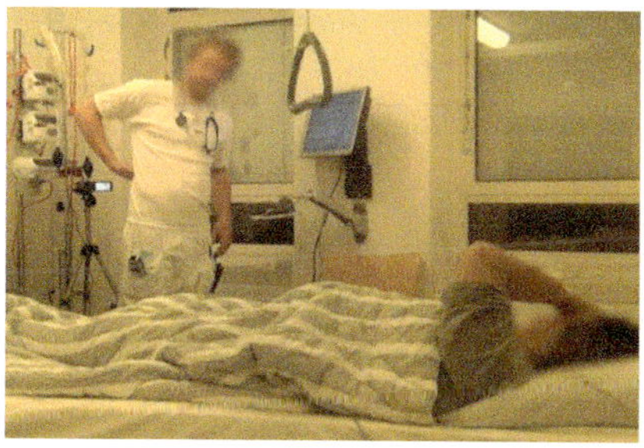

Pic G: 08:23:20
I.18, D: towards the small of your [back around here

as a kind of bodily indexicality, which easily prompts the patient to recall memory and approve the embodied narrative. The direct relationship between the location of the patient's symptoms and her experienced pain and the pointing towards the area on the doctor's body scaffolds the patient's memory. The real-time embodiment in a local visual domain is linked to her past perceptions. Besides, pain which is felt bodily is easy to locate visually since the precise area can be pointed to, or a feeling can be acted out (e.g. breathing pattern). Words, on the contrary, poorly describe symptoms and pain areas in detail. For instance, when relying primarily on words in such tasks, the margin of error increases as misunderstandings are often related to the superficial power of verbal categorisation. With words, we can only represent areas or parts of the body as e.g. the lumbar *area* or the *small of* the back. Alternatively, in this context, the costs of uttering a precise verbal description are too high. It takes time to explain where in the lumbar area the pain is located, or where in your back, leg, foot etc. you have perceived the symptoms. Hence, in such situations, gestures can locate the pain more comprehensively and unambiguously than words in the same time.

This example illustrates how the doctor and the patient co-act and adapt to the shifts in the cognitive system, for instance when the doctor adjusts his perception of the patient's pain area as she shows where she felt the pain. Gestures are important affordances for effective and dialogical problem finding and -solving. The profound use of gestures in this interactivity is unique, and in the coding I have not been able to document similar examples of such systematic and dynamic use of gestures. The embodied actions affect the outcome successfully and the result is achieved much faster compared to situations in which the history taking activity is achieved by prioritising verbal interaction.

5. The need for external success criteria in the assessment of task performance

Overall, the function of embodiment is exemplified in the analyses of the three interactivity trajectories. In order to integrate two different cognitive tasks of typing and dialogue in documentation, it requires a whole-bodied creative strategy, which enhances understanding, precision and patient involvement. It is argued, that the enabling conditions of nested task performance lies in the ability to integrate different cognitive activities through rich embodiment.

In the first case, a static and monological trajectory inhibits dialogical sense-making and shared coaction, which potentially can lead to misunderstanding or even human error. The doctor switches between typing and reading and she interacts with the electronic artefact without being aware of what the patient knows or feels. Paradoxically, the doctor completes the task in accordance with protocols for documentation, but as the situation is compared to alternative strategies of performing this task, her individual-based approach does not seem apt for optimal task performance. In the second case, the doctor meshes two tasks as she multi-performs. Her variation in voice dynamics enables an ongoing interaction with the patient when, at the same time, she completes the documentation task. "Interaction [...] is never 'about' one level of context [...] Rather, it is simultaneously 'about' all of the scales of embodied context the participants bring to bear during the interaction. Embodied action (including speech) always contributes to the sustaining of multiple nested contexts at once" (Streeck and Jordan 2009: 454). Even though Streeck and Jordan separate interaction into various modalities, they focus on how an activity "is one of fluid, multi-scale, joint sustainment *in multiple contexts simultaneously*" (Streeck 2010: 239). Thus, in the second excerpt the doctor's historically developed expertise is played out in different, situated voice dynamics, which have an organising effect on local information gathering. Further, the various voice dynamics enable her to mesh the tasks without letting the computer become the locus of interest. As she types information into the system, she quickly "returns" to the patient and gazes at him, asks more information etc. However, as she does not stray from the computer, the enabling conditions for flexible and dynamical gesturing are partly constrained. In the third case, the doctor meshes the tasks of history taking and documentation, but he does not perform them simultaneously. He moves in and out of the two different activities. When he engages in history taking, he relocates and moves towards the patient. As he does so, he is able to adapt flexibly to the situation. When he perceives changes in the patient's behavioural pattern, he adapts to these changes. For instance, he simulates the patient's gestures and gains a new insight into the patient's symptoms. Further, as the patient shows, feels and visually perceives her medical narrative in the situation, the doctor and the patient jointly make sense of their shared coaction: they co-act by attuning their gestures in interactivity. The result is precise, effective and dialogical task performance. Gestures appeared to have a valuable coordinative function in interactivity. Interactivity enabled the doctor and the patient to coarticulate a functional outcome based on reciprocal, embodied behaviour. Moreover, gestures served as negative feedback mechanisms, which ensure that corrections are made, and understandings are perceived within the local system. Finally, gestures have an important function in the enactment of past perceptions in real-time interaction as self-initiated touch and the perception of the other's self-initiated touch identified areas of pain.

Because various documentation task performances have never been compared, and as negative task results are not immediately perceived, the task baseline is difficult to identify. When the negative outcome remains absent – for instance when the patient does not complain, and the task is completed in accordance with standard procedures – no issues are experienced by the practitioners *in situ*.

The documentation task includes dual cognitive processes, which are optimally integrated in a dialogical way. When the iPatient is prioritised over interaction with the real patient, the task performance is often managed individually. Individual-based documentation impedes the integration of the two cognitively distinct processes (typing and dialogue) as it affords the practitioner to engage in documentation activity based on doctor-artefact interaction. Individual-based trajectories are not necessarily related to dysfunctionality or erroneous outcome *per se*. Nevertheless, such patterns are more likely to cause interpersonal breakdowns, unnecessary frustration amongst patients and relatives, and to minimise recognition of what has been documented. Further, the probability of misunderstanding, and consequently the probability of human error, increases as the tacit conclusions serve as positive feedback-mechanisms: When the doctor's interpretations and conclusions are not validated, nothing causes the practitioner to adjust what he or she is doing. However, in cases where the doctor utters an interpretation, such explication serves as a negative feedback mechanism as the patient is able to adjust, acknowledge or reject the outcome so that clarifications can be made *in situ*.

Finally, understanding the ontological difference between speech and writing is crucial for the design of aiding tools in the documentation process. Thus, the dialogical intentions built into the electronic device must be related to the challenge of balancing the two distinct processes of typing and dialogue with the patient during the overall documentation process. While the computer itself does not have any purpose in itself, its physical location in the room and the way it becomes a central component of the cognitive system, makes it afford a behaviour that easily constrains intended dialogue in situations in which the practitioner is less skilled and therefore less able to prioritise and integrate the patient in the process.

PART III

The aftermath: The scientific enterprise

The phrase "cognition in the wild" refers to human cognition in its natural habitat– that is, to naturally occurring culturally constituted human activity [...]. I hope to evoke with this metaphor a sense of ***an ecology of thinking in which human cognition interacts with an environment rich in organizing resources.***

- Edwin Hutchins, (1995a: xiii–xiv, my emphasis)

CHAPTER 10

The integration of multiple timescales

1. Pursuing careful investigations of natural ecologies

In the first pages of this book, I argued that mainstream models of human errors, interaction and cognition were unsuitable for describing and explaining how error cycles relate to human interactivity in emergency medicine beyond a representational state of cognitive analysis and beyond a micro-sociological perspective on language in interaction. I proposed an alternative ecological approach that takes a different starting point than the above-mentioned approaches as it investigates the cognitive ecology of human errors by turning to the dynamics of cognitive ecosystems (Hodges and Baron 1992; Hutchins 2014) in emergency medicine. Similarly, Gibson has argued that an ecological approach to visual perception, contrary to standard approaches in the field "works from the opposite end. It begins with the flowing array of the observer who walks from one vista to another, moves around an object of interest" (Gibson 1979/86: 303). In line with Gibson, this work extends the object of investigation, not only in space but also in time. An ecological approach prioritises interactivity as it pivots on how local coordination is sense-saturated (Steffensen 2013), i.e., related to lived experience. From this perspective, the slow dynamics of sociocultural coordination mesh with the fast, situated coordinative inter-bodily dynamics.

Therefore, as I pointed out in the introduction, the aim of this qualitative investigation of human error cycles in medical, diagnostic processes has been to provide evidence for the need to deal with multiple timescales in a way that yields new interdisciplinary and analytical methods such as cognitive ethnography and Cognitive Event Analysis. An ecological approach to human error entails a focus on error cycles rather than negative outcomes in isolation. Such an ecological approach renders possible the identification of feedback mechanisms within a cognitive ecosystem and how these mechanisms either intensify errors and result in a system's breakdown or are encountered in a way that leads to recalibration within the system. Part II of this book provides multiple examples of how healthcare practitioners anticipate and counter errors as well as how medical culture affects real-time interaction and finally how the culture itself is shaped by the exact same dynamics.

The overall conclusion is that an ecological approach is suitable to explain how events on multiple timescales are intertwined in here-and-now cognitive task performances because an ecological perspective requires the analyst to zoom in on a system's skilled embodiments. By using cognitive ethnography and CEA, cognitive trajectories have been outlined to show how specific forms of habitual and constrained behaviour are traced to skilled embodiment and cultural patterns. In that sense, culture is constrained, cognitive behaviour, and it manifests itself in how easily and precisely healthcare practitioners adapt to changes in the layout of affordances. Cognitive ethnography provides a methodological framework, which shows promise in its broader general applicability. In line with Hutchins' recommendations, a cognitive ethnographic study gains a deep understanding of the enabling conditions for cognitive events in emergency medicine. Such understanding, I claim, is the prerequisite for enhancing healthcare practices, and eventually it reduces the amount of interaction-based error cycles. In this book I have tried to qualify an account of human interactivity that enables investigations of how the non-local trajectory shapes the local and vice versa. Hutchins argues in similar words that a multi-scalar and integrated view on culture and cognition is necessary:

> [C]ulture was relegated to a peripheral role. As Gardner (1985) pointed out, culture, history, context, and emotion were all set aside as problems to be addressed after a good understanding of individual cognition has been achieved. [...] I am proposing an integrated view on human cognition in which a major component of culture is a cognitive process [...] and cognition is a cultural process.
>
> (Hutchins 1995a: 353ff)

The empirical findings of this book are specific examples of how the multi-scalarity of human cognition in emergency medicine relates to human errors and successes in a socio-cultural environment. It describes what form sociocultural, non-local, dynamics and situational affordances for action take in real-life, (dys)functional diagnostic events. An ecological approach to human action perception changes the understanding of how human errors emerge and develop. Instead of working with a traditional error taxonomy, which identifies errors in relation to negative outcomes, I proposed thinking in terms of error cycles where multiple feedback-mechanisms can be identified and, depending on how they are managed, prevent an erroneous outcome. Thus, the dynamical feedback mechanisms (positive and negative) enrich our understanding of why and how healthcare practitioners are able to solve problems or become fixated. In part II it is argued that, at an overall level, such understanding of the ecology of human cognition can be used to enhance practices. This insight means that one should investigate how cognitive events are managed in naturalistic settings where healthcare practitioners rely on expertise, team members, patients and environmental circumstances rather than look for human errors *per se*. In this book, the analyses of (potential) error cycles and, more generally, how practitioners undertake treatment as a team-based problem-solving activity focusing on thematic aspects related to the systemic function of cognitive behaviour. The analyses demonstrate how team members enact expertise-in-action, and also how lack of coordination and communication can lead to human errors. In particular, it demonstrates that non-routine events are crucial to what goes on in the emergency ward: Anomalous events function as affordances and trigger feedback mechanisms, which prompt team members to anticipate possible changes of plan. Through numerous empirical analyses of how practitioners manage cognitive events, it becomes evident that the concept of multiple timescales is crucial to understanding the enabling conditions of human cognition. The analyses provide insights into how interactivity enables practitioners to manage cognitive events in different settings related to different tasks, different levels of skill, different team constellations and different medical scenarios. Each chapter thus focuses on an aspect related to the systemic function of cognitive activities, e.g., decision-making. Together, a mix of task-related challenges (interruptions, history-taking, documentation etc.) and more general qualities and constraints of interactivity (the function of embodiments, the workings of visual systems, the role of an artefact-rich environment etc.) were investigated.

Several chapters overlap and supplement each other. When comparisons are made between the chapters, the particularities cluster in patterns. A common element unites the chapters and enables a general understanding of the underlying conditions for human error cycles: Each chapter demonstrates that when the observed practitioners are unable to balance the non-local and local constraints within the system, they fixate on one task or phenomenon that increases the risk of the emergence of error cycles and when practitioners are capable of balancing non-local and local constraints within the system, they are able to adapt flexibly to changes in the environment and anticipate what comes next.

2. Practical implications and improvement measures

Hutchins called for an "outdoor psychology" with real impact to contribute to understanding ecologies in new ways based on qualitative cognitive ethnography. This book is an attempt to do this. With a focus on cognitive events and human error cycles, some issues are specifically profound across the analyses. For instance, a difference in novice and expert behaviour was identified and was explained as distinct capabilities to enact skilled embodiment and adapt to the situation at hand. In that process, the functions and roles of teams, artefacts and procedures were important affordances, which served to scaffold functional and dialogical task performance.

Based on these findings, a synthesis of the empirical results forms the basis for a description of their practical implications. I propose three initiatives for healthcare practitioners to work with in order to enhance practice. These initiatives could have an impact on future practical interventions and general challenges in everyday work practice. The initiatives relate to (a) the implementation of a new model of language and cognition in – and beyond – the field of emergency medicine, (b) changing the basic assumptions of what is relevant content in training programmes and (c) dealing with (the design of) material artefacts as flexible artefact environments. The three themes are discussed below.

2.1 The "interactivity turn" in emergency medicine: Beyond laboratory studies

Like other studies, the second part II of the book indicates that adverse events are related to behavioural and non-technical aspects of performance (Yule et al. 2006; Flin and Maran 2004). In the literature on non-technical skills (e.g. Yule et al. 2006; Flin and Maran 2004), there has been a dawning realisation that such skills should be investigated further since human errors are rarely related to technical skills. As a result of this tendency, many training programmes focus on non-technical skills, but they do so in a rather conventional way, which does not correlate with how non-technical skills are developed and used in real life. The consequences of this claim are seen on multiple parameters. First, non-technical skills are separated into multiple demarcated activities. Such a distinction originates in a dualist model that separates cognition from communication, for instance when cognitive skills (e.g. decision-making) are separated from other interpersonal skills (e.g. teamwork). Whilst acknowledging the non-technical turn in emergency medicine, I argue that this field needs to view practitioners' cognition as an ecosystemic activity through which cognitive results are shaped by non-local dynamics and situational affordances for actions within a cognitive, dialogical system. That requires investigations of how task performances are completed as practitioners draw on interactivity. Conventional cognitive and linguistic models are not capable of showing the ecological dynamics of non-technical aspects of task performances. In a similar vein, Hutchins argues:

> In spite of the fact that we engage in cognitive activities every day, our folk and professional models of cognitive performance do not match what appears when cognition in the wild is examined carefully. [...] The study of cognition in the wild may reveal a different sort of task world that permits a different conception of what people do with their minds. (Hutchins 1995a: 371)

Before intervention programmes, rating schemes, protocols and training courses are developed, healthcare institutions would benefit from perceiving non-technical skills as complex activities that do not allow for absolute separation into distinct areas of competence.

Secondly, an ecological perspective on human interactivity suggests a similar ecological perspective on human errors. Since interactivity is sense-saturated, errors are not simply accidental, local achievements. While individuals *can* be held accountable for negative outcomes, the explanations of what enables individual decisions must be investigated within a broader spatio-temporal frame. By emphasising how error cycles are multi-causal and multi-scalar and how non-local dynamics affect local cognition, the seeds for cultural changes are sowed. Thus, cultural changes require that practitioners change their attitudes towards errors (Moser et al. 2011; Mangels et al. 2006), and their understanding of language and cognition as a systemic embodied and distributed activity.

Concurrently, an interactivity-based understanding of cognitive coordination does not just allow for a more realistic, naturalised model of language, it also allows for a deeper understanding of how particulars and peculiarities shape cognitive events in complex, real-life situations such as the emergency ward.

2.2 Developing training programmes on the basis of what happens

When I conducted the cognitive ethnographic study at the emergency department, education and training programmes were developed on the basis of standard procedures and pre-defined hypotheses of where intervention was presumably needed. Such an approach seems to work as the doctors and nurses improve and increase their expertise and skills over time. Yet, it is difficult to show whether such an enhancement is due to a general development of experience that happens regardless of the participation in courses, or whether it is a direct effect of training. Indeed, there are areas of expertise that obviously need further attention. Nevertheless, in the analyses I revealed how some task performances were completed in an undesirable fashion even though such performances were not phenomenologically experienced as error-prone or problematic for task performance (see Chapter 5, 6 and 9). For instance, in Chapter 7, Section 3, the nurse and the doctor jointly and tacitly re-enact a dysfunctional fixed role hierarchy inhibiting them in coming up with the best solution. Further, in Chapter 9 I showed how the documentation process in some cases needs improvement.

Thus, the rapid dynamics of real-time coordination have never been investigated or understood beyond an individual level of subjective experience in the ward. Moreover, when a problem has been identified and addressed, new procedures or protocols are often made. Following Flach (1999), human systems are open systems with an unaccounted variability that cannot be controlled by implementing additional standard procedures (Flach 1999: 111). By adding more control into it, the system becomes less flexible and adaptive, and even more control will constrain flexible behaviour, which seems to be crucial in cases of the unexpected (Flach 1999). The answer to practical implications, is not additional control, rules or standard procedures. I propose that it prioritises the function of medical *teams*. As shown in part II, much is gained from relying on and engaging in the team's sense-making processes in order to develop one's own skills. Thus, coordinated team-performance is crucial in the search for dialogical and functional task performance.

A main challenge is to develop training programmes and educational practices that embrace the complexity of human cognition as distributed. Due to the biased view that existing models of human decision-making etc. provide, a change in the organisational mindset is not straightforward. Finally, as education programmes are biased by the idea that the problem is known in advance, the potential for identifying crucial and latent risks for error cycles is easily overlooked. As proposed by Hutchins (1995a), and in line with the research design of this book, the emergency department is encouraged to work inductively and study what actually happens, before it provides answers and initiates interventions. In fact, the department I studied, has incorporated new procedures into their educational programmes using video-observation on a weekly basis as a means of designing case scenarios that are based on real, contextual needs rather than on general ideas of what is needed.

2.3 Artefact-rich work environments

In the medical ward, the number of material artefacts and tools is massive. They are designed with a specific purpose in mind, and practitioners are taught these purposes. However, Hollan et al. (2000) underline how they, within the field of aviation and ship navigation: "have documented many cases of use of structure that were not anticipated by the designers of the tools involved. Experts often make opportunistic use of environmental structure to simplify tasks" (Hollan et al. 2000: 182). To them the big question is how flexibility can be incorporated into the design of such material structures. They argue that designers should think in terms of work environment rather than the decontextualized function of an artefact (Hollan et al. 2000). As I have argued in the analyses, material artefacts have no intentions. However, their mere physical existence becomes an affordance for certain behavioural actions. As practitioners' level of expertise varies, their visual system allows for different perceptions and actions including how to understand and use an artefact in the situation (cf. Chapter 4, 5 and 9). Thus:

> [W]ork materials are more than mere stimuli for a disembodied cognitive system. Work materials from time to time become elements of the cognitive system itself. Just as a blind person's cane or a cell biologist's microscope is a central part of the way they perceive the world, so well-designed work materials become integrated into the way people think, see, and control activities, part of the distributed system of cognitive control. (Hollan et al. 2000: 178)

The reason why some material artefacts occasionally prove dysfunctional in task performance, relates to designers' propensity to confuse invention, conception and cognition (Hollan et al. 2000). Kirsh (2013) emphasises the opportunities of thinking with material artefacts rather than using them purely as a means of speeding up the cognitive process. That we can think differently with artefacts is important as it can literally change the way human beings think. Thus, Kirsh hypothesises that: "if an object is *cognitively gripped* in the right way then it can be incorporated into our thinking process even if it is not neurally absorbed" (Kirsh 2013: 2–3).

Following Kirsh (2013) and Hollan et al. (2000), educators and designers are not fully aware of the complexity and ambiguity that artefacts can afford in real-life situations. By linking Gibson's ecological theory of visual perception with theories of distributed cognition, understandings of how artefacts afford various options for actions can be clarified. Such information is valuable for designers, educators and practitioners in the ward. Again, by thinking in terms of *artefact-rich work environments*, the ambiguity of artefact interaction in diagnostic settings can be embraced.

3. Particularities and generalisability: Why cognitive ethnography studies are crucial in emergency medicine

Mainstream psychology has for a long time insisted that for psychological phenomena to be studied systematically, they should be performed in controlled, experimental settings unattached to the social practice in which they occur (Dreier 2007). The decontextualised and impersonal "pure" results provide knowledge, Dreier claims, which is very different from the knowledge that qualitative studies of psychological phenomena in their ecological settings provide (Dreier 2007). Similarly, as Hutchins claims: "studying cognition in the wild is difficult, and the outcomes are uncertain" (Hutchins 1995a: 197). However, such studies are uncertain only when they are compared to the kind of results that mainstream psychology produces: "qualitative studies need to promote a different conception of generality than the one which dominates psychology" (Dreier 2007: 188). Yet in this work, I qualitatively investigated the naturalistic *wild* by applying new ecological models of language and cognition that pivoted on changes in interactivity.

With quantitative analyses, one is able to describe general tendencies, but the explanatory power of unique coordination in the object under study is unfeasible. For instance, in the domain of human error in emergency medicine, statistical analyses provide insights about the frequency of human error, where it happens and what the consequences are. But as I have shown with this cognitive ethnographic work, the interactions in which the error cycles emerge vary tremendously. In a similar vein, Steffensen (2016) yields investigations of particulars as ecosystems:

> The ecosystemic emphasis entails that, while the uniqueness of particulars may appear as differences in peripheral details, it is not reducible to such details. Thus, it makes little sense to study specific details in isolation, without considering how they contribute to a specific cognitive system (Steffensen 2016: 30)

The interactivity-based perspective enables studies of how cognitive events are managed *in situ*. The main challenge, in turn, is to move from particularities to some sort of generalisations. This work contributes to the humanities by showing the importance of particulars in medical task performance, not merely by describing these, but crucially by demonstrating *that* particulars matter, *how* particulars matter and *why* particulars matter. Further, it is argued that it is only within the humanities that we find methods that pick out why particulars matter. While a theory of cognitive computation or semiotics, for instance, interprets an agent's capabilities for local representation or his local use of static signs, they are incapable of explaining how the articulation of representations and signs emerge in a complex distributed system (Hollan et al. 2000).

The interactivity-based perspective proposes such ecological investigation of particular events as simultaneously bounded and dynamical. This idea links up with Dreier's insistence that hanging-togetherness should be the locus of interest:

> Insisting on characterising things in isolation is replaced by insisting on characterising the hanging-togetherness of things in social practice. This knowledge leads to insight into the dynamic – contradictory – hanging togetherness of social practice and in social practice (Holzkamp, 1988). Insisting on the concrete hanging togetherness of things does not imply studying everything every time, that is, studying totalities of infinite proportions. It means understanding things by considering them as linked in a pertinent nexus of social practice, that is, the particular hanging togetherness of a particular situation and practice and the relevant hanging togetherness for comprehending the issue of the present study. (Dreier 2007: 3)

Crucial to the ecological perspective on human error, language and cognition, is the fact that local coordination is understood as sense-saturated. As interactivity is sense-saturated, the slow non-local dynamics are identified in local coordination for instance when a nurse enacts her skills in embodied behaviour coordinated with what the doctor does and anticipates, and with what the physical environment offers. Thus, outcomes are results of a synthesis of non-local dynamics and local possibilities for action. As such the analyses present not just a synchronous and unique picture of situated interaction. They also indicate a historical foundation that constrains local possibilities for action, for instance, when procedures and cultural issues related to role hierarchies and the attitude towards emotions affect local coordination and functional cognition. Finally, the empirical findings presented above express multiple dimensions of decision-making – some of them general, others not. However, this is exactly the crucial point in human, flexible, adaptive behaviour. To paraphrase Dennett (2013), human beings are competent in comprehending; in contrast, ants – for instance – are competent too but lack comprehension. Thus, the behaviour of ants is much more generalisable than healthcare professionals' behaviour. Healthcare practitioners' performance is both bounded and dynamical at the same time. This work reflects the point in that it points out that artefacts are used differently in the ward by different groups of people with different levels of skill and expertise. How the artefact is used depends on situated capabilities for action just as non-local, sociocultural patterns and expectations affect the outcome. The book does not provide a complete account of the entire ecology of human cognition. Rather, it offers an ecological account of pivotal elements in functional and dysfunctional cognition. The aim was not to provide generalisations of human errors, but instead to explain the dynamic and complex condition for error cycles in general by providing detailed examples of how they emerge, and how they are avoided. Thus, a cross-section of the ecology was investigated to demonstrate the complexity, spatial extension and multitemporality of human cognition in complex organisations.

When healthcare practitioners engage in dialogue, perform with rich embodiment, rely on the team's sense-making and make decisions based on a value heterarchy, they are more likely to anticipate latent conditions for errors and adapt to these particular changes. This knowledge is valuable in the search for safer, more caring and dialogical healthcare practices. Hence, this study of particularities is an attempt to bridge the gap between the literature on human errors and the reality in which they emerge. It is my hope that the analyses will inform practice in a useful way and that future studies within the field add to this line of research. The ecological approach to real-life emergency wards presented here, involves cognitive ethnography and CEA. This approach makes real contributions by pushing in new directions the analysis of interactivity. It does so in a setting that is not only deeply consequential, but which also provides a perspicuous site for demonstrating the relevance of such an approach far more generally.

4. Future projects and methodological innovations: Adopting cognitive ethnography, interactivity and Cognitive Event Analysis

Altogether, this work reveals what is gained by applying an ecological approach to human interactivity in the field of emergency medicine. Theoretically, it proposed to work with an interactivity-based perspective, which allows for investigations of multi-scalar ecosystems. At a methodological level, it showed how it is possible to account for non-local dynamics in the local by using cognitive ethnography as a framework for investigations of how people adapt, think, move and coordinate. The situations in which healthcare practitioners enact cultural-cognitive patterns are investigated with the method of Cognitive Event Analysis, which allows for systematic annotation of actions that lead to output. Such a scientific enterprise is rather radical. According to Hutchins (2014), only few works have been based on cognitive ethnography (cf. Hutchins 2014, 1995a), but those studies are first lonely exceptions, and second, they do not provide explicit analytical procedures for how to study the ecology of cognitive events (Hutchins, 2014). Studying human behaviour from an ecological perspective requires an integration of interdisciplinary methods and theories, and this is not a simple or easy task. Intellectually, linking the humanities and the cognitive sciences allows for a naturalised view on language and thus to cutting-edge theories in the language sciences, which both enrich the humanities and solve real-life difficulties. Arguing against cognitive and linguistic compartmentalisation, an ecological approach treats cognition and language as embodied biosocial phenomena that can be investigated in human interaction (Cowley 2010, 2011, 2014a, 2014b; Steffensen 2013; Steffensen and Pedersen 2014; Pedersen and Steffensen 2014; Pedersen 2012; Linell 2009, 2015). As mentioned in Chapters 1 and 2, the traditional assumptions within language and cognitive sciences were that cognition is an internal representational process, and language was the means of communicating and articulating thoughts. To overcome the dichotomy, the interactivity-based perspective enriches the humanities by basing a naturalised theory of language on the study of how language is grounded in human coordination in complex sociocultural settings, or, specifically, how healthcare professionals cognitively and interactionally manage high-pressure work practices in a department of emergency medicine.

In Chapter 2 I have argued that the interactivity-based perspective provides rich explanations of how language is cognitive: "Coordinated sense-making embodies thoughts: we depend on *dynamics first and symbols afterwards*" (Cowley 2011: 11). Multiple challenges follow as one opens up for the ecology of human cognition. However, this book does not claim to provide a complete account of human interactivity. Rather it takes the implications of a process ontology seriously, and it seeks to investigate real-life settings as ecological, dynamical and complex ecosystems. The analyses thus provide an ecological account of decisive elements in functional and dysfunctional decision-making and problem-solving. The process of determining the precise extent of cognitive ecosystems can explain the dynamic and bounded possibilities individuals have for producing cognitive results. This insight connects to the scientific interest concerning which methodological innovations can be derived from an ecological perspective. Thus, crucial to the ecological perspective on human error, language and cognition is the fact that local coordination is understood to be sense-saturated. Activities are shaped by sense-saturated coordination rather than being local instantiations of individual logical choices. Treating human language and cognition as perspectives on interactivity challenges traditional approaches in linguistics and cognitive science to adapt their methods in accord with these foundational assumptions.

In a recent chapter that reviews qualitative methods in cognitive psychology, Ormerod and Ball (2017: 587) argue that there is a need for future methodological developments and that:

> [i]t is qualitative approaches that are rising to the fore in relation to the analyses of real-world, embodied cognition in the context of complex task-performance, where **interactivity** with external artefacts is paramount. **An example of a powerful new method for investigating how cognition reflects an embodied coalition between internal and external resources is Cognitive Event Analysis.**
>
> (my emphasis)

The interactivity-based perspective was presented in order to emphasise the underlying assumptions of language and cognition as well as how these concepts are intertwined and relate to multiple timescales. As the cognitive ethnography study took its starting point in how cognitive events are managed *in situ*, CEA became the main analytical approach to frame such events. Hence, starting in the enchronic timescale, CEA was able to work with connections of relevant event pivots rather than a step by step temporal analysis of what happens. The organising principle of the analysis is defined by a criterion of cognitive function and thus multiple transition phases and event pivots, which relate to multiple timescales, are extrapolated from interaction data. However, this work was not just interested in defining local connections of what leads to outcome, but also interested in explaining how connections are possible in a complex organisation. With CEA we can show what happens (not only what subjects perceive or think happens) and define local constraints and possibilities for problem-solving. However, it does not equip us with a comprehensive basis for answering why an incoming phone call prompts practitioners to either ignore or respond to the call.

I argue that the theoretical concepts presented within the analytical section (in particular Hodges and Baron's (1992) ecological account of values, Linell's (2005, 2007, 2009, 2015) dialogism perspective, Gibson's (1979/86) ecological approach to visual perception, Goodwin's (1994) concept of professional vision, and Streeck's (2010) ecological theory of gesture add explanatory power to why connections in the cognitive event trajectory link up as they do. CEA in itself does not explain what makes an enabling condition an enabling condition, but it can point to them as enabling for local cognitive problem-solving. Finally, CEA-investigations of the bio-cognitive dynamical coordination go on beyond the enchronic, conversational scale of interaction. Such investigations can be enriched with perspectives on human cognitive, emotional and linguistic capabilities and moral obligations for actions. Thus, CEA's main quality is its ability to link pivots in cognitive systems to relevant situated actions, which lead to results not only using a step-by-step or turn-by-turn analytic procedure. It studies what real human beings do together and it zooms in on relevant transition phases that are not ordered by a temporal criterion but by one of systemic function.

Finally, the method is in its infancy as a methodology, but its merits have been acknowledged and, more crucially, the need for developing it further is asked for:[1]

> The method's richness and flexibility in terms of levels and modalities of data annotation indicate that CEA is applicable in studying most cognitive behaviours and correlated measures [...], which attests to its future value in the qualitative investigations of cognitive phenomena. To date CEA has primarily been used for generating novel hypotheses [...] whereas in the future the method will no doubt be used to test hypotheses deductively, which will be important for advancing a fully fledged ecological understanding of embodied and situated cognition in real-world cognitive ecosystems." (Ormerod and Ball 2017: 588ff)

With a focus on systemic function and cognitive results, CEA has its shortcomings if one wishes to add another perspective on interactivity. In Chapter 2, interactivity is defined as an "ontological substrate" (Steffensen 2013: 196), and language and cognition, in turn, are characterised as perspectives one can take on interactivity. However, as CEA focuses on pivots that lead to cognitive results, it adds little to situations where no such results occur in a cognitive system. Steffensen et al. (2016) argue that CEA deals with event pivots that are "functionally defined as a transition point which is a *conditio sine qua non* for identifying a segment of a cognitive trajectory as a specific (kind of) event" (Steffensen et al. 2016: 82). Thus, as the model aims at specific kinds of events, it ignores non-cognitive events. In this project, I aimed at more than strict cognitive event analysis, and I thus

1. A method book on CEA is in preparation (Steffensen and Trasmundi (forth.))

combined CEA with other perspectives and theories in the analyses. I will argue that some moral aspects of dialogue (Linell 2009, 2015; Hodges and Baron 1992), have a positive effect on interpersonal relationship, but they do not necessarily affect the cognitive output in a functional sense. Further, as I showed previously in Chapter 9, Section 2, no event pivots were identified as the doctor completed the documentation task without experiencing any "suspended nexts" (Steffensen et al. 2016). The dysfunctionality of this case was only identified through comparative analysis of event trajectories. Thus, CEA has its shortcomings when problems beyond members' experiences emerge. The way out, I suggest, is through comparative analysis and the interactivity-based perspective, which provide the observer with explanatory power beyond situated cognitive events.

Regardless of the perspective in terms of human error, they appear to be part of the livelihood and *raison d'etre* of our species. In other words, human error is a symbol of the evolutionary scars of battles won in the fight for survival (Lents 2018) and let alone a necessary aspect of developing organisations. We therefore revisit the beginning, but hopefully with a richer understanding of the nature of human errors by emphasising that:

> *as strange as it may sound, there is beauty in our imperfections. How boring would our lives be if each of us were a purely rational, perfect specimen? Our flaws are what make us who we are.* - Nathan H. Lents (2018: xiii)

References

Adams, Douglas. 2002. *The Ultimate Hitchhiker's Guide to the Galaxy, Mostly harmless*. New York: Ballantine Books.

Amalberti, René. 2013. "Human Error at the Centre of the Debate on Safety." In *Navigating Safety: Nessecary Compromises and Trade-offs: Theory and Practice*, ed. by René Amalberti, 19–52. Amsterdam: Springer.

Anderson, Michael L. 2014. *After phrenology: Neural reuse and the interactive brain*. Cambridge, MA: The MIT Press. https://doi.org/10.7551/mitpress/10111.001.0001

Anderson, Michael L., Michael J. Richardson, and Anthony Chemero. 2012. "Eroding the Boundaries of Cognition: Implications of Embodiment." *Topics in Cognitive Science* 4(4): 717–730. https://doi.org/10.1111/j.1756-8765.2012.01211.x

Angeli, Elizabeth L. 2015. "Three types of Memory in Emergency Medical Services Communication." *Written Communication* 32(1): 3–38. https://doi.org/10.1177/0741088314556598

Angoff, Nancy R. 2002. "Making a Place for Emotions in Medicine." *Yale Journal of Health Policy, Law, and Ethics* 2(2) Article 8: 447–454.

Baber, Chris, Paul Smith, James Cross, John Hunter, and Richard McMaster. 2006. "Crime scene investigation as distributed cognition." *Pragmatics and Cognition* 14(2): 357–385. https://doi.org/10.1075/pc.14.2.14bab

Baggs, Edward and Anthony Chemero. 2018. "Radical embodiment in two directions." *Synthese*: 1–16.

Ball, Linden J., and Thomas C. Ormerod. 2000. "Putting ethnography to work: The case for a cognitive ethnography of design." *International Journal of Human Computer Studies* 53: 147–168. https://doi.org/10.1006/ijhc.2000.0372

Bang, Jørgen C., and Jørgen Døør. 2007. *Language, Ecology and Society – a dialectical approach* (ed. by S. V. Steffensen and J. Nash). London: Continuum.

Bateson, Gregory. 1972. *Steps to an ecology of mind*. New York: Ballantine Books.

Benne, Christian. 2017. "Rephilologisation: Toward the Integration of Linguistics and Literary Scholarship." In *Creativity and Continuity: Perspectives on the Dynamics of Language Conventionalization*, ed. By Dorthe Duncker and Bettina Perregaard, 73–105). Berlin: Mouton de Gruyter.

Benne, Christian. 2015. *Die Erfindung des Manuskripts: Zu Theorie und Geschichte literarischer Gegenständlichkeit*. Berlin: Suhrkamp Verlag Berlin.

Berg, Lena M., Ann-Sofie Källberg, Katarina E. Göransson, Jan Östergren, Jan Florin, and Anna Ehrenberg. 2013. "Interruptions in emergency department work: an observational and interview study." *BMJ Qual Saf*, 22(8): 656–663. https://doi.org/10.1136/bmjqs-2013-001967

Bergson, Henri. 1911. *Creative Evolution*. New York: Henry Holt and Company. https://doi.org/10.5962/bhl.title.166289

Bernstein, Nicholai A. 1996. *On Dexterity and its development*. In *Dexterity and its development*, ed. by Mark L. Latash and Michael T. Turvey, 3–244). Mahwah, NJ: Lawrence Erlbaum.

Bertalanffy, Ludwig von. 1968. *General System Theory. Foundations, Development, Applications.* New York: George Braziller.

Boden, Magaret A. 2006. *Mind As Machine: a History of Cognitive Science*, Volume 1&2. Oxford: Oxford University Press.

Carman, Taylor. 2008. *Merleau-Ponty*. New York: Routledge. https://doi.org/10.4324/9780203461853

Chapman, Jake. 2004. *System Failure: Why Governments Must Learn to Think Differently*, 2nd ed. London: Demos.

Chemero, Anthony. 2000. "What events are." *Ecological Psychology*, 12: 37–42. https://doi.org/10.1207/S15326969ECO1201_3

Chemero, Anthony. 2003. "An Outline of a Theory of Affordances." *Ecological Phsychology*, 15(2): 181–195. https://doi.org/10.1207/S15326969ECO1502_5

Chemero, Anthony. 2009. *Radical embodied cognitive science*. MIT Press. https://doi.org/10.7551/mitpress/8367.001.0001

Chrisholm, Carey D., Edgar K. Collison, David R. Nelson, and William G. Cordell. 2000. "Emergency Department Workplace Interruptions: Are Emergency Physicians "Interrupt-driven" and "Multitasking"?" *Academic Emergency Medicine* 7(11): 1239–1243. https://doi.org/10.1111/j.1553-2712.2000.tb00469.x

Chisholm, Carey D., Amanda M. Dornfeld, David R. Nelson, and William G. Cordell. 2001. "Work interrupted: a comparison of workplace interruptions in emergency departments and primary care offices." *Ann Emerg Med* 38(2): 146–151. https://doi.org/10.1067/mem.2001.115440

Clark, Andy. 2008. *Supersizing the Mind: Embodiment, Action, and Cognitive Extension*. Oxford: Oxford University Press. https://doi.org/10.1093/acprof:oso/9780195333213.001.0001

Clark C. 2011. "Risk of Medical Errors by ED Doctors Linked to Interruptions." *HealthLeaders Media*. http://www.healthleadersmedia.com/content/QUA-262256/Risk-of-Medical-Errors-by-ED-Doctors-Linked-to-Interruptions

Coan, James A., Hillary S. Schaefer, and Richard J. Davidson. 2006. "Lending a hand: social regulation of the neural response to threat." *Psychol Sci*, 17(12): 1032–1039. https://doi.org/10.1111/j.1467-9280.2006.01832.x

Coiera, Enrico W., Rohan A. Jayasuriya, and Jennifer Hardy. 2002. "Communication loads on clinical staff in the emergency department." *Med J*, 176: 415–418.

Colombetti, Giovanna. 2010. "Enaction, sense-making and emotion." In *Enaction: Toward a new paradigm for cognitive science*, ed. by John Stewart, Olivier Gapenne and Ezequiel. A. Do Paolo, 145–64. Cambridge, MA: MIT Press. https://doi.org/10.7551/mitpress/9780262014601.003.0006

Cowley Stephen J. 1998. "Of timing, turn-taking, and conversations." *Journal of Psycholinguistic Research* 27(5): 541–71. https://doi.org/10.1023/A:1024948912805

Cowley, Stephen J. 2007. "Cognitive dynamics and distributed language." *Language Sciences* 29(5): 575–583. https://doi.org/10.1016/j.langsci.2007.01.002

Cowley, Stephen J. 2009. "Distributed language and dynamics." *Pragmatics & Cognition* 17(3): 495–507. https://doi.org/10.1075/pc.17.3.01cow

Cowley, Stephen J. 2010. "Beyond symbols: Interaction and the enslavement principle." In *New Adventures in Language and Interaction*, ed. by Jürgen Streeck, 47–70. Amsterdam: John Benjamins. https://doi.org/10.1075/pbns.196.03cow

Cowley, Stephen J. 2011. *Distributed Language*. Amsterdam: John Benjamins. https://doi.org/10.1075/bct.34

Cowley, Stephen J. 2014a. "The integration problem: interlacing language, action and perception." *Cybern. Hum. Knowing* 21: 53–65.

Cowley, Stephen J. 2014b. "Human Language and Sensorimotor Contingency." In *Contemporary Sensorimotor Theory*, ed. by Mark, J. Bishop and Andrew O. Martin, 235–255. Dordrecht: Springer. https://doi.org/10.1007/978-3-319-05107-9_16

Cowley, Stephen J. and Luarina Nash. 2013. "Language, interactivity and solution probing: Repetition without repetition." *Adaptive Behavior* 21: 187–198. https://doi.org/10.1177/1059712313482804

De Jaegher, Hanne. 2007. "Participatory Sense-Making: An Enactive Approach to Social Cognition." *Phenomenology and the cognitive sciences* 6(4): 485–507. https://doi.org/10.1007/s11097-007-9076-9

Dekker, Sidney W. A. 2002. "Reconstructing human contributions to accidents: the new view on error and performance." *Journal of Safety Research* 33: 371–385. https://doi.org/10.1016/S0022-4375(02)00032-4

Dennett, Daniel C. 2013. *Intuition Pumps and other Tools for Thinking*. New York: W.W. Norton & Co.

Dewey, John. 1910. *How We Think*. Boston, New York, Chicago: D.C.Heath & Co Publishers. https://doi.org/10.1037/10903-000

Dewey, John. 1929. *Experience and nature*. London: George Allen & Unwin, LTD.. https://doi.org/10.1037/13377-000

Di Paolo, Ezequiel. A., Elena C. Cuffari, and Hanne De Jaegher. 2018. *Linguistic Bodies: The Continuity Between Life and Language*. Cambridge, MA: MIT Press. doi: https://doi.org/10.7551/mitpress/11244.001.0001

Dreier, Ole H. 2007. "Generality and Particularity of Knowledge." In *Citizen City. Between Constructing Agent and Constructed Agent*, ed. by Vasi van Deventer, Martin, T. Blanche, Eduard Fourie, and Puleng Segalo, 188–196. Concord, Canada: Captus University Publ.

DuBrin, Andrew J. 2004. *Leadership Research Findings, Practice, and Skills*, 4th ed. Indianaphlis: Houghlon Mifflin Company.

Dunbar, Roger L. M. and Raghu Garud. 2007. "Distributed Knowledge and Indeterminate Meaning: The Case of the Columbia Shuttle Flight." *Organization Studies* 30(4): 397–421. https://doi.org/10.1177/0170840608101142

Edmondson, Amy C. 2012. "Teamwork On the Fly." *Harvard Business Review* 90(4): 72–80.

Eisenberg, Eric, Alexandra G. Murphy, Kathleen Sutcliffe, Robert Wears, Stephen Schenkel, Shawna Perry, and Mary Vanderhoef. 2007. "Communication in emergency medicine: Implications for patient safety." *Communication Monographs* 72(4): 390–413. https://doi.org/10.1080/03637750500322602

Elstein, Arthur S. and Alan Schwarz. 2002. "Clinical problem solving and diagnostic decision making: selective review of the cognitive literature." *BMJ 23*;324(7339): 729–32. https://doi.org/10.1136/bmj.324.7339.729

Enfield, Nick P. 2014. "Causal dynamics of language." In *Cambridge Handbook for Linguistic Anthropology*, ed. by Nick J. Enfield, Paul Kockelman and Jack Sidnell, 319–335. Cambridge: Cambridge University Press. https://doi.org/10.1017/CBO9781139342872.015

Engel, George L. 1977. "The need for a new medical model: A challenge for biomedicine." *Science* 196(4286): 129–136. https://doi.org/10.1126/science.847460

Fairclough, Norman. 1992. *Discourse and Social Change*. Cambridge: Polity Press.

Fauconnier, Gilles and Mark Turner. 2002. *The Way We Think*. New York: Basic Books.

Ferguson, Charles M. (1990). "Inspection, Auscultation, Palpation, and Percussion of the Abdomen." In *Clinical Methods: The History, Physical, and Laboratory Examinations*. 3rd edition, ed. by H. Kenneth Walker, W. Dallas Hall, and J. Willis Hurst, chapter 93. Boston: Butterworth.

Fioratou, Evridiki, Rhona Flin, Ronnie Glavin, and Rona Patey. 2010. "Beyond monitoring: Distributed situation awareness in anaesthesia." *British Journal of Anaesthesia*. 105(1): 83–90. https://doi.org/10.1093/bja/aeq137

Flach, John M. 1999. "Beyond Error: The Language of Coordination and Stability." In *Handbook of Perception and Cognition: Human Performance and Ergonomics*, ed. by Peter A. Hancock, 106–129). New York: Academic Press. https://doi.org/10.1016/B978-012322735-5/50006-3

Flin, Rhona. and Nicola Maran. 2004. "Identifying and training non-technical skills for teams in acute medicine." *Quality & Safety in Health Care*, 13(suppl II): 180–184.

Foucault, Michelle. 1973. *The Birth of the Clinic*. London and New York: Routledge.

Fowler, Carol. 2010. "Embodied, embedded language use." *Ecological Psychology* 22: 286–303. https://doi.org/10.1080/10407413.2010.517115

Gallagher, Shaun and Daniel Hutto. 2008. "Understanding others through primary interaction and narrative practice." In *The Shared Mind: Perspectives on intersubjectivity*, ed. by Jordan Zlatev, Timothy P. Racine, Chris Sinha, and Esa Itkonen, 17–38. Amsterdam: John Benjamins. https://doi.org/10.1075/celcr.12.04gal

Galosia, Margarita, Sune V. Steffensen, Stephen J. Cowley, and G. Alinier. 2010. "When life hangs on biosemiosis: tracking expertise in a medical simulation centre." In *Signifying bodies: Biosemiosis, interaction and health*, ed. by Stephen J. Cowley, Sune V. Steffensen, Joao C. Major and Alfredo Dinis, 179–206). Braga, Portugal: Portuguese Catholic University Press.

Gardner, Howard. 1985. *The Mind's New Science*. Basic Books.

Geertz, Clifford. 1973. *The Interpretation of Cultures*. London: Fontana.

Geertz, Clifford. 1983. *Local Knowledge: Further Essays in Interpretive Anthropology*. USA: Basic Books.

Gibson, James J. 1966. *The senses considered as perceptual systems*. Boston: Houghton Mifflin.

Gibson, James J. 1979/86. *The ecological approach to visual perception*. Hillsdale, NJ: Lawrence Erlbaum Associates.

Gibson, James J., and Crooks, Laukince E. 1938. "A theoretical field analysis of automobile-driving." *American Journal of Psychology* 51: 453–471. https://doi.org/10.2307/1416145

Giere, Ronald N. 2004. "The Problem of Agency in Scientific Distributed Cognitive Systems." *Journal of Cognition and Culture* 4(3/4): 759–774. https://doi.org/10.1163/1568537042484887

Glaser, Susan R. 1994. "Teamwork and Communication: A 3-Year Case Study of Change." *Management Communication Quarterly* 7(3): 282–296. https://doi.org/10.1177/0893318994007003003

Goffman, Erving. 1959. *The Presentation of Self in Everyday Life*. New York: Doubleday.

Goffman, Erving. 1974. *Frame Analysis: An Essay on the Organization of Experience*. London: Harper & Rowe.

Goffman, Erving. 1983. "The interaction order." *American Sociological Review* 48(1): 1–17. https://doi.org/10.2307/2095141

Goodwin, Charles. 1994. "Professional vision." *American Anthropologist* 96(3): 606–633. https://doi.org/10.1525/aa.1994.96.3.02a00100

Goodwin, Charles. 2000a. "Action and embodiment within situated human interaction." *Journal of Pragmatics* 32: 1489–1522. https://doi.org/10.1016/S0378-2166(99)00096-X

Goodwin, Charles. 2000b. "Practices of color classification." *Mind, Culture and Activity* 7(1–2): 19–36. https://doi.org/10.1080/10749039.2000.9677646
Goodwin, Charles. 2002. "Time in action." *Current Anthropology* 43: 19–35. https://doi.org/10.1086/339566
Goodwin, Charles. 2003. "The body in action." In *Discourse, the body and identity*, ed. by Justin Coupland and Richard Gwyn, 19–42). New York: Palgrave/Macmillan. https://doi.org/10.1057/9781403918543_2
Goodwin, Charles. 2007. "Language, culture, social organization and the material world: Why a five field approach is necessary." *Teaching Anthropology: SACC Notes* 13(2): 5–9.
Goodwin, Charles. 2013. "The co-operative, transformative organization of human action and knowledge." *Pragmatics* 46: 8–23. https://doi.org/10.1016/j.pragma.2012.09.003
Goodwin, Charles. 2014. "The intelligibility of gesture within a framework of co-operative action." In *From Gesture in Conversation to Visible Action as Utterance: Essays in honor of Adam Kendon*, ed. by Mandana Seyfeddinipur and Marianne Gullberg, 199–216. Amsterdam: Benjamins.
Goodwin, Charles. 2018. *Co-Operative Action*. New York: Cambridge University Press.
Goodwin, Marjorie. H. and Asta Cekaite. 2018. *Family Choreography: Practices of Control, Care, and Mundane Creativity*. London and New York: Routledge. https://doi.org/10.4324/9781315207773
Goodwin, Marjorie, Asta Cekaite, Charles Goodwin. 2012. "Emotion as Stance". In *Emotion in Interaction*, ed. by Anssi Perakyla and Marja-Leena Sorjonen, 6–41. Oxford: Oxford University Press. https://doi.org/10.1093/acprof:oso/9780199730735.003.0002
Grumbach, Kevin and Thomas Bodenheimer. 2004. "Can Health Care teams Improve Primary Care Practice?" *JAMA* 291(10): 1246–1251. https://doi.org/10.1001/jama.291.10.1246
Grundgeiger, Tobias, Penelope M. Sanderson, Hamish G. MacDougall, and Balasubramanian. 2010. "Interruption management in the intensive care unit: Predicting resumption times and assessing distributed support." *Journal of Experimental Psychology* 16: 317–334.
Halpern, Jodi. 2001. *From Detached Concern to Empathy: Humanizing Medical Practice*. Oxford: Oxford University Press. https://doi.org/10.1093/acprof:osobl/9780195111194.001.0001
Hammersley, Martyn and Paul Atkinson. 1983. *Ethnography: Principles in Practice*. London: Tavistock.
Hammersley, Martyn and Paul Atkinson. 1995. *Ethnography: Principles in Practice*, 2nd edition. London: Routledge.
Hazlehurst, Brian, Carmit K. McMullen, and Paul N. Gorman. 2007. "Distributed cognition in the heart room: How situation awareness arises from coordinated communications during cardiac surgery." *Journal of Biomedical Informatics* 40(5): 539–551. https://doi.org/10.1016/j.jbi.2007.02.001
Hazlehurst, Brian, Paul N. Gorman and Carmit K. McMullen. 2008. "Distributed Cognition: An alternative model of cognition for medical informatics." *International Journal of Medical Informatics* 77: 226–234. https://doi.org/10.1016/j.ijmedinf.2007.04.008
Heath, Christian, Jon Hindmarsh, and Paul Luff. 2010. *Video in Qualitative Research*. London: Sage.
Heritage, John. 1984. "A change-of-state token and aspects of its sequential placement." In *Structures of Social action*, ed. by James M. Atkinson and John Heritage, 299–345. Cambridge, UK: Cambridge University.
Heritage, John and Steven Clayman. 2010. *Talk in Action: Interactions, Identities, and Institutions*. Chichester: Wiley Blackwell. https://doi.org/10.1002/9781444318135

Hindmarsh, Jon and Alison Pilnick. 2002. "The tacit order of teamwork: Collaboration and embodied conduct in anesthesia." *Sociological Quarterly* 43(2): 139–163. https://doi.org/10.1111/j.1533-8525.2002.tb00044.x

Hodges, Bert H. 2007a. "Values Define Fields: The intentional Dynamics of Driving, Carrying, Leading, Negotiating, and Conversing." *Ecological Psychology* 19(2): 153–178.

Hodges, Bert H. 2007b. "Good prospects: ecological and social perspectives on conforming, creating, and caring in conversation." *Language Sciences* 29: 584–604. https://doi.org/10.1016/j.langsci.2007.01.003

Hodges, Bert H. 2009. "Ecological pragmatics: values, dialogical arrays, complexity and caring." *Pragmatics & Cognition* 17(3): 628–652. https://doi.org/10.1075/pc.17.3.08hod

Hodges, Bert H. and Ruben M. Baron. 1992. "Values as constraints on affordances: Perceiving and acting properly." *Journal for the Theory of Social Behaviour* 22: 263–294. https://doi.org/10.1111/j.1468-5914.1992.tb00220.x

Hollan, Jim, Edwin Hutchins, and David Kirsh. 2000 "Distributed cognition: Toward a new foundation for human-computer interaction." In *Human-Computer Interaction in the New Millenium*, ed. by John M. Carroll, 75–94. New York: Addison-Wesley.

Hollnagel, Erik. 2004. *Barriers and Accident Prevention*. Aldershot: Ashgate.

Hollnagel, Erik. 2012. *FRAM: The functional resonance analysis method: modeling complex socio-technical systems*. Burlington: Ashgate.

Holzkamp, Klaus. 1988. *Grundlegung der Psychologie*. Frankfurt am Main: Campus Verlag.

Horsky, Jan, Jiajie Zhang, and Vimla V. Patel. 2005. "To err is not entirely human: Complex technology and user cogntion." *J Biomed Inform* 38: 264–266. https://doi.org/10.1016/j.jbi.2005.05.002

Husebø, Sissel E., Hans Rystedt, and Febe Friberg. 2011. "Educating for teamwork– nursing students' coordination in simulated cardiac arrest situations." *J Adv Nurs* 67(10): 2239–2255. https://doi.org/10.1111/j.1365-2648.2011.05629.x

Hutchby, I. and Wooffitt, R. (2011). *Conversation Analysis*. Cambridge: Polity Press.

Hutchins, Edwin. 1995a. *Cognition in the wild*. Cambridge MA: MIT Press.

Hutchins, Edwin. 1995b. "How a cockpit manages its speed." *Cognitive Science* 19: 265–288. https://doi.org/10.1207/s15516709cog1903_1

Hutchins, Edwin. 2003. "Cognitive ethnography." In *Proceedings of the twenty-fifth annual conference of the cognitive science society, Pts 1 and 2*: 18–18.

Hutchins, Edwin. 2005. "Material anchors for conceptual blends." *Journal of Pragmatics* 37: 1555–1577. https://doi.org/10.1016/j.pragma.2004.06.008

Hutchins, Edwin. 2014. "The cultural ecosystem of human cognition." *Philosophical Psychology* 27: 34–49. https://doi.org/10.1080/09515089.2013.830548

Hutchins, Edwin and Tove Klausen. 1996. "Distributed cognition in an airline cockpit." In *Cognition and Communication at Work*, ed. by Yrjo Engeström and David Middleton, 15–34. New York: Cambridge University Press. https://doi.org/10.1017/CBO9781139174077.002

Hutchins, Edwin and Leysia Palen. 1997. "Constructing meaning from space, gesture, and speech." In *Tools, and Reasoning: Essays in Situated Cognition*, ed. by Lauren B. Resneck, Roger Saljo, Clotilde Pontecorvo, and Barbara Burge, 23–40. Vienna, Austria: Springer-Verlag. https://doi.org/10.1007/978-3-662-03362-3_2

Hutchins, Edwin and Saeko Nomura. 2011. "Collaborative construction of multimodal utterances." In *Embodied Interaction: Language and Body in the Material World*, ed. by Jürgen Streek, Charles Goodwin and Curtis LeBaron, 29–43. Cambridge: Cambridge University Press.

Ito, John P. 2011. "Repetition without repetition; Bernsteinian Perspectives on Motor Learning for Musicians." *College Music Symposium* 51.

Järvilehto, Timo. 1998. "The theory of the organism-environment system: I. Description of the Theory." *Integrative Physiological and Behavioral Science* 33(4): 321–334. https://doi.org/10.1007/BF02688700

Järvilehto, Timo. 2009. "The Theory of the Organism-Environment System as a Basis of Experimental Work in Psychology." *Ecological Psychology* 21: 112–120. https://doi.org/10.1080/10407410902877066

Jeanmonod, Rebecca, Molly Boyd, Melanie Loewenthal, and Wayne Triner. 2010. "The nature of emergency department interruptions and their impact on patient satisfaction." *Emerg Med J* 27: 376–379. https://doi.org/10.1136/emj.2008.071134

Jefferson, Gail. 1983. "Issues in the Transcription of Naturally-Occuring Talk: Caricature versus Capturing Pronounciational Particulars." *Tilburg Papers in Languge and Literature* 34: 1–12.

Jefferson, Gail. 1985. "An exercise in the transcription and analysis of laughter." In *Handbook of Discourse Analysis*, Volume 3: Discourse and Dialogue, ed. by Teun van Dijk, 25–34. London: Academic Press

Jefferson, Gail. 2005. "Glossary of transcript symbols with an introduction." In *Conversation Analysis: Studies from the First Generation*, ed. by Gene H. Lerner, 13–31. Amsterdam: Benjamins.

Jensen, Thomas W. 2014a. "Emotion in languaging: languaging as affective, adaptive, and flexible behaviour in social interaction." *Front Psychol* 5(720): 1–14.

Jensen, Thomas W. 2014b. "New perspectives on language, cognition, and values." *Journal of Multicultural Discourses* 9(1): 71–78. https://doi.org/10.1080/17447143.2013.861841

Jensen, Thomas W. and Sarah B. Pedersen. 2016. "Affect and affordances– The role of action and emotion in social interaction." *Cognitive Semiotics* 9(1): 79–103. https://doi.org/10.1515/cogsem-2016-0003

Kahneman, Daniel and Gary Klein. 2009. "Conditions for intuitive expertise: a failure to disagree." *American Psychol* 64(6): 515–526. doi: https://doi.org/10.1037/a0016755.

Kirsh, David. 1997. "Interactivity and MultiMedia Interfaces." *Instructional Sciences* 25: 79–96. https://doi.org/10.1023/A:1002915430871

Kirsh, David. 2009. "Problem solving and situated cognition." In *The Cambridge Handbook of Situated Cognition*, ed. by Philip Robbins and Murat Aydede, 264–306. Cambridge: Cambridge University Press

Kirsh, David. 2013. "Embodied cognition and the magical future of interaction design." *ACM Transactions on Computer-Human Interaction* 20(1) Article 3: 1–30. https://doi.org/10.1145/2442106.2442109

Kirsh, David and Paul Maglio. 1994. "On distinguishing epistemic from pragmatic action." *Cognitive Science* 18: 513–549. https://doi.org/10.1207/s15516709cog1804_1

Klein, Gary. 2015. "A naturalistic decision making perspective on studying intuitive decision making." *Journal of Applied Research in Memory and Cognition* 4: 164–168. DOI: https://doi.org/10.1016/j.jarmac.2015.07.001

Klein, Gary. 1998. *Sources of Power: How People Make Decisions*. Cambridge, MA: MIT Press.

Klein, Gary. 2008. "Naturalistic Decision Making." *Human Factors and Ergonomics Society* 50(3): 456–460. DOI https://doi.org/10.1518/001872008X288385.

Kohn, Linda T, Janet M. Corrigan, and Molla S. Donaldson. (eds.). 2000. *To Err is Human: Building a Safer Health System*. Washington, D.C: National Academy Press.

Korzybski, Alfred. 1931. "A Non-Aristotelian System and its Necessity for Rigour in Mathematics and Physics." (paper presentation before the American Mathematical Society at the New Orleans, Louisiana, meeting of the American Association for the Advancement of Science, December 28, 1931. *Reprinted in* Science and Sanity, 1933, 747–761.

Kravchenko, Alexander V. 2007. "Essential properties of language, or, why language is not a code." *Language Sciences* 26: 650–671. https://doi.org/10.1016/j.langsci.2007.01.004

Kravchenko, Alexander V. 2011. "The experimental basis of speech and writing." In *Distributed language*, ed. By Stephen J. Cowley, 33–55. Amsterdam: John Benjamins. https://doi.org/10.1075/bct.34.03kra

Kushniruk, Andre, Vimla L. Patel, and J. J. Cimino. 1997. "Usability testing in medical informatics: Cognitive approaches to the evaluation of information systems and user interfaces." In *Proceedings of the 1997 AMIA Annual Fall Symposium*, 218–222.

Laland, Kevin N., John Odling-Smee, William Hoppitt and Tobias Uller. 2013. "More on how and why: a response to commentaries." *Biol Philos* 28: 793–810. https://doi.org/10.1007/s10539-013-9380-4

Lave, Jean and Etienne Wenger. 1991. *Situated Learning: Legitimate Peripheral Participation.* Cambridge: Cambridge University Press. https://doi.org/10.1017/CBO9780511815355

Leape, Lucian L., Ann G. Lawthers, Troyen A. Brennan, and William Johnson. 1993. "Preventing medical injury." *Qual Rev Bull* 19(5): 144–149. https://doi.org/10.1016/S0097-5990(16)30608-X

Leape Lucian L. 1994. "Error in medicine." *JAMA* 272(23): 1851–1857. https://doi.org/10.1001/jama.1994.03520230061039

Lents, Nathan H. 2018. *Human Errors. A Panorama of Our Glitches, from Pointless Bones to Broken Genes.* New York: Houghton Miifflin Harcourt Publishing Company.

Lewis, Simon J. and Kenneth W. Heaton. 1997. "Stool form scale as a useful guide to intestinal time." *Scandinavian Journal of Gastroenterology* 32: 920–924. https://doi.org/10.3109/00365529709011203

Lichtfield, Damien and Linden J. Ball. 2011. "Rapid communication: Using another's gaze as an explicit aid to insight problem solving." *Quarterly Journal of Experimental Psychology* 64(4): 649–656. https://doi.org/10.1080/17470218.2011.558628.

Liddicoat, Anthony J. 2011. *An Introduction to Conversation Analysis.* London: Continuum.

Linell, Per. 2005. *The Written Language Bias in Linguistics: Its Nature, Origins and Transformations.* London: Routledge.

Linell, Per. 2007. "Dialogicality in languages minds and brains: is there a convergence between dialogism and neuro-biology?" *Language Sciences* 29: 605–620. https://doi.org/10.1016/j.langsci.2007.01.001

Linell, Per. 2009. *Rethinking language, mind, and world dialogically: Interactional and contextual theories of human sense-making.* Charlotte, NC: Information Age Publishing.

Linell, Per. 2015. "Dialogism and the distributed language approach: a rejoinder to Steffensen." *Language Sciences* 50: 120–126. https://doi.org/10.1016/j.langsci.2015.01.003

Loaiza, M. Juan, Sarah B. Trasmundi, and Sune V. Steffensen. forth. "Multiscalar Temporality in Human Behaviour: A Case Study of Constraint Interdependence in Psychotherapy." A special issue on "Enaction and Ecological Psychology: Convergences and Complementarities" in *Frontiers in Psychology*.

Love, Nigel. 2004. "Cognition and the language myth." *Language Sciences* 26: 525–544. https://doi.org/10.1016/j.langsci.2004.09.003

Love, Nigel. 2007. "Are languages digital codes?" *Language Sciences* 29: 690–709. https://doi.org/10.1016/j.langsci.2007.01.008

Lundberg, Jonas, Carl Rollenhagen, and Eik Hollnagel. 2009. "What-You-Look-For-Is-What-You-Find – The consequences of underlying accident models in eight accident investigation manuals." *Safety Science* 47(10): 1297–1311. https://doi.org/10.1016/j.ssci.2009.01.004

Madsen, Jens K. 2014. "Bayesian Subjectivity from a Temporal Perspective." *Cybernetics & Human Knowing* 21: 98–112.

Mangels, Jennifer A., Brady Butterfield, Justin Lamb, Catherine Good, and Carol S. Dweck. 2006. "Why do beliefs about intelligence influence learning success? A social cognitive neuroscience model." *Soc Cogn Affect Neurosci* 1(2): 75–86. https://doi.org/10.1093/scan/nsl013

Manser, Tanja. 2009. "Teamwork and patient safety in dynamic domains of healthcare: A review of the literature." *Acta Anaesthesiol Scand* 53(2): 143–151. https://doi.org/10.1111/j.1399-6576.2008.01717.x

Manser, Tanja, T. Kyle Harrison, David M. Gaba, and Steven K. Howard. 2009. "Coordination Patterns related to High Clinical Performance in a Simulated Anesthetic Crisis." *Anesth Analg* 108: 1606–1615. https://doi.org/10.1213/ane.0b013e3181981d36

Martina, Kelley, Tink Wendy, and Lara Nixon. 2014. "Keeping the Human Touch in Medical Practice." *Academic Medicine* 89(10): 1314. https://doi.org/10.1097/ACM.0000000000000454

Maturana, Humberto R. and Francisco J. Varela. 1987. *The Tree of Knowledge: The Biological Roots of Human Understanding*. Boston: Shambala Press and New Science Library.

Merleau-Ponty, Maurice. 2012. *Phenomenology of Perception*. (Translation of French Original [1945]) New York: Routledge.

Merry, Alan and Alexander M. Smith. 2001. *Errors, Medicine and the Law*. Cambridge: Cambridge University Press. https://doi.org/10.1017/CBO9780511806063

Meyer, Christian, Jürgen Streeck, J. Scott Jordan (eds.). 2017. *Intercorporeality: Emerging Socialities in Interaction*. Oxford: Oxford University Press. https://doi.org/10.1093/acprof:oso/9780190210465.001.0001

Miller, Robert H. and Ida Sim. 2004. "Physicians' Use of Electronic Medical Records: Barriers And Solutions." *Health Aff* 23(2): 116–126. https://doi.org/10.1377/hlthaff.23.2.116

Moser, Jason S., Hans S. Schroder, Carriee Heeter, Tim P. Moran, and Yu-Hao Lee. 2011. "Mind Your Errors: Evidence for a Neural Mechanism Linking Growth Mind-Set to Adaptive Posterror Adjustments." *Psychological Science* 22(12): 1484–1489. https://doi.org/10.1177/0956797611419520

Mylopoulos, Maria and Walid Farhat. 2014. ""I can do better": Exploring purposeful improvement in daily clinical work." *Adv. Health. Sci. Educ. Theory. Pract* 20(2): 237–283.

Nemeth, Christopher P., Richard I. Cook, Michael O'Connor, and P. Allan Klock. 2004. "Using cognitive artifacts to understand distributed cognition." *Systems, Man and Cybernetics, Part A: Systems and Humans, IEEE Transactions* 34(6): 726–735. https://doi.org/10.1109/TSMCA.2004.836798

Newell, Allen, J. C. Shaw, and Herbert A. Simon. 1958. "Elements of a Theory of Human Problem-Solving." *Psychological Review* 65: 151–166. https://doi.org/10.1037/h0048495

Noë, Alva. 2004. *Action in perception*. Cambridge, MA: The MIT Press.

Noë, Alva. 2010. *Out of Our Heads: Why You Are Not Your Brain, and Other Lessons from the Biology of Consciousness*. New York: Hill and Wang.

Norman, Donald A. 1993. *Things That Make Us Smart*. New York: Doubleday/Currency.

O'Daniel, Michelle and Alan H. Rosenstein. 2008. "Professional Communication and team Collaboration." In *Patient Safety and Quality: An Evidence-based Handbook for Nurses*, ed. by Ronda G. Hughes (chapter 33), http://www.ncbi.nlm.nih.gov/books/NBK2637/.

Ormerod, Thomas C. and Linden J. Ball. 2017. "Cognitive Psychology." In *The SAGE Handbook of Qualitative Research in Psychology*, ed. by Carla Willig and Wendy Stainton-Rogers, 574–591. London: SAGE Publications LTD.. https://doi.org/10.4135/9781526405555.n33

Paradis, Elise, Myles Leslie, Kathleen Puntillo, Michael Gropper, Hanan J. Aboumatar, Simon Kitto, and Scott Reeves. 2014. "Delivering Interprofessional Care in Intensive Care: A Scoping Review of Ethnographic Studies." *AJCC American Journal of Critical Care* 23(3): 230–238. https://doi.org/10.4037/ajcc2014155

Pedersen, Sarah B. 2010. "Towards dialogical health care practices: Human errors as a result of cultural affordances." In *Signifying bodies: Biosemiosis, interaction and health*, ed. by Stephen J. Cowley, Sune V. Steffensen, Joao C. Major and Alfredo Dinis, 245–276. Braga, Portugal: Portuguese Catholic University Press.

Pedersen, Sarah B. 2012. "Interactivity in health care: Bodies, values and dynamics." *Language Sciences* 34(5): 532–542. https://doi.org/10.1016/j.langsci.2012.03.009

Pedersen, Sarah B. 2015 *The Cognitive Ecology of Human Errors in Emergency Medicine: An Interactivitybased Approach*. PhDdissertation. Odense: University of Southern Denmark.

Pedersen, Sarah B. and Sune V. Steffensen. 2014. "Temporal Dynamics in Medical Visual Systems." *Cybernetics & Human Knowing* 21: 143–157.

Perry, Mark. 2010. "Socially distributed cognition in loosely coupled systems." *Ai & Society* 25(4): 387–400. https://doi.org/10.1007/s00146-010-0267-5

Port, Robert. 2010. "Rich memory and distributed phonology." *Language Sciences* 32(1): 43–55. https://doi.org/10.1016/j.langsci.2009.06.001

Putsch, Robert W. and Marlie Joyce. 1990. "Dealing with patients from other cultures." In *Clinical Methods: The History, Physical and Laboratory Examinations*, ed. by H. Kenneth Walker, W. Dallas Hall and J. Willis Hurst, 1050–1065. Boston: Butterworths.

Rączaszek-Leonardi, Joanna. 2011. "Symbols as constraints: The structuring role of dynamics and self-organization in natural language." In *Cognition beyond the brain: Computation, interactivity and human artifice*, ed. by Stephen J. Cowley and Frederic Vallée-Tourangeau, 161–184. Dordrecht: Springer.

Rajkomar, Atish, and Ann Blandford. 2012. "A distributed cognition model for analysing interruption resumption during infusion administration." *Proceedings of European Conference on Cognitive Ergonomics (ECCE 2012)*, 108–111. New York: ACM. https://doi.org/10.1145/2448136.2448159

Reason, James. 1990. *Human Error*. New York: Cambridge University Press. https://doi.org/10.1017/CBO9781139062367

Reason, James. 1995. "A System Approach to Organizational Error." *Ergonomics* 38: 1708–1721. https://doi.org/10.1080/00140139508925221

Reason, James. 1997. *Managing the risks of organizational accidents*. Aldershot: Ashgate.

Reason, James. 2000. "Human Error: models and management." *BMJ* 320: 768–770. https://doi.org/10.1136/bmj.320.7237.768

Reason, James. 2001. "Heroic Compensations: The benign face of the human factor." *Flight Safety Australia*, jan-feb: 28–31.

Reason, James. 2005. "Safety in the operating theatre– Part 2: Human error and organisational failure." *Quality and safety in health care* 14: 56–60.

Reason, James. 2008. *The Human Contribution: Unsafe Acts, Accidents and Heroic Recoveries.* Farnham Surray: Ashgate.

Reed, Edward S. 1996. *Encountering the World: Toward an Ecological Psychology.* Oxford: Oxford University Press.

Rockville, MD: Agency for Healthcare Research and Quality.

Ross, Don. 2004. "Metalinguistic signalling for coordination amongst social agents." *Language Sciences* 26(6): 621–642. https://doi.org/10.1016/j.langsci.2004.09.008

Ryle, Gilbert. 1949. *Concept of Mind.* London: Hutchinson's University Library.

Sacks, Harvey, Emanuel A. Schegloff, and Gail Jefferson. 1974. "A simplest systematics for the organization of turn-taking for conversation." *Language* 50(4): 696–735. https://doi.org/10.1353/lan.1974.0010

Salomon, Gavriel. 1993. *Distributed Cognitions.* Cambridge: Cambridge University Press.

Sandars, John. and Aneez Esmail. 2003. "The frequency and nature of medical error in primary care: understanding the diversity across studies." *Family Practice* 20: 231–236. https://doi.org/10.1093/fampra/cmg301

Seale, Clive. 2012. *Researching Society and Culture.* London: Sage.

Secchi, Davide. 2011. *Extendable Rationality: Understanding Decision Making in Organizations.* New York: Springer. https://doi.org/10.1007/978-1-4419-7542-3

Senge, Peter M. 2006. *The Fifth Discipline. The Art and Practice of the Learning Organization.* USA: Doubleday.

Shappell, Scott A. and Douglas A. Wiegmann. 2001. "Applying reason: the human factors analysis and classification system. *(HFACS)" Human Factors and Aerospace Safety* 1(1): 59–86.

Sloetjes, Han and Peter Wittenburg. 2008. "Annotation by category – ELAN and ISO DCR." In *Proceedings of the 6th International Conference on Language Resources and Evaluation* (LREC 2008).

Smith, Richard. 2003. "Thoughts for new medical students at a new medical school." *BMJ* 327(7429): 1430–1433. https://doi.org/10.1136/bmj.327.7429.1430

Steffensen, Sune V. 2011. "Beyond mind: an extended ecology of languaging." In *Distributed language*, ed. by Stephen J. Cowley, 185–210. Amsterdam: John Benjamins. https://doi.org/10.1075/bct.34.10ste

Steffensen, Sune V. 2012. "Care and conversing in dialogical systems." *Language Sciences* 34: 513–531. https://doi.org/10.1016/j.langsci.2012.03.008

Steffensen, Sune V. 2013. "Human interactivity: Problem-solving, solution-probing, and verbal patterns in the wild." In *Cognition beyond the brain: Computation, interactivity and human artifice*, ed. by Stephen J. Cowley and Frederic Vallée-Tourangeau, 195–221. Dordrecht: Springer. https://doi.org/10.1007/978-1-4471-5125-8_11

Steffensen, Sune V. 2015. "Distributed Language and Dialogism: notes on non-locality, sense-making and interactivity." *Language Sciences* 50: 105–119. https://doi.org/10.1016/j.langsci.2015.01.004

Steffensen, Sune V. 2016. "Cognitive probatonics: towards an ecological psychology of cognitive particulars." *New Ideas in Psychology* 42: 29–38. https://doi.org/10.1016/j.newideapsych.2015.07.003

Steffensen, Sune V. and Stephen J. Cowley. 2010. "Signifying bodies and health: a non local aftermath." In *Signifying bodies: Biosemiosis, interaction and health*, ed. by Stephen J. Cowley, Sune V. Steffensen, Joao C. Major and Alfredo Dinis, 331–356. Braga: Portuguese Catholic University Press.

Steffensen, Sune V. and Alvin Fill. 2014. "Ecolinguistics: the state of the art and future horizons." *Language Sciences* 41, Part A: 6–25. https://doi.org/10.1016/j.langsci.2013.08.003

Steffensen, Sune V. and Sarah B. Pedersen. 2014. "Temporal Dynamics in Human Interaction." *Cybernetics & Human Knowing* 21: 80–97.

Steffensen, Sune V., Frederic Vallée-Tourangeau, and Gaëlle Vallée-Tourangeau. 2016. "Cognitive events in a problem-solving task: a qualitative method for investigating interactivity in the 17 Animals problem." *Journal of Cognitive Psychology* 28: 79–105. https://doi.org/10.1080/20445911.2015.1095193

Steffensen, Sune V. and Sarah B. Trasmundi. (forth.) *Cognitive Event Analysis.*

Streeck, Jürgen. 2010. *New Adventures in Language and Interaction.* Amsterdam: Benjamins. https://doi.org/10.1075/pbns.196

Streeck, Jürgen and J. Scott Jordan. 2009. "Communication as a dynamical system: The importance of time-scales and nested contexts." *Communication Theory* 19: 445–464. https://doi.org/10.1111/j.1468-2885.2009.01351.x

Streeck, Jürgen, Charles Goodwin, and Curtis LeBaron. 2011. *Embodied Interaction: Language and Body in the Material World.* Cambridge: Cambridge University Press.

Thibault, Paul J. 2011. "First-order languaging dynamics and second-order language: the distributed language view." *Ecological Psychology* 23(3): 210–245. https://doi.org/10.1080/10407413.2011.591274

Thibault, Paul J. 2014. "Events and Affordances: Ecosocial Time Scales and the Two Orders of Language." *Cybernetics & Human Knowing* 21: 23–36.

Thomas, William I. and Dorothy Thomas. 1928. *The child in America: Behavior problems and programs.* New York: Knopf.

Thompson, Evan. 2007. *Mind in Life: Biology, Phenomenology, and the Sciences of Mind.* Cambridge, MA: Harvard University Press.

Torre, Enrico. 2014. "Digital Inscriptions as Material Anchors for Future Action: Multi-scalar Integration and Dynamic Systems." *Cybernetics & Human Knowing* 21: 128–142.

Trasmundi, Sarah B. 2016. "Distribueret kognition og distribueret sprog: analyse af kognitive events i en akutmedicinsk social praksis." *NyS* 50: 55–85. https://doi.org/10.7146/nys.v1i50.23798

Trasmundi, Sarah B. 2017. "The Ecological Subject and Visual Perception." *RASK, the International Journal of Language and Communication* 46: 15–42.

Trasmundi, Sarah B. 2019. "Skilled embodiment in emergency medicine: The "interactivity turn" and its implication for theory and practice." *Chinese Semiotic Studies* 15(4): 627–651. https://doi.org/10.1515/css-2019-0032

Trasmundi, Sarah B. and Per Linell. 2017. "Insights and their Emergence in Everyday Practices: The Interplay between Problems and Solutions in emergency medicine." *Pragmatics & Cognition* 24(1): 64–92. https://doi.org/10.1075/pc.17002.tra

Trasmundi, Sarah B. and Sune V. Steffensen. 2016. "Meaning emergence in the ecology of dialogical systems." *Psychology of Language and Communication* 20(2): 154–181. https://doi.org/10.1515/plc-2016-0009

Trasmundi, Sarah B. and Matthew Harvey. 2018. "A Blended Quantitative-Ethnographic Method for Describing Vocal Sonofication in Dance Coaching." *the Psychology of Language and Communication* 22(1): 198–229. https://doi.org/10.2478/plc-2018-0009

Uryu, Michiko, Sune V. Steffensen, and Claire Kramsch. 2014. "The ecology of intercultural interaction: Timescales, temporal ranges and identity dynamics." *Language Sciences* 41(part A): 41–59. https://doi.org/10.1016/j.langsci.2013.08.006

Valleé-Tourangeau, Frederic. 2013. "Interactivity, efficiency, and individual differences in mental arithmetric." *Exp. Psychol* 60: 302–311. https://doi.org/10.1027/1618-3169/a000200

van Someren, Maarten W., Yvonne F. Barnard, Jacobijn A. C. Sandberg. 1994. *Think Aloud Method: A practical guide to modelling cognitive processes*. London: Academic Press.

Verghese, Abraham. 2009. "Touch Of Sense." *Health Affairs* 28(4): 1177–1182. https://doi.org/10.1377/hlthaff.28.4.1177

Wilson, Andrew. D. and Sabrina Golonka. 2013. "Embodied Cognition is not What You Think." *Frontiers in Psychology* 4:58. https://doi.org/10.3389/fpsyg.2013.00058.

Wittgenstein, Ludwig. 1963. *Philosophical Investigations*. Oxford: Basil Blackwell Oxford.

Yule, Steven, Rhona Flin, Simon Paterson-Brown, Nicola Maran, and David Rowley. 2006. "Non-technical skills for surgeons in the operating room: A review of the literature." *Surgery* 139: 140–149. https://doi.org/10.1016/j.surg.2005.06.017

Index